Handbook of Oral Pathology and
Oral Medicine

Handbook of Oral Pathology and Oral Medicine

S. R. Prabhu BDS; MDS (Oral Path); FFDRCS (Oral Med); FDSRCS(Edin); FDSRCPS (Glas); FDSRCS (Eng), FFGDPRCS(UK); MOMed RCS (Edin); FICD.

Honorary Associate Professor
School of Dentistry
University of Queensland
Brisbane, Australia

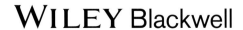

Registered Offices
John Wiley & Sons, Inc., 111 River Street, Hoboken, NJ 07030, USA
John Wiley & Sons Ltd, The Atrium, Southern Gate, Chichester, West Sussex, PO19 8SQ, UK

Editorial Office
9600 Garsington Road, Oxford, OX4 2DQ, UK

For details of our global editorial offices, customer services, and more information about Wiley products visit us at www.wiley.com.

Wiley also publishes its books in a variety of electronic formats and by print-on-demand. Some content that appears in standard print versions of this book may not be available in other formats.

Library of Congress Cataloging-in-Publication Data applied for
[ISBN: 9781119781127]

Cover Design: Wiley
Cover Images: Courtesy of S. R. Prabhu

Set in 9.5/12.5pt STIXTwoText by Straive, Pondicherry, India

Printed in Singapore
M114809_050821

To the victims of COVID-19 infection and all those frontline healthcare workers who are engaged in the fight against the disease with utmost courage and dedication.

Contents

Foreword

This is an amazing work. Professor SR Prabhu has touched constructively on almost every "issue", every decision required, in the day-to-day practice of oral medicine and to a considerable extent, oral/maxillofacial pathology. He has laid out the material in a very logical set of chapters. The extensive illustrations are of uniformly high quality: many of these have been donated by colleagues around the world and I join in thanking them for their generosity: many have become personal friends to us both.

I initially was hesitant to contribute this Foreword. As a quantitative scientist, I always wish to see the evidence base for every diagnosis, test and treatment presented. This is deliberately not the intention here - indeed it is the opposite of Prof Prabhu's intent. As he put it in response to my challenge "My intention is not to compete with great authors of international repute. The material presented is truly a compilation of what is known in the scientific papers, books and case reports that are (*I might interpolate with much hard work*) available. This is a humble attempt to provide students and busy practitioners with a source that provides quick access to information". I see the value of this: indeed, I wish my current undergraduate and postgraduate students came to clinics with a copy in their pockets!

Professor SR Prabhu is a remarkable professional in the autumn of a remarkable career. This has impacted the dental profession, and particularly dental students, across the globe, for decades, beginning with his first teaching appointment in India in 1971. We first met when he was Commonwealth Medical Scholar in my department in London in 1974. Chronologically since then he has taught and led teaching [including from positions as Head of Department or Dean in several institutions] in universities in India, Kenya, Sudan, Australia, Papua New Guinea, West Indies, Malaysia, Saudi Arabia, West Indies (again), United Arab Emirates, and several Australian universities, again. His vast knowledge reflects this.

I have learned much from his global experience and it was particularly educative for me to work with him, as co-editor and co-author of his largest work *Oral Diseases in the Tropics* (Oxford University Press 1992; Revised reprint, Jaypee Bros. 2017). Beyond that his bibliography is extensive.

We are fortunate that he has maintained the drive and passion to give us this valuable work at this time: one positive outcome of Covid-2019.

Newell W Johnson, CMG
Emeritus Professor of Oral Health Sciences,
Kings' College London, &
Dean Emeritus and Honorary Professor of Dental Research,
Griffith University, Queensland, Australia
Brisbane, June 2021

Preface

The *Handbook of Oral Pathology and Oral Medicine* is primarily targeted at undergraduate dental students and practitioners. Dental students find the available prescribed textbooks of oral pathology and oral medicine loaded with information and are not user friendly, particularly at the time of preparation for examinations. Teachers and students alike feel that there is a need for a book that offers information in a concise manner for quick reference. This handbook aims to fill this need by providing a highly illustrated succinct guide presented as bulleted lists for easy reference. Text style used in this handbook allows the reader to quickly gather essential information relevant to the disease without scanning through lengthy paragraphs. For further information, a recommended reading list is provided at the end of each chapter.

Topics included in this book are in accordance with the universally followed curricula in oral pathology and oral medicine. The text is divided in seven parts: pathology of teeth, pulp, and supporting structures, pathology of jawbones, pathology of the oral mucosa, pathology of the salivary glands, clinical presentation of mucosal disease, orofacial pain, and miscellaneous topics of clinical relevance. Many international clinicians and teachers have generously contributed clinical, radiographical and photomicrographic images to this handbook.

The author and the publishers feel that the format, design, style, and content of the text used in this handbook will assist dental students and clinicians in dentistry and other healthcare professions. Accompanying this handbook is a website containing case scenarios and MCQs especially designed for dental students preparing for examinations.

S. R. Prabhu
Brisbane
June 2021

Acknowledgements

I wish to thank Professor Newell Johnson for the Foreword and his inspirational role in shaping my academic career in oral pathology and oral medicine.

I also wish to express my grateful thanks to many colleagues who have shared their teaching material to this book. Every effort has been made to trace and acknowledge copyright material for the images used. If someone's name has been inadvertently missed or infringement of copyright has occurred accidentally, I tender my sincere apologies.

My great appreciation goes to guidance provided by Associate Commissioning Editor for Veterinary and Dentistry books Miss Loan Nguyen and Managing Editor for Health and Life Sciences Miss Tanya McMullin of John Wiley & Sons (UK). Others at Wiley publishing who deserve my grateful thanks include Adalfin Jayasingh, Fathima Shaheen, and Susan Engelken.

Finally, I am indebted to my wife Uma Prabhu for her unconditional support during the COVID-19 stay-at-home period when the preparation of manuscripts for this handbook was started and completed.

S. R. Prabhu
Brisbane
June 2021

About the Companion Website

Don't forget to visit the companion web site for this book:

www.wiley.com/go/prabhu/oral_pathology

There you will find valuable materials, including:

- 240 multiple choice questions
- 36 clinical case scenarios
- Images from the book as downloadable PowerPoint slides

Scan this QR code to visit the companion website

Nomenclature Used in The Study of Human Disease

Nomenclature of diseases:

- **Disease:** impairment of normal physiological function affecting all or part of an organism manifested by signs and symptoms.
- **Disorder:** deviation from the usual way the body functions.
- **Condition:** an abnormal state of health that interferes with the usual activities or feeling of wellbeing.
- **Risk factor:** something that increases a person's chances of developing a disease.
- **Aetiology:** the study of the underlying cause of the disease/disorder.
- **Pathogenesis:** the development and chain of events leading to a disease.
- **Epidemiology:** a branch of medical science that deals with the incidence, distribution, and control of disease in a population.
- **Incidence:** the measure of the probability of occurrence of new cases of a disease over a certain period.
- **Prevalence:** total number of individuals in a population who have a disease or health condition at a specific period, usually expressed as a percentage of the population.
- **Prognosis:** prediction of the likely course and outcome of a disease.
- **Morbidity:** the extent to which a patient's overall health is affected by a disease.
- **Mortality:** the likelihood of death from a particular disease.
- **Acute and chronic illnesses:**
  - Acute illnesses are of rapid onset.
  - Chronic conditions usually have a gradual onset and are more likely to have a prolonged course.
- **Syndrome** refers to a collection or set of signs and symptoms that characterize or suggest a particular disease.

Clinical nomenclature of oral mucosal lesions:

- **Lesion:** clinically detectable surface changes in the skin or mucous membranes can be termed 'lesions'. They include the following:
  - **Macule:** a macule is a change in surface colour, without elevation or depression and therefore nonpalpable, well- or ill-defined, but generally considered less than 1.5 cm in diameter at the widest point.
  - **Patch:** a patch is a large macule equal to or greater than 1.5 cm across. Patches may have some subtle surface change, such as a fine scale or wrinkling but although the consistency of the surface is changed, the lesion itself is not palpable.
  - **Papule:** a papule is a circumscribed, solid, palpable elevation of skin/mucous membrane with no visible fluid, varying in size from a pinhead to less than 1.5 cm in diameter at the widest point.

- **Plaque:** a plaque is a broad, flat-topped papule, or confluence of papules, equal to or greater than 1.5 cm in diameter, or alternatively as an elevated, plateau-like lesion that is often greater in its diameter than in its depth.
- **Nodule:** a nodule is morphologically similar to a papule and is a palpable spherical lesion in all three directions: length, width, and depth. A nodule is usually a solid lesion of 1.5 cm or less in diameter. It may be sessile (attached directly by the base) or pedunculated (attached by a peduncle – a stem).
- **Tumour:** similar to a nodule but larger than 1.5 cm in diameter.
- **Vesicle:** a vesicle is a small blister; a circumscribed, fluid-filled, epithelial elevation generally less than 1.5 cm in diameter at the widest point. The fluid is a clear serous fluid.
- **Bulla:** a bulla is a large, rounded or irregularly shaped blister of the skin or mucous membrane containing serous or seropurulent fluid. Bullae are greater than 1.5 cm in diameter.
- **Pustule:** a pustule is a small elevation of the skin or mucous membrane containing cloudy or purulent material (pus) usually consisting of necrotic inflammatory cells. When haemorrhagic, the colour of the pustule may be red or blue.
- **Cyst:** a cyst is an epithelial-lined pathological cavity containing liquid, semisolid, or solid material.
- **Pseudocyst:** a cyst-like lesion that is not lined by epithelium.
- **Fissure:** a fissure is a crack in the skin or mucous membrane that is usually narrow and deep.
- **Erosion:** an erosion is a lesion that lacks the full thickness of the overlying epithelium and is moist, circumscribed, and usually depressed.
- **Ulcer:** an ulcer is a discontinuity of the skin or mucous membrane exhibiting complete loss of the epidermis or epithelium, with some amount of destruction of the subepithelial connective tissue.
- **Telangiectasia:** a telangiectasia represents an enlargement of superficial blood vessels in the skin or mucous membrane to the point of being visible.
- **Scale:** a skin lesion that consists of dry or greasy laminated masses of keratin.
- **Crust:** a skin lesion that is dried sebum, pus, or blood, usually mixed with epithelial and sometimes bacterial debris. Can occur on the vermilion as well.
- **Lichenification:** epidermal thickening of the skin characterized by visible and palpable thickening with accentuated skin markings.
- **Excoriation:** a punctate or linear abrasion of the skin produced by mechanical means (often scratching), usually involving only the epidermis, but commonly reaching the papillary dermis.
- **Induration:** dermal or mucosal thickening causing the cutaneous or mucosal surface to feel thicker and firmer.
- **Atrophy:** a loss of epithelial or submucous tissue. With epithelial atrophy, the mucous membrane appears thin, translucent, and wrinkled. Atrophy should be differentiated from erosion.
- **Maceration:** in maceration, the skin softens and turns white, due to being consistently wet.
- **Umbilication:** formation of a depression at the top of a papule, vesicle, or pustule.
- **Rash:** presence of multiple non-vesicular skin eruptions.
- **Sinus/fistula:** a sinus or fistula is a tract connecting cavities to each other or to the surface.
- **Sessile lesion:** a lesion attached to the underlying tissues with a broad base.
- **Pedunculated lesion:** a lesion attached to the underlying tissues with a narrow base, such as a stalk or pedicle.
- **Serpiginous lesion:** a lesion with a wavy border.
- **Discoid lesion:** a round or disc-shaped lesion.
- **Annular** or **circinate lesion:** a ring-shaped lesion.
- **Herpetiform lesions:** lesions resembling those of herpes.

- **Reticular** or **reticulated lesion:** a lesion resembling a net or lace.
- **Verrucous lesion:** a wart-like lesion.
- **Stellate lesion: a** star-shaped lesion.
- **Target lesion** or '**bull's eye lesion:** named for its resemblance to the bullseye of a shooting target. Also referred to as an 'iris' lesion.
- **Purpura:** haemorrhage into the surface of the skin or mucous membrane. Purpura measure 3–10 mm whereas petechiae measure less than 3 mm, and ecchymoses greater than 10 mm. The appearance of an individual area of purpura varies with the duration of the lesions. Early purpura is red and becomes darker, purple, and brown, yellow as it fades. Purpuric spots do not blanch on pressure.
- **Petechiae:** petechiae are small sharply outlined and slightly elevated red- or purple-coloured purpuric macules of about 1–3 mm in diameter. They contain extravasated blood.
- **Ecchymoses:** ecchymoses are larger purpuric lesions that are macular and deeper in origin than petechiae. They are to be distinguished from hematoma caused by extravasation of blood.
- **Hematoma:** a localized swelling that is filled with blood caused by a break in the wall of a blood vessel.
- **Hamartoma:** a benign (non-neoplastic) tumour-like growth consisting of a disorganized mixture of cells and tissues normally found in the body where the growth occurs.
- **Epulis:** a nonspecific exophytic gingival mass.

Histological nomenclature of oral mucosal lesions:

- **Hyperplasia:** an increase in the amount of organic tissue that results from cell proliferation.
- **Parakeratosis:** a mode of keratinization characterized by the retention of nuclei in the stratum corneum.
- **Hyperkeratosis:** thickening of the stratum corneum associated with the presence of an abnormal quantity of keratin.
- **Orthokeratosis:** hyperkeratosis without parakeratosis. No nucleus is seen in the cells as in the normal epidermis (skin) or epithelium (mucous membrane).
- **Acanthosis:** a benign abnormal thickening (hyperplasia) of the stratum spinosum, or prickle cell layer of the epidermis (skin) or epithelium (mucous membrane).
- **Acantholysis:** the loss of intercellular connections (desmosomes), resulting in loss of cohesion between keratinocytes in the skin or mucous membrane.
- **Spongiosis:** intercellular oedema (abnormal accumulation of fluid) in the epidermis in the skin or the epithelium in the mucous membrane.
- **Dyskeratosis:** abnormal keratinization occurring prematurely within individual cells or groups of cells below the stratum granulosum.
- **Vacuolization:** the formation of vacuoles within or adjacent to cells and often confined to the basal cell-basement membrane zone area.
- **Cellular** or **epithelial dysplasia:** an epithelial anomaly of growth and differentiation often indicative of an early neoplastic process.
- **Metaplasia:** cells of one mature, differentiated type are replaced by cells of another mature, differentiated type.
- **Atypia:** deviation from normal or a state of being not typical. Atypical cells are not necessarily cancerous.
- **Colloid bodies (also called Civatte bodies):** these apoptotic keratinocytes are oval or round, immediately above or below the epidermal or epithelial basement membrane.
- **Hydropic (liquefaction) degeneration:** basal cells become vacuolated, separated, and disorganized.
- **Hyaline bodies:** necrotic keratocytes; also termed colloid bodies, Civatte bodies, and apoptotic bodies.

Standard Abbreviations for Prescribers

ac (before meals)

ad lib (as desired)

ASAP (as soon as possible)

bid (twice a day)

btl (bottle)

c (with)

cap (capsule)

crm (cream)

disp (dispense on a prescription label)

elix (elixir)

g (gram)

gtt (drop)

h (hour)

hs (at bedtime)

iu (international units)

IV (intravenous)

l (litre)

liq (liquid)

loz (lozenge)

mg (milligram)

min (minute)

ml (millilitre)

NaF (sodium fluoride)

prn (as needed)

q (every)

q2h (every 2 hours)

q4h (every 4 hours)

q6h (every 6 hours)

q8h (every 8 hours)

q12h (every 12 hours)

qam (every morning)

qd (every day)

qhs (every bedtime)

qid (four times a day)

qod (every other day)

qpm (every evening)

qsad (add a sufficient quantity to equal)

qwk (every week)

Rx (prescription)

s (without)

sig (patient dosing instructions on prescription label)

sol (solution)

stat (Immediately)

syr (syrup)

tab (tablet)

tbsp (ttablespoon)

tid (three times a day)

top (topical)

tsp (teaspoon)

oint (ointment)

OTC (over the counter)

oz (ounce)

p (after)

pc (after meals)

PO (by mouth)

U (unit)

ut dict (as directed)

visc (viscous)

wk (week)

yr (year)

Part I

Pathology of Teeth and Supporting Structures

1

Disorders of Tooth Development and Eruption

1.1   Anodontia, Hypodontia and Oligodontia

1.1.1   Definition/Description

- Anodontia: All teeth are developmentally (congenitally) missing
- Hypodontia: one to six developmentally (congenitally) missing teeth except the third molars
- Oligodontia: more than six developmentally (congenitally) missing teeth

1.1.2   Frequency

- Anodontia: extremely rare
- Hypodontia: incidence: 4.4–13.4%. The most common developmental anomaly
- Oligodontia: incidence: 0.25%
- Hypodontia of the deciduous teeth affects less than 1% of children

Handbook of Oral Pathology and Oral Medicine, First Edition. S. R. Prabhu.
© 2022 John Wiley & Sons Ltd. Published 2022 by John Wiley & Sons Ltd.
Companion website: www.wiley.com/go/prabhu/oral_pathology

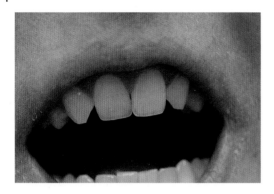

Figure 1.1 Hypodontia: clinical photograph of missing maxillary lateral incisors (*source:* Bin im Garten, https://commons.wikimedia.org/wiki/File:Hypodontie_der_zweiten_oberen_Schneidz%C3%A4hne_IMG_1726.JPG. Licensed under CC BY-SA 3.0).

1.1.3   Aetiology/Risk Factors

- Anodontia: mutations in *EDA*, *EDAR* and *EDARADD* genes
- Hypodontia: mutations in *MSX1*, *PAX9*, *IRF6*, *GREM2*, *AXIN2*, *LRP6*, *SMOC2*, *LTBP3*, *PITX2* and *WNT10B. WNT10A* genes
- Oligodontia: mutations in *MSX1*, *PAX9*, *IRF6*, *GREM2*, *AXIN2*, *LRP6*, *SMOC2*, *LTBP3*, *PITX2* and *WNT10B. WNT10A* genes
- Environmental factors: hypodontia can result from trauma to the developing dental tissues such as chemotherapy or radiotherapy

1.1.4   Clinical Features

- The most common missing multiple teeth (other than third molars) are:
  - Maxillary lateral incisors (Figure 1.1). This is followed by the mandibular second premolars and maxillary second premolars
  - Skin/nails/hair/sweat glands may be affected in some cases of hypodontia
  - Morphology of teeth may be defective (microdontia/peg-shaped laterals) in hypodontia
  - In Down syndrome oligodontia is common
  - Hypodontia/oligodontia might also be associated with cleft lip and palate
  - Over retention of the overlying deciduous tooth (because of the missing permanent tooth germ) occurs frequently

1.1.5   Radiographical Features

- In many cases routine radiography may reveal developmentally missing teeth

1.1.6   Diagnosis

- History
- Clinical examination
- Radiography

1.1.7   Management

- Prosthodontic treatment/implants or orthodontic treatment for edentulous spaces

1.2 Hyperdontia (Supernumerary Teeth)

1.2.1 Definition/Description

- Hyperdontia/supernumerary teeth: excess number of teeth beyond the expected 20 deciduous and 32 permanent teeth
- The shape of the supernumerary tooth may resemble a tooth of the normal series. In this case, the extra tooth is called supplemental tooth

1.2.2 Frequency

- 98% of supernumerary teeth occur in the maxilla
- In 1% of the population, a supernumerary tooth occurs in the midline in anterior maxilla; this is called mesiodens

1.2.3 Aetiology/Risk Factors

- Budding of the dental lamina: stimulus for budding is not known

1.2.4 Clinical Features

- Asymptomatic: supernumerary teeth may be detected incidentally on radiography for other reasons
- Supernumerary teeth are five times more common in the permanent dentition than in the deciduous dentition
- Supernumerary teeth may be single or multiple, unilateral or bilateral, and may be present in one or both jaws.
- The most common single supernumerary tooth: midline of the anterior maxilla, known as a mesiodens. This is also an example of microdontia
- Other supernumerary teeth: maxillary fourth molars, maxillary lateral incisors, mandibular fourth molars and mandibular premolars
- The most common site for multiple supernumerary teeth is the mandibular premolar region (Figure 1.2)

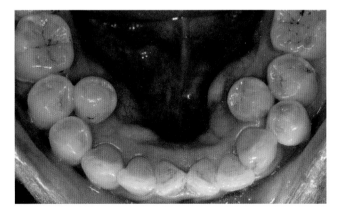

Figure 1.2 Supernumerary premolars located lingual to the mandibular first and second premolars.

- A supernumerary tooth lingual or buccal to a molar is called a paramolar
- A supernumerary tooth located distal to a third molar is called a distomolar
- Supernumerary teeth are common in patients with cleidocranial dysplasia and Gardner syndrome
- Complications of supernumerary teeth may include:
  - Delayed or ectopic eruption of adjacent teeth
  - Root resorption of adjacent teeth
  - Crowding
  - Malocclusion
  - Diastema
  - Pericoronal cyst or infection

1.2.5 Radiographical Features

- Cone beam computed tomography (CBCT) precisely defines the location of the tooth and its proximity to vital anatomical structures such as the nasal floor and nasopalatine canal

1.2.6 Diagnosis

- History
- Clinical examination
- Radiography

1.2.7 Management

- Extraction in most cases

1.3 Microdontia and Macrodontia

1.3.1 Definition/Description

- Microdontia: size of the tooth unusually smaller than average
- Macrodontia: size of the tooth unusually larger than average

1.3.2 Frequency

- Differences in prevalence rates exist
- Approximate prevalence in general population:
  - 1.58% for microdontia
  - 0.03% for macrodontia
  - Microdontia in maxillary lateral incisors ('peg laterals') is common (0.8–8.4%)

1.3.3 Aetiology/Risk Factors

- Maternal influences, genetic and environmental factors.
- Deciduous teeth are affected more due to intrauterine maternal influences
- Permanent teeth are affected more due to environmental factors

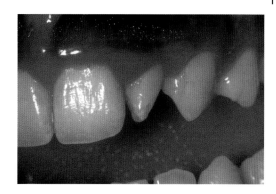

Figure 1.3 Microdontia: maxillary left lateral incisor ('peg lateral') is cone shaped and smaller than average for lateral incisor (*source:* by kind permission of Professor Charles Dunlap, Kansas City, USA).

1.3.4 Clinical Features

- Generalized microdontia involving all teeth is extremely rare
- Generalized macrodontia is rare: often seen in pituitary gigantism
- Generalized microdontia may be a feature of Down syndrome and pituitary dwarfism
- Microdontia may be associated with hypodontia
- Macrodontia may be associated with hyperdontia
- Microdontia is more frequent in females
- Macrodontia is more frequent in males
- Maxillary lateral incisor is commonly involved in microdontia (peg lateral; Figure 1.3)
- Isolated microdontia is frequently seen in third molars
- Isolated macrodontia is occasionally seen in incisors, canines, second premolars and third molars (fused and geminated teeth to be differentiated from macrodontia)

1.3.5 Diagnosis

- History
- Clinical examination
- For macrodontia, radiography is useful to rule out gemination or fusion

1.3.6 Management

- No treatment is required unless for aesthetic purposes.
- Porcelain crown for peg lateral is often used

1.4 Gemination, Fusion and Concrescence

1.4.1 Definition/Description

- Gemination: attempt at a single tooth bud to divide, resulting in a tooth with bifid crown and a common root and root canal (clinically seen as double teeth)
- Fusion: union of two normally separated tooth buds resulting in a joined tooth with confluent dentine (clinically seen as double teeth) and separate root canals
- Concrescence: union of two teeth by cementum without confluence of dentine

1.4.2 Frequency

- Varies; approximate prevalence rates are:
  - Gemination: 0.22%
  - Fusion: 0.19%
  - Concrescence: 0.8% in permanent teeth and 0.2–3.7% in deciduous teeth

1.4.3 Aetiology/Risk Factors

- Gemination and fusion: evolution, trauma, heredity and environmental factors
- Concrescence: inflammation around roots

1.4.4 Clinical Features

- Tooth count:
  - Individuals with gemination have a normal tooth count. Clinically seen as double teeth but radiograph shows common root canal (Figure 1.4a,b)
  - Individuals with fusion show a missing tooth due to the union of two teeth. Clinically seen as a large tooth crown (Figure 1.4c)
  - Individuals with concrescence have a normal tooth count. Roots of two teeth are joined by cementum (Figure 1.4d)
- Gemination: more common in the maxilla
- Fusion: more common in the mandible
- Concrescence: common in posterior maxillary region. Often, second molar roots are joined with adjacent impacted third molar roots
- Gemination and fusion in deciduous teeth may cause crowding, abnormal spacing or delayed eruption of permanent teeth

1.4.5 Radiographical Features

- Gemination: common root, common root canal
- Fusion: separate roots and root canals
- Concrescence: roots joined at cementum of two adjoining teeth. CBCT is useful for concrescence (gives a three-dimensional image)

1.4.6 Diagnosis

- History
- Clinical examination
- Radiography

1.4.7 Management

- Depends on patient requirement
- Usually not indicated unless symptomatic due to other causes, such as extensive caries, periodontal pathology or interference with tooth eruption

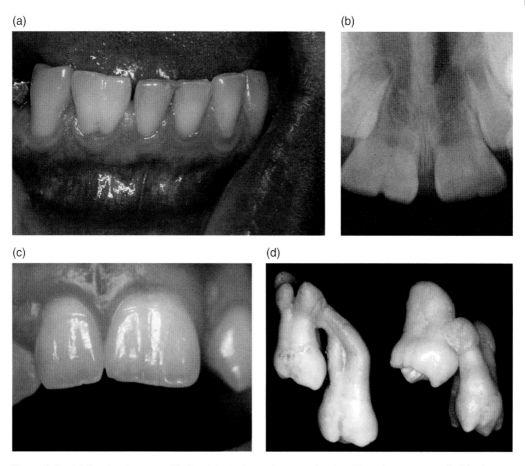

Figure 1.4 (a) Gemination; mandibular right incisors show gemination. Note the presence of all incisors. (b) Radiograph of bilateral gemination in maxillary central incisors. Note incisal notch and common root and root canal. (c) Fusion; shows left maxillary lateral incisor fused with the central incisor. (d) Concrescence; roots of two teeth are joined by cementum. (*sources:* a–c, by kind permission of Professor Charles Dunlap, Kansas City, USA); d, by kind permission of Dental Press Publishing, Brazil.)

1.5 Taurodontism and Dilaceration

1.5.1 Definition/Description

- Taurodontism refers to an enlarged pulp chamber, apical displacement of the pulpal floor and no constriction at the level of the cementoenamel junction
- Dilaceration refers to abnormal angulation or bend in the root

1.5.2 Frequency

- Range:
  - Taurodontism: 0.5–4.6% in general population
  - Dilaceration: 0.3–15% in general population

1.5.3 Aetiology/Risk Factors

- Taurodontism:
  - Failure of Hertwig's epithelial root sheath diaphragm to invaginate at the proper horizontal level
  - No genetic association
- Dilaceration:
  - Idiopathic
  - Injury that displaces the calcified portion of the tooth germ from the uncalcified portion resulting in an abnormal angle of the root

1.5.4 Clinical Features

- Taurodontism:
  - May be unilateral or bilateral
  - Permanent teeth are frequently affected
  - No gender predilection
  - May occur as a part of syndromes such as Klinefelter syndrome, Mohr syndrome and McCune–Albright syndrome
  - Increased frequency in patients with cleft lip, cleft palate and those with hypodontia.
  - Increased chances of pulp exposure in decayed teeth with taurodontism
  - Degree of taurodontism:
    - ○ hypotaurodontism (mild form)
    - ○ mesotaurodontism (moderate form)
    - ○ hypertaurodontism (severe form)

- Dilaceration:
  - Mandibular third molars are frequently involved followed by maxillary second premolars and mandibular second molars
  - Rare in deciduous dentition
  - Asymptomatic in most cases
  - Associated with syndromes (e.g. Ehlers–Danlos syndrome)

1.5.5 Radiographical Features

- Taurodontism:
  - Commonly detected on routine radiography
  - Involved teeth presume a rectangular shape
  - The pulp chamber is exceedingly large with a greater apical–occlusal height than normal
  - The tooth lacks the usual constriction at the cervical region
  - Roots are exceedingly short and trifurcation or bifurcation may be seen a few millimetres above the apices of the roots (Figure 1.5a)
- Dilaceration:
  - Radiographically, detected as mesial or distal bend in the root (Figure 1.5b)
  - Periodontal ligament space is normal
  - Detected on routine radiography

(a)

(b)

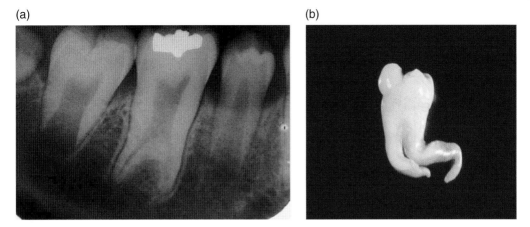

Figure 1.5 (a)Taurodontism of the mandibular first molar shows abnormally large pulp chamber and short roots. (b) Dilaceration of an extracted tooth shows abnormal bend in the roots. (*source:* by kind permission of Professor Charles Dunlap, Kansas City, USA.)

1.5.6 Management

- Taurodontism:
  - No specific treatment required
- Dilaceration:
  - No treatment for mild dilaceration
  - If symptomatic due to gross dilaceration, tooth requires surgical extraction

1.6 Amelogenesis Imperfecta

1.6.1 Definition/Description

- A group of inherited disorders caused by defects in the genes that encode enamel matrix proteins, resulting in defective structure of the enamel involving both dentitions

1.6.2 Incidence/Prevalence

- Global prevalence: 0.5%

1.6.3 Aetiology/Risk Factors

- Caused by mutations or altered expression in five genes:
  - *AMEL* (amelogenin)
  - *ENAM* (enamelin)
  - *MMP20* (matrix metalloproteinase-20)
  - *KLK4* (kallikrein-4)
  - *FAM83H*. 6–16
- Inheritance can be autosomal dominant, recessive or x-linked

1.6.4 Clinical/Radiographical Features

- Three types of amelogenesis imperfecta have been identified – hypoplastic, hypocalcified and hypomaturation:
  - Hypoplastic type:
    - Enamel is of reduced thickness due to a defect in the formation of normal matrix
    - Enamel is pitted, grooved, stained and thin
    - Enamel is normally mineralized; hard and translucent
    - Radiographically, the enamel contrasts normally from dentine
  - Hypocalcified type:
    - Enamel matrix is normal in quantity
    - Enamel calcification is defective
    - Enamel is weak in structure and vulnerable to attrition
    - Teeth become opaque, stained and rapidly wear down (Figure 1.6)
    - Radiographically, enamel is less radio-opaque than dentine
  - Hypomaturation type:
    - Enamel is normal in thickness, shows opaque brownish-yellow patches
    - Enamel mimics fluorotic mottled enamel in appearance
    - Enamel is soft and vulnerable to attrition
- Other features that may occur in any of the above types of amelogenesis imperfecta include:
  - Delay in dental eruption
  - Microdontia
  - Deviant crown and morphology
  - Root resorption
  - Short roots
  - Enlarged pulp chamber
  - Pulp stones
  - Dens in dente (dens invaginatus)
  - Tooth agenesis
  - Crowding of teeth

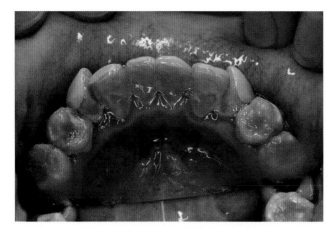

Figure 1.6 Amelogenesis imperfecta (hypocalcified type); the enamel is stained and vulnerable to attrition (*source:* by kind permission of Professor Charles Dunlap, Kansas City, USA).

1.7 Dentinogenesis Imperfecta

1.6.5 Differential diagnosis

- Dental fluorosis
- Dentinogenesis imperfecta
- Enamel hypoplasia
- Trauma
- Molar incisor hypomineralization

1.6.6 Diagnosis

- History including a detailed family history
- Pedigree plotting (family health history tree)
- Clinical examination
- Radiography

1.6.7 Management

- Aesthetic treatment
- Treatment for symptoms if present (e.g. tooth sensitivity)

1.7 Dentinogenesis Imperfecta

1.7.1 Definition/Description

- A group of autosomal dominant genetic conditions characterized by abnormal dentin structure affecting both the primary and secondary dentitions

1.7.2 Frequency

- Incidence of 1 in 6000 to 1 in 8000

1.7.3 Aetiology/Risk Factors

- Mutations in dentin sialoprotein genes

1.7.4 Clinical Features

- Primary and permanent teeth are affected
- Teeth appear amber, brown/blue, or opalescent brown (Figure 1.7a)
- Syndromic form, osteogenesis imperfecta: opalescent dentine, blue sclera and short stature

1.7.5 Radiographical features

- The crowns may appear bulbous (Figure 1.7b)
- Pulp chambers are often small or obliterated
- The roots are often narrow with small or with obliterated root canals

(a)　　　　　　　　　　　　　　(b)

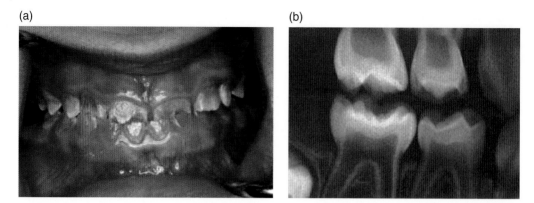

Figure 1.7 Dentinogenesis imperfecta. (a) Note tooth wear and opalescent crowns. (b) Radiograph shows bulbous crowns and cervical constriction of molars. (*source:* by kind permission of Professor Charles Dunlap, Kansas City, USA.)

1.7.6　Differential Diagnosis

- Hypocalcified forms of amelogenesis imperfecta
- Osteogenesis imperfecta
- Congenital erythropoietic porphyria
- Conditions leading to early tooth loss
- Permanent teeth discolouration due to tetracyclines
- Vitamin D-dependent and vitamin D-resistant rickets

1.7.7　Diagnosis

- Family history
- Pedigree construction
- Detailed clinical examination
- Radiography

1.7.8　Management

- The aims of treatment are to remove sources of infection or pain, restore aesthetics and protect posterior teeth from wear
- Preservation of occlusal face height, maintenance of function and aesthetic needs are priorities
- For the primary dentition, stainless steel crowns are recommended

1.8　Dentinal Dysplasia (Dentin Dysplasia)

1.8.1　Definition/Description

- A rare inherited disorder of dentin formation characterized by either absent or short conical roots
- Two types occur: radicular dentin dysplasia (type 1) and coronal dentin dysplasia (type 2)
- Coronal dentin dysplasia is a severe form of dentinogenesis imperfecta

1.8.2 Frequency

- Type 1: 1 in 100 000
- Type 2: 1 in 6000 to 1 in 8000

1.8.3 Aetiology/Risk Factors

- Defective dentin sialoprotein gene for both types

1.8.4 Clinical Features

- Radicular type (type 1):
  - Diffusely affects both dentitions: severe manifestations in deciduous teeth
  - Coronal enamel and dentin are normal
  - Radicular dentin is defective: short roots result in tooth mobility and premature tooth loss
  - Strength of roots is reduced
  - Hypersensitive dentin
  - Loss of pulpal vitality
  - Absent root canals
  - Bifurcation is close to the apex in molars
  - Periapical pathology is common (seen as periapical radiolucency)
- Coronal type (type 2):
  - Primary and permanent teeth are affected
  - Teeth appear amber, brown/blue or opalescent brown

1.8.5 Radiographical features

- Coronal type:
  - The crowns may appear bulbous
  - Pulp chambers are often small or obliterated
  - The roots are often narrow with small or obliterated root canals
  - Roots may be absent (Figure 1.8)

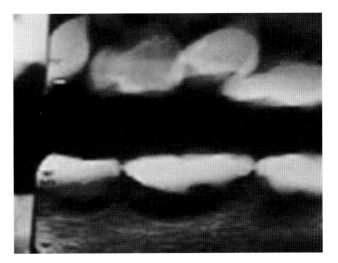

Figure 1.8 Dentinal dysplasia radiograph showing absence of roots (*source:* by kind permission of Professor Charles Dunlap, Kansas City, USA).

1.8.6   Differential Diagnosis

- Dentinogenesis imperfecta
- Osteogenesis imperfecta
- Conditions that cause premature loss of teeth

1.8.7   Diagnosis

- Family history
- Clinical examination
- Radiography

1.8.8   Management

- Symptomatic and preventive care and meticulous oral hygiene

1.9   Regional Odontodysplasia (Ghost Teeth)

1.9.1   Definition/Description

- A rare non-hereditary dental anomaly involving enamel, dentin and cementum of both dentitions, but mostly the teeth of one quadrant

1.9.2   Frequency

- A rare disorder

1.9.3   Aetiology/Risk Factors

- Unknown
- Probably alteration in vascular supply in the jaws around developing teeth

1.9.4   Clinical Features

- Female predilection (female to male ratio 1.7 : 1)
- Both dentitions are involved
- Mostly one but rarely two quadrants are involved
- Age at diagnosis: 2–4 years for deciduous teeth and 7–11 years for permanent teeth
- Maxillary predominance (ratio of maxillary to mandibular width 1.6 : 1)
- Failure of tooth eruption is common
- Erupted teeth exhibit small brown crowns
- Pulp necrosis is common
- Early tooth exfoliation

1.9.5   Radiographical features

- Thin enamel and dentin appear surrounding enlarged radiolucent pulp chamber (hence the name ghost tooth)
- Pulp stones are occasionally detected on radiography

1.9.6   Differential Diagnosis

- Oculodentodigital dysplasia
- Segmental odontomaxillary dysplasia
- Odonto-onychodermal dysplasia
- Odontochondrodysplasia

1.9.7   Diagnosis

- History
- Clinical examination
- Radiography

1.9.8   Management

- Unerupted teeth to remain without any interference
- Erupted teeth: steel crowns
- Non-salvageable teeth to be extracted

1.10   Delayed Tooth Eruption

1.10.1   Definition/Description

- Delayed tooth eruption is the emergence of a tooth into the oral cavity at a time that deviates significantly from norms established for different races, ethnic groups and sexes

1.10.2   Frequency

- Delayed eruption is relatively common; racial and gender variations exist
- Failure of eruption is less common
- Agenesis of teeth cause failure of eruption

1.10.3   Aetiology/Risk Factors

- Local causes associated with delayed tooth eruption:
  - Supernumerary teeth
  - Mucosal barrier scar tissue due to trauma/surgery/gingival hyperplasia
  - Tumours: odontogenic or non-odontogenic tumours
  - Ankylosis of deciduous teeth
  - Enamel pearls
  - Injuries to primary teeth
  - Regional odontodysplasia
  - Ectopic eruption
  - Impacted permanent teeth
  - Embedded primary teeth
  - Oral clefts
  - Radiation damage

- Systemic causes associated with delayed tooth eruption:
  - Nutritional deficiencies
  - Vitamin D-resistant rickets
  - Hypoparathyroidism
  - Hypopituitarism
  - Long-term chemotherapy
  - Cerebral palsy
  - Prematurity or low birth weight
  - Phenytoin use
  - Genetic disorders

1.10.4   Clinical and Radiographical Features

- Local factors causing delayed tooth eruption are frequently detected by radiography
- Systemic factors causing delayed tooth eruption are detected by systemic clinical features and laboratory findings
- Failure of tooth eruption: congenital absence of teeth (third molars, mandibular second premolars and maxillary lateral incisors) results in failure of tooth eruption
- Radiographical evidence of absence of teeth is diagnostic

1.10.5   Diagnosis

- History
- Clinical examination
- Radiography (panoramic view is ideal)
- Laboratory tests if systemic factors are suspected

1.10.6   Management

- Patient with eruption delay of more than 12 months (delayed eruption) of the normal age range should be referred to a paediatric dentist for further evaluation
- Identification of the causes and their elimination is important
- Surgical exposure followed by orthodontic treatment may be required for some patients with delayed eruption

1.11   Tooth Impaction (Impacted Teeth)

1.11.1   Definition/Description

- Teeth that are completely or partially retained in the jaws beyond their normal date of eruption

1.11.2   Frequency

- Common; variations in incidence and prevalence exist
- The mandibular third molars are the most common impacted teeth, with their prevalence ranging from 27% to 68.8% in various parts of the world

- The reported prevalence of impacted teeth of canines and second premolars ranges from 2.9% to 13.7%

1.11.3 Aetiology

- Lack of space for tooth eruption due to inadequate arch length
- Crowding of teeth
- Dense overlying bone
- Excessive soft tissue in the path of eruption
- Genetic abnormalities
- Long tortuous path of eruption (for canines)

1.11.4 Clinical Features

- Frequently impacted teeth: mandibular third molars followed by the maxillary third molars, maxillary canines and mandibular premolars
- Young adults are commonly affected; often detected on routine radiography
- Impacted deciduous teeth are extremely rare
- Impacted permanent first and second molars are rare
- Often supernumerary teeth are impacted (detected on radiography)
- Impacted teeth may or may not be symptomatic
- With no history of extraction, clinically the number of teeth present in the dentition is less than normal
- Impaction can be full or partial
- Symptomatic patients with lower third molar may complain of earache or paraesthesia of the lip
- Pericoronitis may occur (pain, inability to open the mouth, swelling of the pericoronal soft tissue)
- Often, all four third molars may be impacted
- Occasionally impactions are associated with syndromes or odontogenic cysts and tumours

1.11.5 Radiographical Features

- Types of impaction: mesioangular, distoangular, vertical or horizontal impaction for third molars (Figure 1.9 a-d). Canine impaction may be bilateral (Figure 9 e) or inverted
- Proximity of the impacted tooth to the inferior dental nerve for lower third molar impactions may cause paraesthesia
- Impacted teeth may be associated with cysts or odontogenic tumours

1.11.6 Diagnosis

- History
- Clinical examination
- Radiography (panoramic view)

1.11.7 Management

- No treatment is required for asymptomatic impactions
- Surgical removal for symptomatic impacted teeth
- Surgery for impacted teeth associated with cysts or tumours

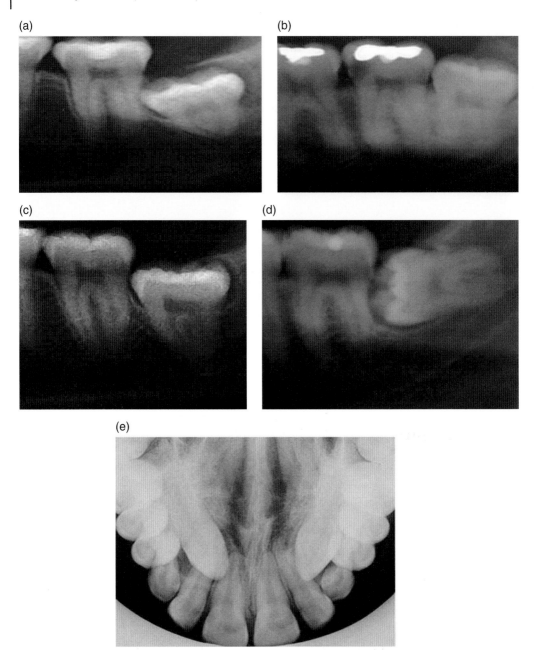

Figure 1.9 (a) Mesioangular impaction of the mandibular third molar. (b) Distoangular impaction of the mandibular third molar (c) Vertical impaction of the mandibular third molar. (d) Horizontal impaction of the mandibular third molar. (e) Bilateral impaction of maxillary canines.

1.12 Dens Invaginatus and Dens Evaginatus

1.12.1 Definition/Description

- Dens invaginatus refers to an exaggeration of the process of formation of lingual pit causing invagination (also called dens in dente or dilated odontome)

- Dens evaginatus refers to an enamel and dentin covered spur extending outward from the occlusal surfaces of molars or premolars and rarely lingual surfaces of lower anterior teeth. This is the opposite of dens evaginatus (also called evaginated odontome)

1.12.2 Frequency

- Dens invaginatus: prevalence: 0.3–10%, affecting more males than females
- Dens evaginatus: more common in people of Asian descent; prevalence: 0.06–7.7%; 15% in Inuit and Native American populations

1.12.3 Aetiology/Risk Factors

- Dens invaginatus:
  - Deepening or invagination of the enamel organ into the dental papilla prior to calcification of the dental tissues
  - Genetics may play a role
- Dens evaginatus:
  - A result of an unusual growth and folding of the inner enamel epithelium and ectomesenchymal cells of dental papilla into the stellate reticulum of the enamel organ

1.12.4 Clinical Features

- Dens invaginatus:
  - The permanent maxillary lateral incisors appear to be the most frequently affected tooth (90% of all cases)
  - Maxillary posterior teeth: 6.5% of all cases
  - Mandibular teeth are very rarely affected
- May be associated with taurodontism, microdontia, gemination, supernumerary tooth and dentinogenesis imperfecta

(a)   (b)

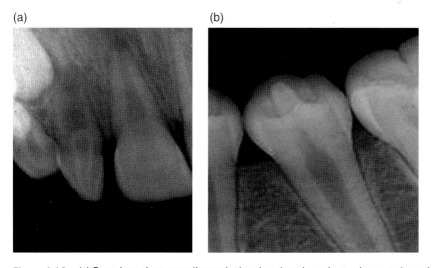

Figure 1.10   (a) Dens invaginatus; radiograph showing dens invaginatus in a peg lateral incisor (*source:* by kind permission of Professor Charles Dunlap, Kansas City, Kansas, USA). (b) Dens evaginatus; radiograph showing dens evaginatus. Note a tubercle extending outward from the occlusal surface of the premolar.

- Causes food debris deposits and renders tooth vulnerable to caries
- Dens evaginatus:
  - More common in mandibular premolar teeth
  - May be bilateral and symmetrical tubercles on the occlusal surfaces of posterior teeth or on lingual surfaces of lower anterior
  - Slight female sex predilection
  - Can cause malocclusion with opposing teeth
  - Abnormal wear and fracture of the tubercle may occur

1.12.5   Radiographical features

- Three types of dens invaginatus occur which can be detected on radiography:
  - Type I: invagination ends in a blind sac, limited to the tooth crown (Figure 1.10a)
  - Type II: invagination extends to the cementoenamel junction extending in a blind sac. It may or may not extend into the root pulp
  - Type III: invagination extends to the interior of the root providing an opening to the periodontium, sometimes this presents another foramen in the apical region of tooth
  - Dens evaginatus shows a tubercle on the occlusal surface (Figure 1.10b)

1.12.6   Diagnosis

- History
- Clinical examination (tooth morphology)
- Radiography (intraoral periapical views)

1.12.7   Management

- Dens invaginatus: placement of sealants and endodontic treatment for severe cases
- Dens evaginatus: removal of the tubercle and application of fluorides

1.13   Fluorosis (Mottled Enamel)

1.13.1   Definition/Description

- Dental fluorosis (mottled enamel) is a qualitative defect of enamel resulting from an increase in fluoride concentration during enamel formation

1.13.2   Frequency

- Fluorosis is extremely common
- Global variations exist. The global prevalence of fluorosis is reported to be about 32%

1.13.3   Aetiology/Risk Factors

- A higher than normal amount of fluoride ingestion while teeth are forming
- When the level of fluoride is above 1.5 mg/l (1.5 ppm) in drinking water, dental fluorosis occurs
- The severity of fluorosis is dependent on the dose and time of exposure to fluoride levels

- Other sources of fluoride: toothpastes, mouth rinses, fluoride supplements, beverages (brick tea, tea and butter tea) and food (infant formula, fish, beans, potatoes and wheat)

1.13.4   Clinical Features

- Severity of fluorosis is dose dependent
- Mild fluorosis: opaque lines following the perikymata
- Moderate fluorosis: the opaque lines merge and more irregular cloudy areas become visible
- Severe fluorosis: enamel is grossly defective with opaque chalky appearance and punched out pits. Extrinsic brown staining in the pits is frequent (Figure 1.11)
- Moderate to severe enamel fluorosis is called mottled enamel
- Teeth with fluorosis are weak but resistant to caries

1.13.5   Differential Diagnosis

- Turner's hypoplasia
- Hypoplastic teeth in systemic disorders
- Amelogenesis imperfecta
- Early carious lesions
- Tetracycline staining of teeth

1.13.6   Diagnosis

- History (residence/ migration, water fluoridation, other sources of fluorides in the diet)
- Clinical examination

1.13.7   Management

- Aesthetic procedures as required

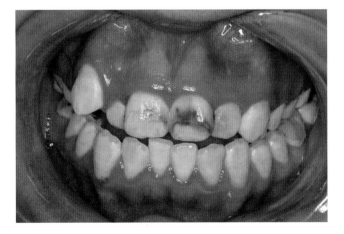

Figure 1.11   Yellow-brown discoloration of maxillary incisors due to fluorosis (*source:* From Mary A. Aubertin. 2014. Common Benign Dental and Periodontal Lesions. In: *Diagnosis and Management of Oral Lesions and Conditions: A Resource Handbook for the Clinician.* ed. Cesar A. Migliorati and Fotinos S. Panagakos. IntechOpen. doi: 10.5772/57597).

- Close monitoring of sources of fluoride during the first three years of age
- Water fluoridation: 0.7–1 ppm recommended
- Use of fluoride tooth paste after 12 months of age
- Infant formula with fluoridated water to be avoided
- Fluoride supplements only in non-fluoridated areas

1.14 Tetracycline-Induced Discoloration of Teeth: Key Features

- Tetracycline is a broad-spectrum antibiotic commonly used for infections
- Tetracycline has several different analogues such as doxycycline, oxytetracycline, minocycline, chlortetracycline, demeclocycline
- Tetracycline can stain teeth if ingested by the mother in the third trimester or by the child during the years of tooth formation of deciduous and permanent dentition
- The discoloration, which is permanent, varies from yellow or grey to brown (Figure 1.12)
- Administration of tetracycline to pregnant women must be avoided during the second or third trimester of gestation and to children up to eight years of age.
- Tetracycline-stained teeth must be differentiated from dentinogenesis imperfecta

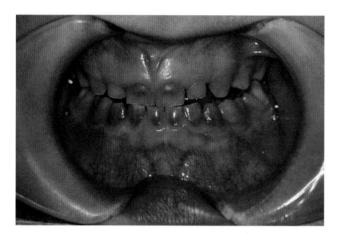

Figure 1.12 Tetracycline-induced grey/brown discolouration of deciduous teeth in a child (*source:* by kind permission of Professor Charles Dunlap, Kansas City, Kansas, USA).

1.15 Enamel Pearl: Key Features

- The enamel pearl is a globule of enamel formation located on the root surface (Figure 1.13)
- It is characterized by a core of dentin covered by enamel and may contain a pulp chamber
- Enamel pearl may cause periodontal pockets and periodontitis

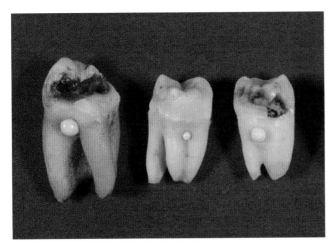

Figure 1.13 Enamel pearl on the cementum (*source:* by kind permission of Professor Charles Dunlap, Kansas City, Kansas, USA).

1.16 Talon Cusp: Key Features

- Talon cusp is a rare developmental anomaly presenting as a wisp-like structure arising from the cervical region of anterior teeth
- Resembles an eagle's talon

Figure 1.14 Periapical radiograph of talon cusp on a partially erupted upper left permanent maxillary incisor in an eight-year-old boy. Note V-shaped radiopaque structure overlapping the affected crown with its apex directed incisally (*source:* Matthew Fergusson, https://en.wikipedia.org/wiki/File:Talon_cusp.png. Licensed under CC BY-SA 4.0).

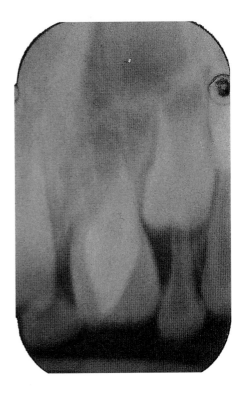

- In canines and incisors, it originates usually in the palatal cingulum as a tubercle projecting from the palatal surface
- Its prevalence varies from less than 1% to approximately 8%
- Radiographically, talon cusp appears as appears as a V-shaped radiopaque structure overlapping the affected crown with its apex directed incisally (Figure 1.14)
- Symptoms include interference with occlusion, irritation of soft tissues, accidental cusp fracture and susceptible to dental caries

1.17   Hutchinson's Incisors and Mulberry Molars: Key Features

- 'Hutchinson's incisors' and 'Mulberry molars' are dental developmental defects seen in children with congenital syphilis; they are rare conditions
- In Hutchinson's incisors, the incisal edge is either notched or screwdriver shaped. The bulbous crown is short and narrow ('barrel shaped'). In the centre of the incisal edge a deep vertical central notch may be present (Figure 1.15a)
- Mulberry molars are characterized by multiple rounded rudimentary enamel cusps on the permanent first molars (Figure 1.15b)
- Hutchinson's incisors and mulberry molars are caused by direct invasion of tooth germs by Treponema organisms during tooth development

(a)   (b)

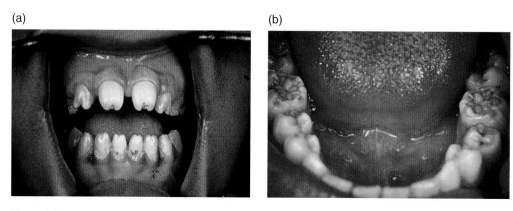

Figure 1.15   (a) Hutchinson's incisors of congenital syphilis. Note screwdriver shape and central notch on the crowns of upper and lower permanent incisors. (b) Mulberry molars of congenital syphilis. Note multiple poorly formed globular cusps on the occlusal surfaces of mandibular permanent first molars. (*source:* images by kind permission of Professor Charles Dunlap, Kansas City, Kansas, USA.)

1.18   Tooth Ankylosis: Key Features

- Anatomical fusion of tooth cementum with the alveolar bone:
    - Mandibular primary first molars are frequently ankylosed
    - Ankylosis of permanent teeth is uncommon
    - A sharp solid note on percussion is noted, suggesting ankylosis
    - Periodontal ligament space is absent on radiography
    - In many examples, the permanent successor is missing

Figure 1.16   An extracted mandibular molar with three roots.

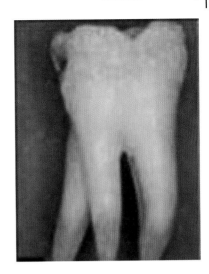

1.19   Supernumerary Roots: Key Features

- Normally, the permanent mandibular first molar has two roots, one mesial and one distal root
- Rarely, an additional third root is seen, which is found distolingually, called the radix entomolaris (Figure 1.16)
- Occasionally, supernumerary roots may be detected in mandibular third molars, mandibular canines and premolars
- No treatment is required
- Detection is critical for endodontic treatment

Recommended Reading

Consolaro, A., Hadaya, O., Oliveira Miranda, D.A., and Colsolaro, R.B. (2020). Concrescence: can the teeth involved be moved or separated? *Dental Press Journal of Orthodontics* 25 (1): 20–25.

Miletich, I. and Sharpe, P.T. (2003). Normal and abnormal dental development. *Human Molecular Genetics* 12 (Suppl 1): R69–R73.

Neville, B.W., Damm, D.D., Allen, C.M., and Chi, C.A. (2016). Developmental alterations of teeth. In: *Oral and Maxillofacial Pathology*, 4ee, 49–92. St. Louis, MO: Elsevier.

Odell, E.W. (2017). Disorders of tooth development. In: *Cawson's Essentials of Oral Pathology and Oral Medicine*, 9ee, 23–42. Edinburgh: Elsevier.

Parsa, A. and Rapala, H. (2016). Endodontic treatment of a mandibular 6 years molar with three roots: a pedodontist perspective. *International Journal of Pedodontic Rehabilitation* 1: 64–67.

Rhoads, S.G., Hendricks, H.M., and Frazier-Bowers, S.A. (2013). Establishing the diagnostic criteria for eruption disorders based on genetic and clinical data. *American Journal of Orthodontics and Dentofacial Orthopaedics* 144 (2): 194–202.

Rosa, D.C.L., Simukawa, E.R., Capelozza, A.L.A. et al. (2019). Alveolodental ankylosis: biological bases and diagnostic criteria. *RGO Revista Gaúcha de Odontologia* 67: e2019003.

Seow, W.K. (2014). Developmental defects of enamel and dentine: challenges for basic science research and clinical management. *Australian Dental Journal* 59 (1 Suppl): 143–154.

2

Dental caries

2.1   Definition/Description

- Dental caries is an infectious, transmissible disease resulting in destruction of tooth structure by acid-forming bacteria found in dental plaque (an intraoral biofilm) in the presence of fermentable carbohydrates
- The infection results in the loss of tooth minerals that begins with the outer surface of the tooth and can progress through the dentin to the pulp, ultimately compromising the vitality of the tooth

2.2   Frequency

- 60–90% of schoolchildren worldwide; the disease is most prevalent in Asian and Latin American countries

2.3   Aetiology/Risk Factors/Pathogenesis

- Biofilm acid-producing bacteria metabolize sugars and produce acids that lower the biofilm pH creating conditions that demineralize tooth enamel and dentin
- Acid-producing bacteria are *Mutans streptococci* and *Lactobacillus* species
- Acids produced include lactic, acetic, formic and propionic acids. These acids are capable of demineralizing enamel and dentin

Handbook of Oral Pathology and Oral Medicine, First Edition. S. R. Prabhu.
© 2022 John Wiley & Sons Ltd. Published 2022 by John Wiley & Sons Ltd.
Companion website: www.wiley.com/go/prabhu/oral_pathology

- Cycles of demineralization and remineralization continue in the mouth in the presence of cariogenic bacteria, fermentable carbohydrates and saliva
- Plaque microorganisms, substrate, susceptible tooth and time are essential factors for the development of caries

2.4 Classification of Caries

- Classification is based on:
  - Rate of progression: acute and chronic caries
  - Affected dental hard tissues: enamel, dentin and cemental (root surface) caries
  - Location on the tooth surface involved: pit and fissure caries, approximal/smooth surface caries and root surface caries (Table 2.1)

Table 2.1   American Dental Association caries classification system: Site Definitions-Origin

Site	Definition
Pit and fissure	The anatomical pits or fissures (clefts or valleys in the tooth surface) of the teeth at the occlusal, facial or lingual surfaces of posterior teeth OR the lingual surfaces of the maxillary incisors or canines
Approximal surface	The contact point(s) between adjacent teeth
Cervical and smooth surface	The cervical area or any other smooth enamel surface of the anatomic crown adjacent to an edentulous space (toothless space); may exist anywhere around the full circumference of the tooth
Root	The root surface apical to the anatomic crown

Source: Based on Ismail, A.I., Tellez, M., Pitts, N.B. et al. (2013). Caries management pathways preserve dental tissues and promote oral health. *Community Dentistry and Oral Epidemiology* 41 (1): e12–e40.

2.5 Clinical Features

- Asymptomatic in the initial stages
- Mild pain, tooth sensitivity when carious lesion gets larger
- Visible cavity in the tooth
- Brown, black or white chalky discoloration
- Oral malodour

2.5.1 Primary Caries

- Decay at a location that has not previously experienced decay

2.5.2 Secondary Caries (Recurrent Caries)

- Appears at a location with a previous history of caries
- Frequently found on the margins of fillings and other dental restorations

2.5.3 Arrested Caries

- A lesion on a tooth that was previously demineralized but was remineralized before causing a cavitation

2.5.4 Rampant Caries

- Severe decay on multiple surfaces of many teeth (Figure 2.1)
- Those at risk: individuals with xerostomia, poor oral hygiene, drug-induced dry mouth, large sugar intake and radiation to the head and neck region
- Treatment options include therapeutic and preventive strategies, including diet modifications

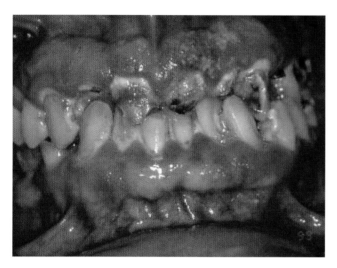

Figure 2.1 Rampant caries (*source:* From Mary A. Aubertin. 2014. Common Benign Dental and Periodontal Lesions. In: *Diagnosis and Management of Oral Lesions and Conditions: A Resource Handbook for the Clinician*, ed. Cesar A. Migliorati and Fotinos S. Panagakos, IntechOpen, doi: 10.5772/57597).

2.5.5 Early Childhood Caries

- Rampant dental caries in infants and toddlers; also known as baby-bottle caries
- Most likely affected teeth: maxillary anterior deciduous teeth (Figure 2.2)
- Cause: allowing children to fall asleep with sweetened liquids in their bottles or feeding children sweetened liquids multiple times during the day
- Education of parents/carers to follow healthy dietary and feeding habits to prevent the development of early childhood caries is important

2.5.6 Methamphetamine-Induced Caries

- Rampant caries often found in methamphetamine users and is often called 'meth mouth'
- The dental symptoms of methamphetamine users include poor oral hygiene, gingival inflammation, xerostomia, rampant caries and excessive tooth wear

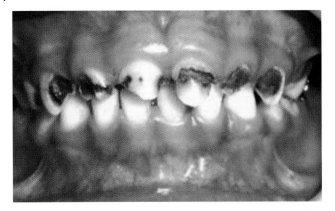

Figure 2.2 Early childhood caries (*source:* by kind permission of Dr Sadashivmurthy Prashanth, JSS Dental College, Mysuru, India).

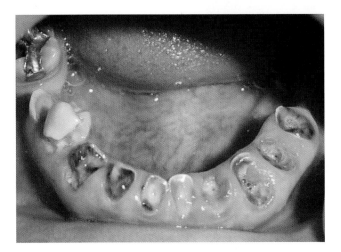

Figure 2.3 Caries in a methamphetamine user (*source:* From Mary A. Aubertin. 2014. Common Benign Dental and Periodontal Lesions. In: *Diagnosis and Management of Oral Lesions and Conditions: A Resource Handbook for the Clinician*, ed. Cesar A. Migliorati and Fotinos S. Panagakos, IntechOpen, doi: 10.5772/57597).

- The pattern of caries is distinctive: it tends to start near the gums and involves the buccal smooth surface of the posterior teeth and the interproximal space of the anterior teeth, and progresses to complete destruction of the coronal portion of the tooth (Figure 2.3)
- The key to successful dental treatment is cessation of methamphetamine use.

2.5.7 Radiation Caries

- Radiation caries is a complication of head and neck cancer radiotherapy
- Typical radiation caries is characterized by enamel erosion and dentin exposure (Figure 2.4)
- Indirect effects of radiotherapy include changes in salivary quantity and composition, together with alteration of the oral flora. These changes are widely regarded as the major causes of radiation caries

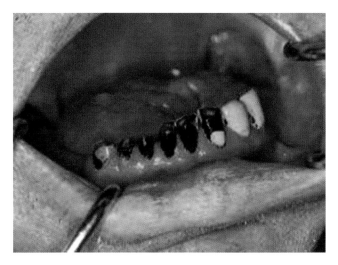

Figure 2.4   Radiation caries (*source:* by kind permission from Dr Vlaho Brailo, School of Dental Medicine, University of Zagreb, Zagreb, Croatia).

- Management of radiation caries includes management of xerostomia and restorative treatment radiation-induced dental caries. Glass ionomer cements have proved to be a better alternative to composite resins in irradiated patients.

2.6   Differential Diagnosis

- Hypoplastic enamel
- Hypocalcified enamel
- Fluorosis
- Stains

2.7   Diagnosis

- History
- Clinical examination: initially a chalky white spot lesion
- Blowing air across the suspected tooth surface is useful
- Later stages cavitation
- Radiography/laser detection

2.8   Microsopic Features

2.8.1   Enamel Caries

- Early enamel lesion shows:
  - Conical lesion with its apex towards dentin
  - Lesion shows four distinct zones of differing translucency (Figure 2.5a and b)
    - Translucent zone (deepest zone)

(a) (b)

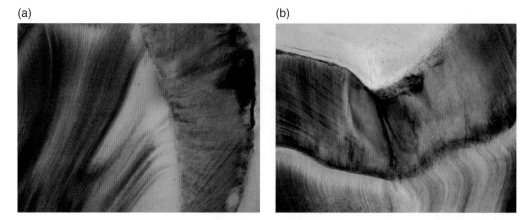

Figure 2.5 (a) Early approximal enamel caries. Undecalcified section of a precavitation stage of enamel caries showing a cone-shaped carious lesion on the proximal surface of the tooth with its apex towards dentine. The intact surface layer and the body of the lesion are visible. Evidence of early demineralization of dentine is seen beneath the amelodentinal junction deep to the carious enamel lesion. This is due to the diffusion of acids from the enamel lesion into the dentine. The dentine also shows numerous dead tracts. (b) Early pit and fissure enamel caries. Undecalcified section showing precavitation stage of enamel caries surrounding an occlusal pit. The dense surface zone, main body of the lesion, dark zone and peripheral translucent zones are visible. (*Source:* by kind permission of David Wilson, Adelaide, Australia.)

  ○ Dark zone (superficial to the translucent zone)
  ○ Body of the lesion (extends from beneath the surface zone to the dark zone)
  ○ Surface zone
 – Caries reaches enamel–dentin junction and spreads laterally, undermining the enamel
- Characteristics of enamel preceding cavitation:
 – Translucent zone:
  ○ 1% mineral loss
 – Dark zone:
  ○ 2-4% mineral loss overall. A zone of remineralization behind the advancing front becomes evident
 – Body of the lesion:
  ○ 5-25% mineral loss
 – Surface zone:
  ○ 1% mineral loss

2.8.2   Dentinal Caries

- Dentin caries shows a conical lesion with broad base at the enamel–dentin junction and apex towards pulp
- Bacterial colonies infiltrate dentinal tubules (Figure 2.6 a and b)
- Three zones of dentinal caries seen:
 – zone of demineralization
 – zone of bacterial penetration
 – zone of dentine destruction

(a)

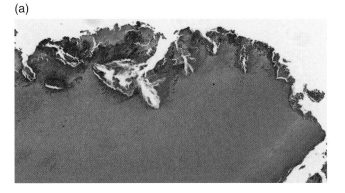

(b)

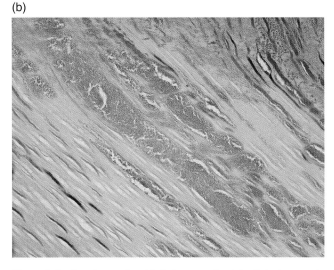

Figure 2.6 Dentine caries. (a) Carious tooth with clinical crown lost to decay. Note bacterial colonies infiltrating dentinal tubules (*source:* by kind permission of Associate Professor Kelly Magliocca, Department of Pathology and Laboratory Medicine, Winship Cancer Institute at Emory University, Atlanta, GA, USA). (b) Decalcified section showing softened dentinal tubules filled with colonies of bacteria. Multiple clefts caused by spreading infection of dentine are visible (*source:* by kind permission of David Wilson, Adelaide, Australia).

2.9   Management

- Goal: preserve tooth structure and prevent further spread
- Non-cavitated lesions: arrest of caries by remineralization (optimum oral hygiene and topical fluoride application) and reduction of frequency of refined sugar intake (non-operative treatment)
- Cavitated lesions: dental restorations with dental amalgam, composite resin, porcelain etc.
- Tooth extraction: non-restorable carious teeth
- Dental sealants

2.10 Prevention

- Oral hygiene maintenance
- Dietary modification
- Use of fluoridated water (0.7–1.0 ppm) during tooth development periods
- Topical fluoride applications (fluoride toothpaste, varnish, and mouth wash)

Recommended Reading

Featherstone, J.D.B. (2008). Dental caries: a dynamic disease process. *Australian Dental Journal* 53: 286–293.

Machiulskiene, V., Campus, G., Carvalho, J.C. et al. (2020). Terminology of dental caries and dental caries management: consensus report of a workshop organized by ORCA and Cariology research group of IADR. *Caries Research* 54: 7–14.

Major, I. (2005). Clinical diagnosis of recurrent caries. *Journal of the American Dental Association* 136 (10): 1426–1433.

Odell, E.W. (2017). Dental caries. In: *Cawson's Essentials of Oral Pthology and Oral Medicine*, 9ee (ed. E.W. Odell), 53–70. Edinburgh: Elsevier.

Petersen, P.E., Bourgeois, D., Ogawa, H. et al. (2005). The global burden of oral diseases and risks to oral health. *Bull World Health Organ* 83: 661–669.

Philip, N., Suneja, B., and Walsh, L.J. (2018). Ecological approaches to dental caries prevention: paradigm shift or shibboleth? *Caries Research* 52: 153–165.

Pitts, N., Zero, D., and Partnership, C.P. (2012). *White Paper on Dental Caries Prevention and Management. A summary of the current evidence and the key issues in controlling this preventable disease*. Geneva: FDI World Dental Federation.

3

Diseases of the Pulp and Apical Periodontal Tissues

CHAPTER MENU

3.1 Classification of Diseases of the Pulp and Apical Periodontal Tissues
3.2 Pulpitis
3.3 Apical Periodontitis and Periapical Granuloma
3.4 Apical Abscess (Dentoalveolar Abscess)
3.5 Condensing Osteitis

3.1 Classification of Diseases of the Pulp and Apical Periodontal Tissues

Disease	Description
Reversible pulpitis	A clinical diagnosis based upon subjective and objective findings indicating that the inflammation should resolve and the pulp return to normal
Symptomatic Irreversible pulpitis	A clinical diagnosis based on subjective and objective findings indicating that the vital inflamed pulp is incapable of healing. Additional descriptors: lingering thermal pain, spontaneous pain, referred pain
Asymptomatic irreversible pulpitis	A clinical diagnosis based on subjective and objective findings indicating that the vital inflamed pulp is incapable of healing. Additional descriptors: no clinical symptoms but inflammation produced by caries, caries excavation, trauma, etc.
Pulp necrosis	A clinical diagnostic category indicating death of the dental pulp. The pulp is usually nonresponsive to pulp testing
Symptomatic apical periodontitis	Inflammation, usually of the apical periodontium, producing clinical symptoms including a painful response to biting and/or percussion or palpation. It may or may not be associated with an apical radiolucent area
Asymptomatic apical periodontitis	Inflammation and destruction of apical periodontium that is of pulpal origin, appears as an apical radiolucent area, and does not produce clinical symptoms
Acute apical abscess	An inflammatory reaction to pulpal infection and necrosis characterized by rapid onset, spontaneous pain, tenderness of the tooth to pressure, pus formation and swelling of associated tissues
Chronic apical abscess	An inflammatory reaction to pulpal infection and necrosis characterized by gradual onset, little or no discomfort, and the intermittent discharge of pus through an associated sinus tract
Condensing osteitis	Diffuse radiopaque lesion representing a localized bony reaction to a low-grade inflammatory stimulus, usually seen at apex of tooth

Source: Based on ENDODONTICS: Colleagues for Excellence, Endodontic Diagnosis, Fall 2013. American Association of Endodontists (2012 update)

Handbook of Oral Pathology and Oral Medicine, First Edition. S. R. Prabhu.
© 2022 John Wiley & Sons Ltd. Published 2022 by John Wiley & Sons Ltd.
Companion website: www.wiley.com/go/prabhu/oral_pathology

3.2 Pulpitis

3.2.1 Definition/Description

- Pulpitis refers to inflammation of the dental pulp. Types include:
  - Reversible pulpitis: pulpal inflammation resolves once the aetiology is removed
  - Irreversible pulpitis: pulpal inflammation does not resolve once the aetiology is removed
  - Chronic hyperplastic pulpitis (pulp polyp)

3.2.2 Frequency

- Prevalence varies from country to country. Ranges from 27%-54% of the population
- Irreversible pulpitis is more common in females

3.2.3 Aetiology/Risk Factors

- Caries
- Traumatic exposure of the pulp
- Fracture of the crown or cusp
- Cracked tooth
- Thermal or chemical irritation

3.2.4 Clinical and Radiographical Features

- Reversible pulpitis:
  - Pain from cold test does not linger for longer than 30 seconds
  - No percussion sensitivity
  - No spontaneous pain
  - No heat sensitivity
- Irreversible pulpitis:
  - Pain from cold test lingers for longer than 30 seconds
  - May get pain from heat test
  - May have spontaneous pain
  - May be percussion sensitive
  - Sleep or work is affected
  - A patient may have difficulty locating the tooth from which the pain originates
  - Radiographically or clinically, deep caries may be visible
- Chronic hyperplastic pulpitis:
  - Presence of a pink fleshy mass filling a carious cavity (pulp polyp; Figure 3.1)
  - Usually single, rarely involving multiple teeth
  - Non-tender or mildly tender
  - Bleeds readily on probing

3.2.5 Microscopic Features

- Acute pulpitis:
  - Pulpal hyperaemia
  - Focus of acute inflammatory cell infiltrate

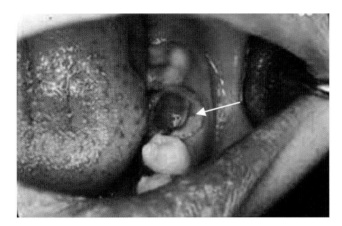

Figure 3.1 Chronic hyperplastic pulpitis (pulp polyp) presenting as a fleshy mass in the carious cavity (white arrow).

- – Destruction of odontoblasts
- – Formation of an abscess in some cases
- Chronic pulpitis:
  - – Mononuclear cell infiltrate (chronic inflammatory cells)
  - – Focus of pulp necrosis
  - – Abscesses and pus formation
  - – Wall of granulation tissue
- Chronic hyperplastic pulpitis:
  - – Mass composed of granulation tissue
  - – Rich vasculature
  - – Chronic inflammatory cell infiltrate
  - – Stratified squamous epithelial lining covers the surface of granulation tissue

3.2.6 Differential Diagnosis

- Periodontal pain
- Dentin hypersensitivity
- Cracked tooth syndrome
- Dental trauma
- Idiopathic orofacial pain
- Pain from restorative procedures
- Pain of non-odontogenic origin

3.2.7 Diagnosis

- Based on history, clinical examination and testing
- Radiography detects carious lesions causing pulpitis
- Thermal tests

- Radiographical examination for clinically visible and non-visible caries and for recurrent carries under restorations, lamina dura and periodontal ligament (PDL) space

3.2.8 Management

3.2.8.1 Reversible Pulpitis
- Remove the irritant or repair tooth structure (caries, exposed dentin, defective restoration)
- Continue to monitor the patient's symptoms
- Advise patient to return if symptoms persist or worsen
- Pain management with analgesics (ibuprofen and paracetamol)
- Antibiotics are not required

3.2.8.2 Irreversible Pulpitis
- Pulpectomy of the offending tooth: complete removal of the pulp
- Root canal treatment
- Pain management with analgesics
- Antibiotics are not recommended
- Extraction if tooth cannot be saved

3.2.8.3 Chronic Hyperplastic Pulpitis
- Extraction of the tooth

3.3 Apical Periodontitis and Periapical Granuloma

3.3.1 Definition/Description

- Apical periodontitis refers to inflammation of the PDL surrounding the apex of the tooth caused by infection, bacterial products, or other irritants through the apex of the root. Usually, this occurs due to acute inflammation (acute apical periodontitis)
- Periapical granuloma, also known as chronic apical periodontitis, refers to formation of granulation tissue surrounding the apex of a non-vital tooth arising in response to pulpal necrosis

3.3.2 Frequency

- Prevalence of apical periodontitis shows variation
- Prevalence increases with age; by 50 years of age, one in two individuals will experience apical periodontitis
- In individuals over 60 years of age, the prevalence rises to 62%

3.3.3 Aetiology/Risk Factors

- Bacterial invasion from the pulp
- Occlusal trauma from the high spots of restorations

- Irritants and inflammatory mediators from the necrotic pulp
- Endodontic procedures (iatrogenic)
- Gingival infection

3.3.4 Clinical Features

- Apical periodontitis:
  - Acute form is common
  - Pain and tenderness of the tooth on slight touch
  - Minutely extruded tooth
  - No changes with hot and cold drinks or food
  - Sequelae: may proceed to dental abscess or chronic apical periodontitis
- Periapical granuloma:
  - Most cases are asymptomatic
  - Tooth involved is non-vital
  - Tooth is slightly tender to percussion

3.3.5 Radiographical Features

- Apical periodontitis:
  - Usually, no significant changes seen
  - Occasionally, lamina dura may show haziness or slightly wide periodontal space
- Periapical granuloma:
  - Presents as a radiolucent lesion
  - A radiolucent lesion of a few millimetres in size is usually indistinguishable from a periapical cyst
  - An affected tooth typically reveals loss of the apical lamina dura
  - Root resorption is not uncommon
  - A radiolucent lesion associated with the root apex often has fuzzy borders (Figure 3.2a)

(a) (b) (c)

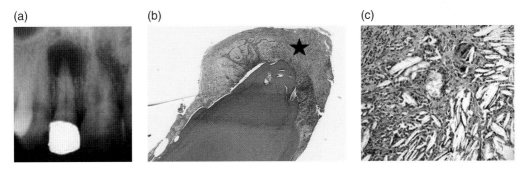

Figure 3.2 Periapical granuloma. (a) Radiolucent lesion of periapical granuloma at the root apex of the non-vital lateral incisor. (b) Photomicrograph showing apical connective tissue (black star) with chronic inflammatory cells and proliferating epithelial cells. Microscopic features demonstrate an evolving periapical cyst arising from periapical granuloma (*source:* by kind permission of Associate Professor Kelly Magliocca, Department of Pathology and Laboratory Medicine, Winship Cancer Institute at Emory University, Atlanta, GA, USA). (c) This photomicrograph shows cholesterol clefts and multinucleated giant cells in a mature periapical granuloma. These features are similar to those of periapical cyst.

3.3.6 Microscopic Features

- Apical periodontitis:
  - Engorged blood vessels
  - Intense infiltration of neutrophils
- Periapical granuloma:
  - Chronically inflamed granulation tissue around apex of a non-vital tooth shows:
    - ○ Lymphocytes, macrophages, and plasma cells intermixed with neutrophils and proliferating epithelial cells (cell rests of Malassez) within the granulation tissue (Figure 3.2b)
    - ○ Cholesterol clefts with multinucleated giant cells, red blood cells, and areas of hemosiderin pigment (Figure 3.2c)
    - ○ Uninflamed layers of fibrous tissue at the periphery
    - ○ Presence of osteoclasts
- Sequelae of periapical granuloma:
  - Acute exacerbation can cause rapid enlargement of the lesion and may progress to abscess formation
  - Proliferation of the epithelial cell rests of Malassez associated with the inflammation may lead to the development of an inflammatory radicular cyst

3.3.7 Differential Diagnosis

- Cracked-tooth syndrome and acute periapical abscess to be differentiated from acute apical periodontitis
- Periapical lesions presenting as radiolucent lesions in the apical region of the roots (e.g. periapical cyst, chronic periapical abscess) to be differentiated from periapical granuloma
- Sometimes nasopalatine duct cyst (in maxillary anterior teeth) presents radiographical features mimicking those of periapical granuloma

3.3.8 Diagnosis

- History
- Clinical examination
- Radiography

3.3.9 Management

- Apical periodontitis:
  - Identify and eliminate the cause: endodontic therapy is effective
  - Extraction of the tooth if exudate is to be drained (apical abscess)
  - Usually, antibiotics are not required for simple (non-suppurative) cases of periodontitis
  - Pain management with analgesics
- Periapical granuloma:
  - Endodontic treatment
  - Extraction of the tooth if tooth cannot be restored

3.4 Apical Abscess (Dentoalveolar Abscess)

3.4.1 Definition/Description

An odontogenic infection characterized by localization of pus in the structures that surround the teeth

3.4.2 Frequency

- Shows a wide range of variation
- Common in children: accounts for 47% of all dental-related attendances at paediatric emergency rooms in the United States

3.4.3 Aetiology/Risk Factors

- Secondary to dental caries, trauma, or failed root canal treatment
- Bacteria and their toxic products enter the periapical tissues via the apical foramen and induce acute inflammation and pus formation
- Polymicrobial odontogenic infection:
  - Anaerobic cocci, *Prevotella* species
  - *Fusobacterium* species
  - Viridans group streptococci

3.4.4 Clinical and Radiographical Features

- Non-vital tooth in most cases
- Involved tooth is tender to percussion
- Lower molars commonly involved
- In the initial stages there is no swelling, only intense, throbbing pain
- Gingiva related to the tooth is red and tender
- In established abscess buccal or labial painful gingival swellings (Figure 3.3a)
- Palatal swelling for maxillary molars is common
- Trismus due to pain and swelling
- Cervical lymphadenopathy is common
- Early dental abscesses, within the first 10 days, may not show any radiographical features
- Mild thickening of apical PDL, loss of lamina dura and loss of trabecular bone become evident as abscess advances (Figure 3.3b)
- Discharge of pus may occur in established abscess; pain subsides after the discharge of pus
- Complications include cellulitis/Ludwig's angina or osteomyelitis
- Life-threatening complications include thrombophlebitis and septicaemia
- Complete blood count for leucocytosis

3.4.5 Differential Diagnosis

- Acute periodontitis
- Infected radicular cyst
- Focal sclerosing osteomyelitis
- Periapical granuloma

(a)   (b)

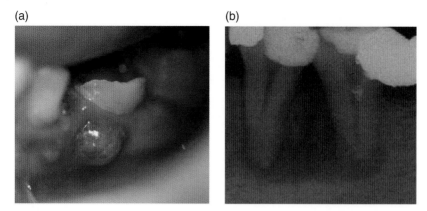

Figure 3.3   Apical abscess. (a) Presenting as a fluctuant gingival swelling; a decayed, broken down tooth with pulpal necrosis has caused this apical (periapical) abscess. Note draining pus via an intraoral sinus (*source:* Damdent, https://commons.wikimedia.org/wiki/File:Abces_parulique.jpg. Licensed Under CC BY-SA 3.0. (b) Radiographical appearance of an established periapical abscess. Note the loss of periodontal ligament, lamina dura, and trabecular bone.

3.4.6 Diagnosis

- History
- Clinical examination
- Radiography (periapical and panoramic views)
- Needle aspirate for aerobic and anaerobic cultures
- Blood culture studies

3.4.7 Management

- Most dental abscesses respond to incision and drainage, root canal, or extraction. These procedures eliminate the source of infection
- Antibiotics are usually not recommended for localized abscesses
- If drainage is not possible or if the patient shows signs of systemic involvement, or is immunocompromised, antibiotics are required for a period of seven days

3.5 Condensing Osteitis

3.5.1 Definition/Description

- Condensing osteitis refers to focal areas of bone sclerosis associated with apices of teeth with pulpitis or pulpal necrosis
- Also known as focal sclerosing osteitis and focal sclerosing osteomyelitis

3.5.2 Frequency

- Occurs in 4–7% of population

3.5.3 Aetiology

- Low-grade inflammatory stimulus from an inflamed dental pulp

3.5.4 Clinical Features

- Most frequently in young adults
- Asymptomatic
- Most lesions are discovered on routine radiography

3.5.5 Radiographical Features

- Localized increased radiodensity adjacent to the apex of the tooth (Figure 3.4)
- Widened periodontal ligament space

3.5.6 Microscopic Features

- Normally bone biopsy is not indicated unless significant pathology (other than condensing osteitis) is suspected
- The following microscopic features confirm the diagnosis of condensing osteitis:
  - Replacement of marrow spaces and cancellous bone by dense, sclerotic compact bone
  - Bone may show prominent incremental lines
  - May see fibrosis replacing fatty marrow or scant connective tissue
  - Inflammatory changes are absent or minimal

3.5.7 Differential Diagnosis

- Differential diagnoses on radiography include:
  - Periapical cemental dysplasia
  - Osteoma
  - Complex odontoma
  - Cementoblastoma
  - Osteoblastoma
  - Hypercementosis

Figure 3.4 Condensing osteitis. Note the increased radiodensity around the roots of a carious molar (black arrow). (*Source:* by kind permission of Professor Charles Dunlap, Kansas City, USA.)

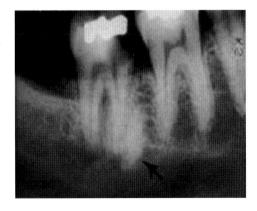

3.5.8 Diagnosis

- Clinical history is non-contributory since condensing osteitis is asymptomatic
- Most cases of condensing osteitis are incidentally detected on routine radiography

3.5.9 Management

- No treatment is required for asymptomatic bony lesions
- Tooth that caused the condensing osteitis needs to be identified and treated

Recommended Reading

Abbott, P.V. (2004). Classification, diagnosis, and clinical manifestations of apical periodontitis. *Endodontic Topics* 8: 36–54.

Abbott, P.V. and Yu, C. (2007). A clinical classification of the status of the pulp and the root canal system. *Australian Dental Journal* 52 (1 Suppl): S17–S31.

Braz-Silva, P.H., Bergamini, M.L., Mardegan, A.P. et al. (2019). Inflammatory profile of chronic apical periodontitis: a literature review. *Acta Odontologica Scandinavica* 77: 173–180.

Dabuleanu, M. (2013). Pulpitis (reversible/irreversible). *Journal of the Canadian Dental Association* 79: d90.

Neville, B.W., Damm, D.D., Allen, C.M., and Chi, C.A. (2016). Pulpal and periapical disease. In: *Oral and Maxillofacial Pathology*, 4ee, 111–136. St Louis, MO: Elsevier.

Odell, E.W. (2017). Pulpitis and apical periodontitis. In: *Cawson's Essentials of Oral Pathology and Oral Medicine*, 9ee, 73–81. Edinburgh: Elsevier.

4

Tooth Wear, Pathological Resorption of Teeth, Hypercementosis and Cracked Tooth Syndrome

4.1   Tooth wear: Attrition, Abrasion, Erosion, and Abfraction

4.1.1   Definition/Description

- Attrition is a normal physiological process characterized by tooth wear caused by tooth-to-tooth contact. Usually this affects the tips of cusps of canines and posterior teeth and incisal edges of incisor teeth
- Abrasion is tooth wear caused by an abrasive external agent. It affects both enamel and dentin
- Erosion is a process characterized by progressive solubilization of tooth substance, usually by exposure to external or gastric acids
- Abfraction is the pathological loss of hard tooth substance caused by biomechanical loading forces

4.1.2   Frequency

- Prevalence of tooth wear varies from region to region
- A universal agreement on prevalence of attrition, abrasion, and erosion does not exist
- The most prevalent type of tooth wear is attrition, followed by abrasion and erosion

4.1.3   Aetiology/Risk Factors

- Attrition is the physiological wearing of the tooth due to masticatory forces
- Bruxism is a known cause of attrition
- Abrasion is caused by abrasive dentifrices, cigars, pipes, smokeless tobacco use, improper tooth brushing techniques, and inappropriate use of dental floss or toothpicks

Handbook of Oral Pathology and Oral Medicine, First Edition. S. R. Prabhu.
© 2022 John Wiley & Sons Ltd. Published 2022 by John Wiley & Sons Ltd.
Companion website: www.wiley.com/go/prabhu/oral_pathology

- Erosion is caused by dietary acids from soft drinks, fruit juices and wine, chronic regurgitation of gastric contents (as in oesophageal reflux disorder, bulimia, and pregnancy), and chewable vitamin C and aspirin tablets
- Abfraction occurs when occlusal forces are eccentrically applied to a tooth

4.1.4 Clinical Features

- Attrition:
  - Deciduous and permanent dentitions are affected
  - Incisal and occlusal surfaces are commonly affected and rarely the entire dentition may be involved (Figure 4.1a)
  - Other teeth may include lingual surfaces of the maxillary anterior teeth and labial surfaces of the lower anterior teeth
  - Flat large wear facets corresponding to the pattern of occlusion are commonly seen
  - Interproximal contact points are also affected
  - Usually asymptomatic
  - Attrition is a slow process
  - Dental pulp is usually protected by reactionary dentin and dentinal tubular sclerosis

(a)

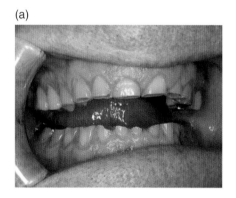

(b)   (c)

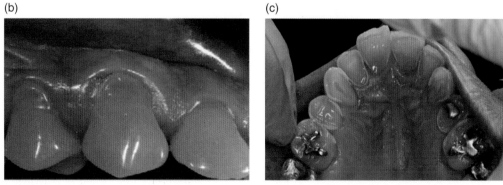

Figure 4.1 (a) Generalized attrition of the incisal and occlusal surfaces. (b) Abrasion of the labial surfaces of maxillary canine and premolars. (c) Erosion of the palatal surfaces in a patient with bulimia (*Source:* by kind permission of Associate Professor N. Narayana, UNMC Nebraska, USA.)

- Abrasion:
  - Incisal and occlusal wear is related to abrasive diet
  - Cervical wear of posterior teeth is related to faulty brushing techniques
  - A horizontal V-shaped groove is commonly seen at the cervical margin of teeth in those who brush teeth vigorously or use abrasive dentifrice (Figure 4.1b)
  - V-shaped notches on the incisal edges of anterior teeth are seen in those who use pipes or bobby pins, and in thread biting
  - Abrasion of the interproximal surfaces is seen in those who use dental floss or toothpicks inappropriately
- Erosion:
  - Palatal, occlusal, and labial surfaces of maxillary teeth are commonly affected
  - Common among those with bulimia and gastroesophageal reflux disease (Figure 4.1c)
  - Concave facets on palatal and buccal surfaces are seen
  - Cusps are dimpled
  - Incisal labial enamel is seen with thin, sharp, and translucent ridge
  - Dentinal hypersensitivity is common
- Abfraction:
  - Wedge-shaped deep defects limited to cervical area like those of abrasion
  - Occasionally subgingival defects
  - Facial surfaces of premolars and molars are involved

4.1.5 Differential diagnosis

- Amelogenesis imperfecta
- Dentinogenesis imperfecta
- Tooth defects from trauma

4.1.6 Diagnosis

- History: diet, habits (clenching/bruxism), use of pipes and smokeless tobacco, tooth-brushing techniques, regurgitation of gastric contents (bulimia, gastro-oesophageal reflux disease), etc.
- Clinical examination: location and type of wear facets and tooth defects

4.1.7 Management

- Attrition: no treatment is required unless symptomatic or aesthetically unpleasant
- Abrasion: restorative treatment for tooth defects to avoid abrasion
- Switch to a minimally abrasive toothpaste
- Erosion: removal of the cause
  - Fluoride application for dentinal hypersensitivity and use of a straw for soft drinks
  - Medical referral for those with a history of bulimia or gastro-oesophageal reflux disease

4.1.8 Prognosis

- Prognosis is good with appropriate restorative treatment

4.2 Pathological Resorption of Teeth

4.2.1 Definition/Description

- Resorption of teeth:
  - A condition associated with either a physiological or a pathological process resulting in the loss of dentin, cementum, and/or bone
  - Physiological resorption is a feature of shedding of deciduous teeth
    Only pathological resorption of permanent teeth is discussed in this chapter
- External resorption:
  - Resorption is initiated in the periodontium and initially affects the external surfaces of the tooth
  - External resorption may be further classified as surface, inflammatory, or replacement resorption, or by location as cervical, lateral, or apical resorption
- Internal resorption:
  - A defect of the internal aspect of the root following necrosis of odontoblasts because of chronic inflammation and bacterial invasion of the pulp tissue

4.2.2 Frequency

- External resorption: common
- Internal resorption: rare

4.2.3 Aetiology/Risk Factors

- Causes of external resorption:
  - Periapical periodontitis
  - Impacted tooth pressing on the root of an adjacent tooth as evidenced on radiography
  - Unerupted teeth over time may show signs of resorption
  - Replanted teeth
  - Pressure from periapical granuloma, cysts or tumours
  - Orthodontic treatment (common)
- Causes of internal resorption:
  - Unknown (idiopathic)

4.2.4 Clinical Features

- External resorption:
  - Asymptomatic in most cases
  - Localized to one tooth or a group of teeth
  - May occur on any surface of the root and occasionally on the crown of an unerupted tooth
- Internal resorption:
  - Asymptomatic
  - Clinically, a 'pink spot' may be seen at the centre of the crown

4.2.5   Radiographical features

- External resorption:
  - Apex of the root is shortened (Figure 4.2a)
  - Opening of the apical foramen may be visible
  - Resorbed areas may show irregular margins
  - Radiodensity of the resorbed area shows variation
- Internal resorption:
  - May be an incidental finding on radiographs
  - Root canal or pulp chamber shows enlarged radiolucent area (Figure 4.2b)
  - Resorbed area may be symmetrical and the walls may balloon out
  - Margins of the resorbed area are smooth and clearly defined

4.2.6   Microscopic Features

- External resorption:
  - Numerous multinucleated dentinoclasts near the resorbed surface
  - Resorbed areas may show deposition of osteodentin (sign of repair)
  - Granulation tissue in large areas of resorption
- Internal resorption:
  - Cellular and vascular fibrous connective tissue
  - Multinucleated dentinoclasts
  - Inflammatory cells: lymphocytes, histiocytes and polymorphonuclear leukocytes
  - Presence of woven bone as a sign of repair process

(a)   (b)

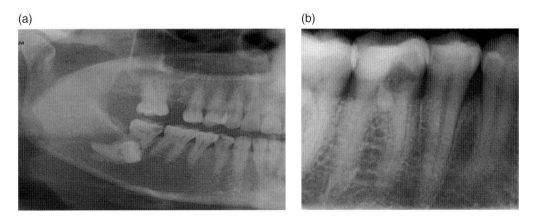

Figure 4.2   Resorption. (a) External: cropped orthopantomograph shows external resorption of roots of 47 caused by impacted 48. (b) Internal: radiograph showing radiolucency in the dentinal wall of the pulp chamber of first mandibular molar. (*Source:* by kind permission of Dr Amar Sholapurkar, James Cook University School of Dentistry, Cairns, Australia.)

4.2.7 Differential diagnosis

- Carious lesions for internal resorption and periapical lesions for external root resorption should be considered in the differential diagnosis

4.2.8 Diagnosis

- History of dental procedures (orthodontic treatment in particular)
- Radiography (cone beam computed tomography preferred)

4.2.9 Management

- External resorption:
  - Identification and elimination of the cause
- Internal resorption:
  - Root canal treatment

4.2.10 Prognosis

- Good prognosis if the cause has been identified and eliminated and appropriate treatment is carried out

4.3 Hypercementosis

4.3.1 Definition/Description

- Apposition of excess amounts of normal cementum on the root surface
- Also called cemental hyperplasia
- Two types occur: isolated and diffuse

4.3.2 Frequency

- The prevalence of hypercementosis is not well established

4.3.3 Aetiology/Risk Factors

- Isolated (single or a group of teeth) hypercementosis:
  - Most cases are idiopathic and age related
  - Some cases show periapical pathosis, parafunctional occlusal trauma, and lack of functional opposition
- Diffuse or generalized (involving all teeth) hypercementosis:
  - May be associated with various syndromes and systemic diseases, such as Paget's disease of bone, acromegaly, thyroid goitre, calcinosis, arthritis, and rheumatic fever

4.3.4 Clinical Features

- Asymptomatic in the majority of cases
- May involve single tooth, several teeth or generalized

Figure 4.3 Hypercementosis; extracted tooth with hypercementosis at the tip of the roots (*source:* by kind permission of Professor Charles Dunlap, Kansas City, USA).

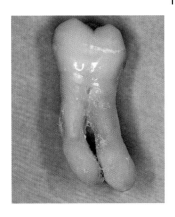

- Isolated hypercementosis involves mandibular molars, followed by maxillary and mandibular second premolars, and mandibular first premolars
- An extracted tooth shows blunt root tips (Figure 4.3)

4.3.5 Radiographical features

- Detected on routine radiography
- Widening of roots
- Apical third shows a blunt root tip surrounded by radiolucent periodontal ligament space
- Occasionally, fusion of the roots of the adjacent roots caused by hypercementosis (concrescence) is seen

4.3.6 Microscopic Features

- Deposition of excessive cementum (mostly acellular) over the original layer of primary cementum
- Concentric layers of cementum deposition are seen
- May include the entire root or limited to the root tip

4.3.7 Differential Diagnosis

- Cemento-osseous dysplasia
- Cementoblastoma

4.3.8 Management

- No treatment required
- Problems with extraction
- Systemic conditions associated with hypercementosis should be treated by specialists

4.4 Cracked Tooth Syndrome

4.4.1 Definition/Description

- An incomplete fracture of a vital posterior tooth that involves the dentine and occasionally extends into the pulp

4.4.2 Frequency

- Common
- Incidence rate of 34–74%

4.4.3 Aetiology/Risk factors

- Teeth grinding (bruxism/habitual clenching)
- Large restorations
- Chewing or biting hard food
- Trauma: blows to the teeth (violence or accident related)

4.4.4 Clinical Features

- Majority of patients are 30–50 years of age
- Men and women are equally affected
- Most affected teeth are the mandibular second molars, followed by mandibular first molars, and maxillary premolars
- Deep cracks may involve pulp (Figure 4.4)
- Patient complains of pain on biting that ceases after the masticatory pressure has been withdrawn
- Pain on tooth grinding and with cold drinks or food
- Difficulty in identifying offending tooth (by the patient)
- Vitality test is usually positive
- Tenderness can be elicited when pressure is applied to an individual cusp
- Pain/tenderness increases as the occlusal force increases, and relief occurs once the pressure is withdrawn

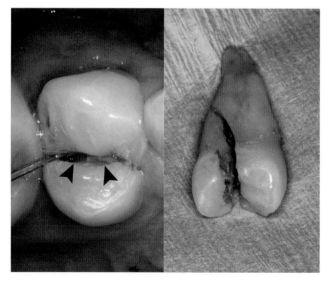

Figure 4.4 Cracked tooth syndrome; fractured premolar tooth (black arrows) viewed in the mouth (left) and after extraction (right). (*Source:* Coronation Dental Specialty Group Canada; Wikipediahttps://en.wikipedia.org › wiki. Creative Commons Attribution-Share Alike 3.0 Unported license

4.4.5 Differential Diagnosis

- Acute periodontal diseases
- Reversible pulpitis
- Dentinal hypersensitivity
- Galvanic pain associated with silver amalgam restorations
- Sensitivity following microleakage from recently placed composite resin restorations
- Areas of hyperocclusion from dental restorations
- Occlusal trauma from parafunctional habits
- Orofacial pain arising from conditions such as trigeminal neuralgia and atypical facial pain

4.4.6 Diagnosis

- Detailed history:
  - Recent dental restorations, occlusal adjustments
  - Parafunctional habits (bruxism)
  - Pain history: character, intensity, relation to chewing, etc.
- Clinical examination:
  - Periodontal probing
- Bite tests:
  - Patient is asked to bite on various items such as a toothpick, cotton roll, rubber abrasive wheels, or wooden stick
  - Pain/tenderness increases as the occlusal force increases, and relief occurs once the pressure is withdrawn (diagnostic)
- Dye test:
  - Special stains such as methylene blue or gentian violet are frequently used to highlight the cracks
- Vitality tests for individual tooth are usually positive
- Radiographs are not reliable (since cracks usually occur in a mesiodistal direction)
- Transillumination is an important aid in diagnosing the cracks

4.4.7 Management

- Depends on the site, direction, size, or the degree of the crack
- Minor cracks: restored with a filling or a crown
- Deep cracks with pulp involvement: root canal treatment and a crown
- Pain management by analgesics
- Crack extending into the root of the tooth beneath the bone: extraction of the tooth

4.4.8 Prognosis

- Prognosis is good for most cases with endodontic treatment and crown
- Where vertical cracks occur or where the crack extends through the pulpal floor or below the level of the alveolar bone, the prognosis is not favourable, and extraction is the treatment of choice.

Recommended Reading

Odell, E.W. (2017). Tooth wear, tooth resorption, hypercementosis and osseointegration. In: *Cawson's Essentials of Oral Pathology and Oral Medicine*, 9e, 85–91. Edinburgh: Elsevier.

Imfeld, T. (1996). Dental erosion: definition, classification, and links. *European Journal of Oral Sciences* 104: 151–154.

Neville, B.W., Damm, D.D., Allen, C.M., and Chi, C.A. (2016). Abnormalities of teeth. In: *Oral and Maxillofacial Pathology*, 4e, 49–66. St Louis, MO: Elsevier.

Schlueter, N., Amaechi, B.T., Bartlett, D. et al. (2020). Terminology of erosive tooth wear: consensus report of a workshop organized by the ORCA and the cariology research group of the IADR. *Caries Research* 54: 2–6.

5

Gingival and Periodontal Diseases

Handbook of Oral Pathology and Oral Medicine, First Edition. S. R. Prabhu.
© 2022 John Wiley & Sons Ltd. Published 2022 by John Wiley & Sons Ltd.
Companion website: www.wiley.com/go/prabhu/oral_pathology

5.1   Classification of Gingival and Periodontal Diseases

Disease type	Diseases
Gingival	
	Gingivitis associated with dental plaque only
Dental plaque induced	Gingivitis modified by systemic factors:
	Puberty associated
	Menstrual cycle associated
	Pregnancy associated
	Diabetes mellitus associated
	Down syndrome associated
	Gingivitis associated with leukaemia and other blood disorders
	Gingival diseases modified by medications:
	Drug modified gingival enlargement (e.g. calcium channel blockers and antiepileptic drugs)
	Gingival diseases modified by malnutrition:
	Ascorbic acid deficiency gingivitis
Non-plaque induced lesions	Infections: bacterial, viral and fungal
	Genetic conditions (e.g. hereditary gingival fibromatosis)
	Gingival manifestations of dermatological disease:
	Mucocutaneous disease (desquamative gingivitis as a manifestation of vesiculoerosive diseases)
	Allergic reactions (e.g. plasma cell gingivitis)
Traumatic lesions	Fictitious, iatrogenic (e.g. overhanging restorations)
	Accidental trauma
Foreign body reactions	
Necrotizing gingival diseases	
Local predisposition	
Periodontal	
Chronic	Plaque induced (localized or generalized)
Aggressive periodontitis	Localized or generalized
Manifestation of systemic disease	Associated with hematologic disorders
	Associated with genetic disorders
Combined periodontal–endodontic lesions	

From 1999 International Workshop for a Classification of Periodontal Disease, simplified version. *Source:* Odell, E.W. (2017). Gingival and periodontal diseases. In. *Cawson's Essentials of Oral Pathology and Oral Medicine*, 9e, 96. Edinburgh: Elsevier.

5.2   Chronic Gingivitis

5.2.1   Definition/Description

- Gingivitis is defined as a reversible gingival inflammatory condition mostly induced by plaque
- According to duration, gingivitis can be classified as acute and chronic
- Chronic gingivitis is the most common form of gingivitis

5.2.2 Frequency

- Chronic gingivitis is common in children and adolescents
- Prevalence is estimated to be as high as 80% among children and adolescents

5.2.3 Aetiology/Risk Factors

- Aetiology of bacterial plaque:
  - Gram-positive bacteria in initial stages (*Actinomyces* species predominate)
  - Gram-negative bacteria in later stages (anaerobic plaque: *Veillonella, Fusobacterium* and *Campylobacte*r species predominate)
- Risk factors:
  - Poor oral hygiene
  - Mouth-breathing during sleep
  - Medications and conditions that cause xerostomia
  - Tobacco/smokeless tobacco habits
  - Stress
  - Mental health issues such as depression
  - Pre-existing conditions such as diabetes
  - Pregnancy/puberty
  - Down syndrome
  - HIV disease
  - Poor nutrition (vitamin C deficiency)

5.2.4 Clinical Features

- Gingival margins: red and slightly swollen, oedematous (Figure 5.1)
- Bleeding gums during tooth brushing/flossing (this is the most common complaint)
- Bleeding gums associated with biting on fruits
- Halitosis

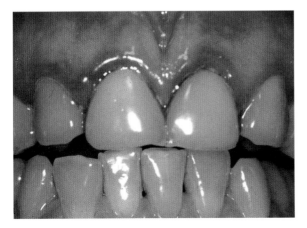

Figure 5.1 Chronic gingivitis: clinical appearance of chronic marginal gingivitis with erythema, oedema, and loss of stippling (*source:* by kind permission of Adj. Associate Professor John Highfield, University of Sydney, Australia).

- Gingival pockets may occur without involving the bone (false pocketing: no radiographical changes)
- Tooth mobility is not affected

5.2.5 Microscopic Features

- Early stages:
  - Vasodilation
  - Infiltration by neutrophils
  - Leakage of exudate into gingival sulcus
- Over time:
  - Plasma cell infiltrate predominate limited to interdental papillae
  - Destruction of superficial connective tissue fibres

5.2.6 Differential Diagnosis

- Puberty gingivitis
- Pregnancy gingivitis
- Plasma cell gingivitis
- Necrotizing gingivitis
- Linear gingival erythema
- Chronic periodontitis
- Early stages of leukaemic gingival infiltration

5.2.7 Diagnosis

- History
- Clinical examination including probing
- Radiography (to rule out periodontitis)

5.2.8 Management

- Calculus removal
- Oral hygiene maintenance (tooth brushing and interdental cleaning habits)
- Attention to local exacerbating factors
- Attention to systemic predisposing factors

5.2.9 Prognosis

- Good

5.3 Necrotizing Periodontal Diseases

5.3.1 Definition/Description

- Necrotizing periodontal disease is a spectrum of conditions that affect the periodontium (gingiva, periodontal ligament, and alveolar bone) through necrosis and ulceration

- Clinical entities in this group include:
  - necrotizing ulcerative gingivitis (NUG)
  - necrotizing ulcerative periodontitis (NUP)
  - necrotizing ulcerative stomatitis (NUS):
- NUG is limited to the gingiva
- When progression of NUG involves destruction of gingival tissues, periodontal ligament, and loss of alveolar bone, the condition is known as NUP
- When destruction of structures occurs beyond the mucogingival junction the condition is known as NUS, which is also called noma or cancrum oris. It is prevalent among malnourished children in developing countries
- Only NUG and NUP are discussed below

5.3.2 Frequency

- The prevalence rate of NUG varies over a wide range: 0.11–6.7%
- NUP occurs in young adults (aged 18–30 years) and is more common in malnourished children or immunocompromised individuals

5.3.3 Aetiology/Risk Factors

- NUG and NUP are infectious diseases caused by mixed bacterial flora. Microorganisms involved include *Fusobacterium nucleatum*, *Borrelia vincentii*, *Prevotella intermedia*, *Porphyromonas gingivalis*, and *Selenomonas sputigena*
- Malnutrition, viral infections, immune defects (HIV), stress, leukaemia, lymphoma, lack of sleep, and smoking are predisposing factors

5.3.4 Clinical Features

- NUG is characterized by necrotic, crater-like 'punched-out' ulcerations of the interdental papilla, typically covered with grey pseudomembranous slough (Figure 5.2a)
- NUP is characterized by localized or generalized periodontitis, with rapid/sudden onset with excruciating intense pain, necrosis of gingival tissues, and loss of periodontal ligament and alveolar bone. Deep periodontal pockets are usually absent (Figure 5.2b)
- Other features common to both include spontaneous pain, haemorrhage, halitosis, fever, lymphadenopathy, and malaise
- When necrotic ulcerative lesions progress beyond mucogingival tissue, the condition is called NUS.
- NUG commonly affects children, young adults, and those with HIV infection

5.3.5 Microscopic Features

- Four histological layers (from the superficial to the deepest) are recognized in NUG:
  - The bacterial area with a superficial fibrous mesh, composed of degenerated epithelial cells, leukocytes, cellular rests, and a wide variety of bacterial cells, including rods, fusiform organisms and spirochetes
  - The neutrophil-rich zone, composed of a high number of leukocytes, especially neutrophils, and numerous spirochetes of different sizes

(a)   (b)

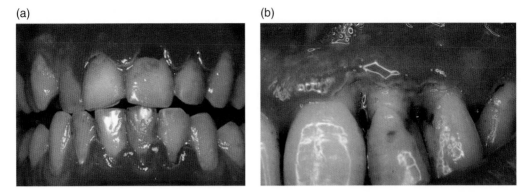

Figure 5.2 (a) Necrotizing ulcerative gingivitis shows papillary and gingival ulcers. (b) Necrotizing ulcerative periodontitis. This condition is characterized by the loss of periodontal ligament and alveolar bone. (*Source:* by kind permission of Adj. Associate Professor John Highfield, University of Sydney, NSW, Australia.)

- The necrotic zone, containing disintegrated cells, together with medium- and large-size spirochetes and fusiform bacteria
- The spirochaetal infiltration zone, where the tissue components are adequately preserved

5.3.6 Differential Diagnosis

- Herpetic gingivostomatitis and infectious mononucleosis
- Gonococcal or streptococcal gingivitis
- Desquamative gingivitis
- Chronic periodontitis
- Aggressive periodontitis
- Agranulocytosis
- Necrotizing stomatitis
- Leukaemia

5.3.7 Diagnosis

- History (including HIV status)
- Clinical examination
- Microbial culture (smears from the ulcers show fusospirochaetal bacteria and leukocytes)

5.3.8 Management

- Treatment includes debridement of necrotic debris under local anaesthesia, mouth rinses with chlorhexidine, warm salt water, or diluted hydrogen peroxide (local oxygen therapy)
- Metronidazole (250 mg every 8 hours) is the drug of first choice because it is active against strict anaerobes
- Penicillin, tetracyclines, clindamycin, amoxicillin, or amoxicillin plus clavulanate are also effective
- Antifungal agents are indicated in immunodepressed patients who are undergoing antibiotic therapy
- Analgesics/antipyretics for pain and fever
- Soft nutritious diet, fluid intake and bed rest, oral hygiene instruction, and tobacco counselling
- If the patient is immunocompromised, close communication with the physician is essential

5.3.9 Prognosis

- Signs and symptoms resolve within a week of adequate therapy

5.4 Plasma Cell Gingivitis

5.4.1 Definition/Description

- Plasma cell gingivitis is a rare inflammatory condition characterized by dense plasma cell infiltrate in the gingival connective tissue secondary to hypersensitive reaction

5.4.2 Frequency

- Rare
- More prevalent in females

5.4.3 Aetiology/Risk Factors

- Not clearly understood. Possible cause includes:
  - Hypersensitivity to a variety of agents used in chewing gums or toothpastes
  - Allergens, including mint, cinnamon, cloves, cardamom, red chilli peppers, khat, colocasia leaves, and pumice used in prophy paste

5.4.4 Clinical Features

- Asymptomatic in some cases
- Appears as a diffuse reddening and oedematous swelling of the gingiva with a sharp demarcation along the mucogingival border (Figure 5.3a)
- Anterior gingival segment is commonly involved
- Gingiva bleeds readily

5.4.5 Microscopic Features

- Dense infiltration of plasma cells with scattered lymphocytes in the lamina propria
- Dilated vasculature (Figure 5.3b)
- Histologically can be mistaken for multiple myeloma and extramedullary plasmacytoma

5.4.6 Differential Diagnosis

- Leukaemic infiltration of leukaemia
- Extramedullary plasmacytoma
- Multiple myeloma

5.4.7 Diagnosis

- History of onset, duration, and dietary history
- Clinical examination

(a)   (b)

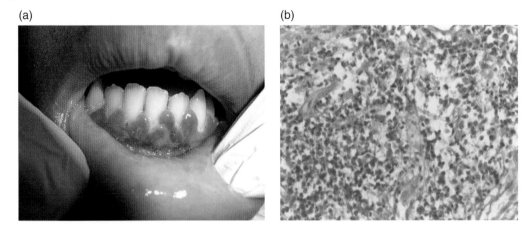

Figure 5.3 (a) Plasma cell gingivitis. Note swollen, oedematous red gingiva (b) Photomicrograph shows dense sheets of plasma cells in the lamina propria. (*Source:* by kind permission of Dr Susmitha HR, Farooqia Dental College and Hospital, Mysuru, India.)

- Microscopic examination of the gingival tissue
- Haematological screening to rule out myeloma and plasmacytoma is required

5.4.8 Management

- Identification and elimination of allergen
- Topical or systemic immunosuppressive agents
- Topical agents: betamethasone rinses, fluocinonide gel, and triamcinolone
- Systemic prednisone is effective
- Surgery, cryosurgery, electrocoagulation, and CO_2 lasers have been tried with varying success

5.4.9 Prognosis

- Favourable

5.5 Foreign Body Gingivitis

5.5.1 Definition/Description

- Inflammation of the gingival tissues associated with the presence of foreign material in the gingival connective tissues

5.5.2 Frequency

- Uncommon
- Prevalence is not known
- More common in females

5.5.3 Aetiology/Risk Factors

- Dental materials implanted in the gingival connective tissue during dental procedures (iatrogenic)

5.5.4 Clinical Features

- Symptomatic: pain and swelling in the affected tissues
- Solitary or multiple red or red and white lesions, which may resemble and be mistaken for lichen planus
- Marginal and attached gingiva and interdental papilla are inflamed

5.5.5 Microscopic Features

- Infiltration with lymphocytes, plasma cells and macrophages
- Occasionally particles of foreign material can be detected

5.5.6 Differential Diagnosis

- Lichen planus (desquamative gingivitis)
- Lichenoid lesions

5.5.7 Diagnosis

- History
- Clinical features
- Microscopic features

5.5.8 Management

- Surgical resection of the affected tissues

5.5.9 Prognosis

- Good

5.6 Desquamative Gingivitis

5.6.1 Definition/Description

- Desquamative gingivitis is not a specific diagnosis. It is a descriptive term used for nonspecific gingival manifestation characterized by formation of vesicles, atrophy, erosion, and desquamation seen as diffuse erythema of the marginal and keratinized gingiva
- It is associated with different dermatological and vesiculoerosive diseases

5.6.2 Frequency

- Global prevalence is unknown
- Varies depending on the underlying disorder

5.6.3 Aetiology/Risk Factors

- Unclear aetiology
- Desquamative gingivitis represents a manifestation of one of several different diseases such as mucous membrane pemphigoid, pemphigus vulgaris, systemic lupus erythematosus, lichen planus, linear immunoglobulin A disease, dermatitis herpetiformis, psoriasis and erythema multiforme
- Oral lichen planus, mucous membrane pemphigoid and pemphigus vulgaris account for 88–98% of desquamative gingivitis cases
- Contact allergic reactions to various oral hygiene products are also known to cause desquamative gingivitis

5.6.4 Clinical Features

- Desquamation of the free and keratinized gingival epithelium
- Labial/buccal surfaces are commonly involved
- Can be seen on the edentulous alveolar ridge
- More common in females (female to male ratio: 80% : 20%)
- Symptoms: chronic pain/burning sensation; rarely asymptomatic
- Intolerance to spicy food
- Epithelium is fragile and peels off readily
- Gingiva is erythematous, shiny, and smooth (Figure 5.4)
- Vesicles may precede desquamation
- White streaks on the red background are seen if condition is due to lichen planus
- Associated with signs and systems of systemic/mucocutaneous conditions

5.6.5 Microscopic Features

- Histological features of the underlying disorder (e.g. mucous membrane pemphigoid/pemphigus vulgaris/lichen planus) that has caused desquamative gingivitis becomes evident (see microscopic features of these lesions in Chapter 16)
- Direct and indirect immunofluorescence studies are also useful in the diagnosis

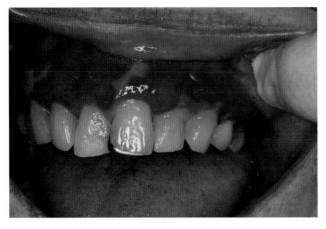

Figure 5.4 Desquamative gingivitis in a patient with mucous membrane pemphigoid. Note shiny red gingival surfaces with evidence of desquamation of the gingival epithelium.

5.6.6 Differential Diagnosis

- The differential diagnosis of desquamative gingivitis must be made with other forms of gingivitis:
  - Plaque-induced gingivitis
  - Herpetic gingivostomatitis
  - Gingivitis in haematological diseases (e.g. leukaemic gingivitis)
  - Diabetes-induced gingivitis
- Systemic disorders to be considered include:
  - Mucous membrane pemphigoid
  - Pemphigus vulgaris
  - Lichen planus

5.6.7 Diagnosis

- History: onset and duration of symptoms, medical history
- Clinical examination
- Histopathology and direct immunofluorescence testing of biopsied perilesional intact tissue specimen to identify the underlying disorder

5.6.8 Management

- Symptomatic treatment for pain/burning sensation
- Topical corticosteroid application
- Identification and treatment of the underlying disorder is important

5.6.9 Prognosis

- Good

5.7 Chronic Periodontitis

5.7.1 Definition/Description

- Chronic periodontitis refers to chronic inflammation of the periodontal tissues arising from pre-existing gingival inflammatory process and resulting in destruction of periodontal ligament and resorption of crestal bone

5.7.2 Frequency

- Chronic periodontitis is one of the most prevalent diseases
- Varies in its prevalence rate
- 10–15% of the population suffers from severe periodontitis

5.7.3 Aetiology/Risk Factors

- Long term persistence of gingivitis (chronic gingivitis)
- Risk factors/predisposing factors:
  - Chronic periodontitis is associated with:

  - ○ Advancing age
  - ○ Poor oral hygiene
  - ○ Local factors: calculus, traumatic occlusion, and poor interdental contact
  - ○ Smoking
  - ○ Diabetes mellitus
  - ○ Osteoporosis
  - ○ Lower socioeconomic strata
  - ○ The disease appears to result from a complex interplay between bacterial infection and the host response, often modified by behavioural factors
- Role of microorganisms:
  - – *Porphyromonas gingivalis*, *Prevotella intermedia*, *Tannerella forsythia*, *Treponema denticola*, *Fusobacterium nucleatum*, and *Campylobacter* species are present in diseased sites and have been implicated in disease progression

5.7.4 Clinical Features

- Begins in youth and early adulthood
- Gingivitis precedes periodontitis
- Initially asymptomatic
- In the early stages: gingival bleeding, unpleasant taste, and oral malodour
- Gingival margins show redness and swelling
- Loss of attachment results in pocketing (pocket depth greater than 3 mm)
- Interdental papillae are destroyed, gingival margins become straight with swollen edges (Figure 5.5a)
- Plaque and calculus fill the pockets
- Bone loss occurs
- Teeth are mobile and drift out of alignment
- Dull note on percussion of teeth
- Bleeding on minimal pressure is common
- Pus may be expressed in severely affected periodontal tissues
- Tooth loss occurs if not treated early

5.7.5 Radiographical features

- Blunting of the tip of the alveolar crest in early stages
- Horizontal bone loss where alveolar bone is thin and vertical or angular bone loss where alveolar bone is thick (Figure 5.5b)

5.7.6 Microscopic Features

- Plasma cells and lymphocytes in the gingival connective tissues along the lining epithelium of the pocket (close to the plaque and calculus)
- Neutrophils migrate into the pockets

5.7.7 Differential Diagnosis

- Aggressive periodontitis
- Periodontitis associated with systemic factors (e.g. diabetes, pregnancy, and puberty)
- Necrotizing ulcerative periodontitis

(a)

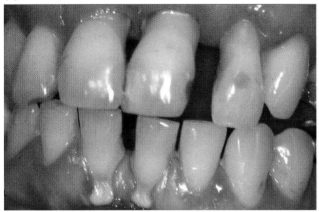

(b)

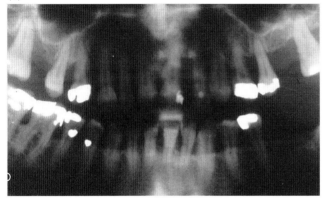

Figure 5.5   Generalized chronic periodontitis. (a) Disease in a 55-year-old woman; note the generalized recession, plaque, calculus, and anterior migration with opening of a diastema. (b) Radiograph showing generalized advanced bone loss which is both horizontal and vertical (*Source:* by kind permission of Adj. Associate Professor John Highfield, University of Sydney, Australia).

5.7.8   Diagnosis

- History
- Clinical examination
- Radiography

5.7.9   Management

- Modification of risk factors (e.g. smoking, diabetic control)
- Non-surgical or surgical root debridement
- Oral hygiene reinforcement and periodontal maintenance therapy
- Additional management may include:
  - Guided tissue regeneration
  - Local or systemic antibiotics

5.7.10 Prognosis

- Prognosis is fair for those treated early
- Much depends on the oral hygiene level maintained by the patients

5.7.11 Complications of Chronic Periodontitis

- Chronic periodontitis can worsen diabetic control in patients with diabetes
- Associated with elevated risk of preterm birth and low birthweight
- Bacterial burden of periodontal infection may have some association with cardiovascular disease

5.8 Aggressive Periodontitis

5.8.1 Definition/Description

- Aggressive periodontitis is characterized by rapid attachment loss and bone destruction in otherwise healthy individuals
- Two types have been identified: generalized and localized
    - Generalized: more than two teeth (other than incisors and molars) are involved. This is also known as generalized juvenile periodontitis
    - Localized: only two permanent teeth (incisor and molar) are involved. This is also known as localized juvenile periodontitis

5.8.2 Frequency

- The prevalence of aggressive periodontitis varies considerably between continents, and differences in race or ethnicity seem to be major contributing factors
- Global prevalence has been estimated as 0.1–3.4%

5.8.3 Aetiology/Risk Factors

- Aggressive periodontitis is a multifactorial disease with many complex interactions including host factors, microbiology, and genetics
- Gram-negative microbes are considered the chief etiological agents of aggressive periodontitis:
    - *Aggregatibacter acitinomycetemcomitans* is commonly associated with the disease
    - In some cases, *Porphyromonas gingivalis* are found

5.8.4 Clinical and Radiographical Features

- In generalized aggressive periodontitis, more than two teeth other than incisors and molars are involved (Figure 5.6a and b)
- Localized type may proceed to generalized aggressive periodontitis by the age of 15 years, and is usually diagnosed before the age of 30 years
- Localized type begins around puberty (11–13 years of age)
- In localized aggressive periodontitis, attachment loss is primarily localized to first molars and incisors (Figure 5.6c and d)

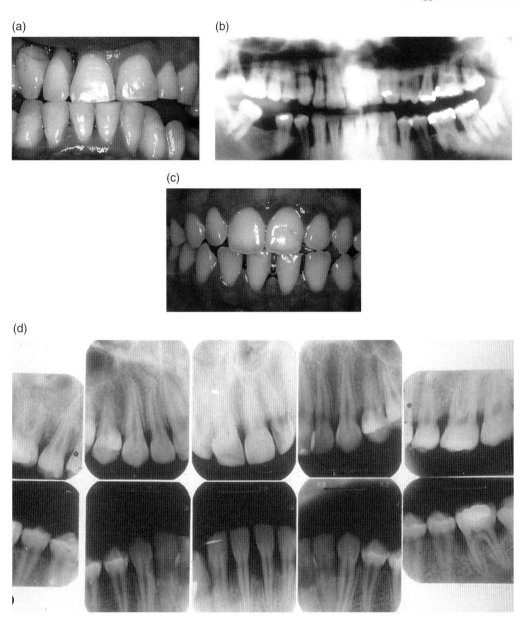

Figure 5.6 (a) Generalized aggressive periodontitis (rapidly progressive periodontitis). Clinical photograph of 21 year-old man showing anterior gingival recession reflecting attachment loss. Inflammation is not marked as the patient had received some treatment and the disease was in remission. (b) Radiograph showing advanced bone destruction. (c) Localized aggressive periodontitis (localized juvenile periodontitis) in a 13-year-old (circumpubertal) otherwise healthy girl. The gingival tissues show marked gingivitis which is not typical. Attachment loss in incisors and molars is a typical feature of this condition. (d) Localized aggressive periodontitis (localized juvenile periodontitis). Radiographs show bone loss in the first molar and incisor teeth. (*Source:* by kind permission of Adj. Associate Professor John Highfield, University of Sydney, Australia.)

- Common features of both types include:
  - Advanced bone loss/vertical bone loss bilateral and symmetrical
  - Diastema may result
  - Sensitive exposed roots seen
  - Individual complains of dull pain radiating to the jaw
  - Lack of signs of inflammation
  - Cervical lymphadenopathy is present
  - Periodontal abscesses may occur
  - Neutrophil dysfunction may be present in both types of the disease

5.8.5   Microscopic Features

- Similar to those of chronic periodontitis:
  - Plasma cell (predominant) and lymphocytes in the gingival connective tissues along the epithelial pocket lining (close to the plaque and calculus)
  - Neutrophils also migrate into the pockets

5.8.6   Differential Diagnosis

- Chronic periodontitis
- Periodontitis associated with systemic diseases
- Necrotizing ulcerative periodontitis

5.8.7   Diagnosis

- History: onset, duration, and family history
- Clinical examination
- Radiography
- Microbiological findings (anaerobic cultures)
- Leukocyte function tests
- Strong antibody response to infecting agents can be detected in local type whereas, in generalized type the antibody response is poor

5.8.8   Management

- Early aggressive treatment with root debridement and antibiotic (tetracyclines or minocycline) administration in early stages of the disease
- Professional prophylaxis once a month for six months for re-evaluation
- Penicillins and metronidazole are highly effective
- Persistent pocketing requires surgical intervention
- Strict oral hygiene maintenance
- Siblings to be screened for the disease (because of the genetic background)

5.8.9   Prognosis

- Favourable

5.9 Fibrous Epulis (Peripheral Fibroma)

5.9.1 Definition/Description

- Fibrous epulis: a common tumour-like lesion of the gingiva, located in the interdental papilla as a hyperplastic response to local irritation
- Also known as peripheral fibroma
- Epulis is the term used for gingival masses only

5.9.2 Frequency

- Common

5.9.3 Aetiology/Risk factors

- Chronic local irritation at the gingival margin; usually carious cavity, calculus, or plaque

5.9.4 Clinical Features

- A firm or rubbery pink, pedunculated or sessile mass located at the interdental gingiva of anterior teeth (Figure 5.7a)
- Slow growing and painless

5.9.5 Microscopic Features

- Hyperplastic covering epithelium
- Hyperplastic lightly inflamed or densely collagenous fibrous tissue (Figure 5.7b)
- Occasional bone formation within the fibrous tissue (mineralizing fibrous epulis)

(a) (b)

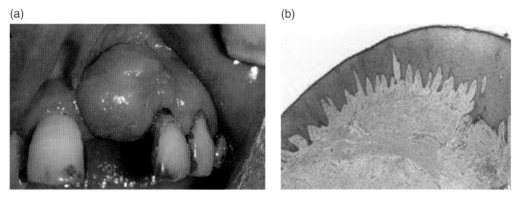

Figure 5.7 Fibrous epulis. (a) Peripheral fibroma presenting as firm, pink, uninflamed mass growing from under the gingiva (*source:* by kind permission of Amit Arvind Agrawal, MGV's KBH Dental College and Hospital, Nashik, Maharashtra, India). (b) Photomicrograph showing hyperplastic covering epithelium and fibrous hyperplasia of the gingiva.

5.9.6 Differential Diagnosis

- Pyogenic granuloma/pregnancy tumour
- Peripheral giant cell epulis
- Peripheral ossifying fibroma

5.9.7 Diagnosis

- History
- Clinical finding
- Microscopic finding

5.9.8 Management

- Surgical excision
- Elimination of the cause (subgingival irritation)
- Recurrence possible if cause is not eliminated

5.9.9 Prognosis

- Good

5.10 Peripheral Ossifying/Cementifying Fibroma

5.10.1 Definition/Description

- A tumour-like non-neoplastic ossifying/cementifying fibrous lesion on the gingiva derived from periodontal ligament

5.10.2 Frequency

- Accounts for 9.6% of gingival lesions

5.10.3 Aetiology/Risk Factors

- Local irritation or low-grade trauma
- Calcifying mature pyogenic granuloma

5.10.4 Clinical Features

- Occurs exclusively on the gingiva; interdental papillae in particular
- Age of occurrence: predominantly in teenage years
- Female preponderance
- Pedunculated or sessile lesion
- Pink or red nodular lesion usually less than 2 cm in diameter (Figure 5.8a)
- Slow growing
- Sometimes ulcerated surface seen

5.10.5 Microscopic Features

- Cellular fibrous tissue covered by stratified squamous epithelium (Figure 5.8b)
- Areas of dystrophic calcification; cementum-like material or woven bone (Figure 5.8c)
- Inflammatory cell infiltrate present

5.10.6 Differential Diagnosis

- Fibrous epulis
- Peripheral giant cell granuloma
- Pyogenic granuloma
- Peripheral odontogenic fibroma

5.10.7 Diagnosis

- History
- Clinical findings
- Microscopic findings

(a)

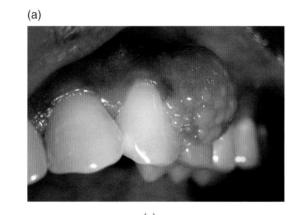

(b)   (c)

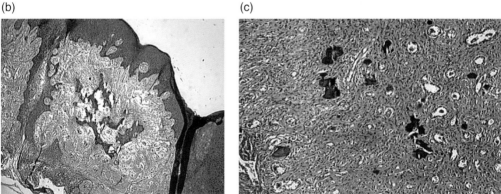

Figure 5.8 Peripheral ossifying/cementifying fibroma. (a) Pink nodular lesion. (b) Photomicrograph reveals a highly cellular connective tissue with ossifications in the form of irregular trabeculae of woven bone (c) Note highly cellular connective tissue with acellular basophilic cementum-like material (*source:* (a) courtesy of Amit Arvind Agrawal, MGV's KBH Dental College and Hospital, Nashik, Maharashtra, India; (b,c) by kind permission of Dr Amberkar VS, College of Dental Sciences, Davangere, Karnataka, India).

5.10.8 Management

- Surgical excision and scaling of teeth

5.10.9 Prognosis

- Good
- 8–16% of lesions recur
- Does not recur if completely removed

5.11 Peripheral Giant Cell Granuloma (Giant Cell Epulis)

5.11.1 Definition/Description

- A tumour-like reactive hyperplastic lesion of the gingival margin located anterior to the permanent molars

5.11.2 Frequency

- Common

5.11.3 Aetiology/Risk Factors

- Local irritation or trauma

5.11.4 Clinical Features

- Mean age group affected: 30–45 years of age
- Slight female preponderance
- Exclusively on the gingiva, mandibular in particular
- Site predilection: anterior to permanent molars or alveolar ridge
- Red or red-blue nodular sessile or pedunculated lesion (Figure 5.9a)

5.11.5 Microscopic Features

- Highly cellular lesion covered by stratified squamous cell epithelium
- Presence of osteoclast like multinucleated giant cells in a cellular vascular stroma (Figure 5.9b)
- Chronic inflammatory cell infiltrate
- Haemorrhagic areas and haemosiderin deposits common

5.11.6 Differential Diagnosis

- Pyogenic granuloma
- Peripheral ossifying fibroma
- Fibrous epulis

(a) (b)

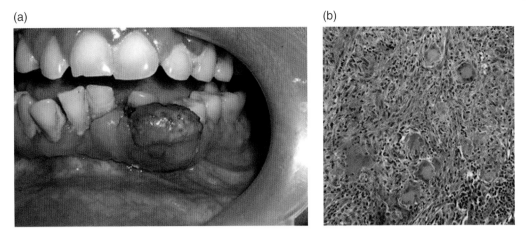

Figure 5.9 (a) Peripheral giant cell granuloma (giant cell epulis). This highly vascular lesion is clinically characterized by purplish red-colour and its tendency to bleed (*source:* by kind permission of Amit Arvind Agrawal, MGV's KBH Dental College and Hospital, Nashik, Maharashtra, India). (b) Photomicrograph shows highly cellular connective tissue stroma with numerous multinucleated giant cells.

5.11.7 Diagnosis

- History
- Clinical finding
- Microscopic findings

5.11.8 Management

- Surgical excision and curettage

5.11.9 Prognosis

- Good to excellent
- Recurrence in 10–18% of cases

5.12 Angiogranuloma (Pyogenic granuloma/pregnancy epulis)

5.12.1 Definition/Description

- A highly vascular, localized inflammatory tumour-like lesion with abundant granulation tissue
- Pyogenic granuloma is a misnomer since there is no pus associated with this lesion
- Angiogranuloma in pregnant women is called pregnancy epulis or pregnancy tumour

5.12.2 Frequency

- Common

5.12.3 Aetiology/Risk Factors

- Local low-grade irritation or trauma
- Female hormones in pregnancy can be precipitating factor

5.12.4 Clinical Features

- Common in females
- Children and young adults commonly affected
- Pedunculated fleshy mass with a predilection for facial surfaces of gingival tissues (75–85% of all cases)
- Anterior maxillary gingiva more commonly involved
- Lips, tongue, and buccal mucosa occasionally affected
- Painless or mildly painful or tender
- Often bleeds easily
- Smooth surface or lobulated, and red or purple in colour (Figure 5.10a and b)
- Surface ulcerated in most cases
- Occasional history of rapid growth

5.12.5 Microscopic Features

- Lesion covered by stratified squamous epithelium, some showing ulceration
- Thin-walled blood vessels in a loose connective tissue stroma with varying amount of predominantly chronic inflammatory cell infiltrate (Figure 5.10c)
- Occasionally presence of trabeculae of woven bone

5.12.6 Differential Diagnosis

- Fibrous epulis
- Peripheral ossifying fibroma
- Peripheral giant cell epulis

5.12.7 Diagnosis

- History
- Clinical findings
- Microscopic findings

5.12.8 Management

- Conservative surgical excision with a wide margin
- Scaling adjacent teeth
- Recurrences occurs in about 16% of cases

5.12.9 Prognosis

- Excellent

(a)

(b)

(c)

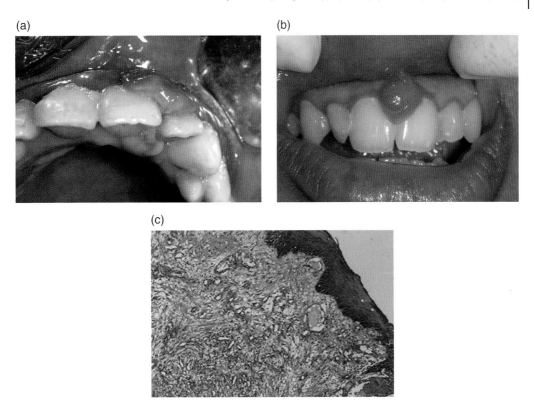

Figure 5.10 Angiogranuloma. (a) a red lobulated mass is connected through the col area seen labially and palatally around the left maxillary central and lateral incisors. (b) Angiogranuloma in pregnancy (pregnancy epulis/pregnancy tumour) involving the interdental papilla between the maxillary central incisors. Note signs of marginal gingivitis (pregnancy gingivitis). (c) Photomicrograph shows parakeratinized stratified squamous epithelium, loose connective tissue stroma, numerous endothelial lined blood vessels and varying amount of inflammatory cell infiltrate. (*Source:* (a,b) by kind permission of Amit Arvind Agrawal, MGV's KBH Dental College and Hospital, Nashik, Maharashtra, India; (c) by kind permission of Dr Ravi Sharma, Centre for Excellence in Esthetics and Dentistry, Jaipur, Rajasthan, India.)

5.13 Inflammatory Gingival Hyperplasia (Inflammatory Gingival Enlargement)

5.13.1 Definition/Description

- Inflammatory gingival hyperplasia is a chronic inflammatory process resulting in generalized gingival enlargement

5.13.2 Frequency

- Common

5.13.3 Aetiology

- Poor oral hygiene
- The irritant could be microbial deposits in dental plaque and calculus

- Systemic factors include hormonal disturbances or blood dyscrasias, which can render gingiva susceptible to the microbial flora and can contribute to inflammatory gingival enlargement

5.13.4   Clinical Features

- Interdental papillae and marginal gingiva have a mildly painful onset and appear diffusely red, oedematous, enlarged with a tendency to bleed easily (Figure 5.11)
- Long-standing inflammatory gingival enlargement shows a significant fibrotic component and is generally painless
- Chronic inflammatory enlargement causes loss of stippling and pseudopockets
- May lead to periodontitis

5.13.5   Microscopic Features

- Granulation tissue: endothelial cells and chronic inflammatory cells and as lesion matures fibroblasts proliferate

5.13.6   Differential Diagnosis

- Pregnancy gingivitis
- Puberty gingivitis
- Drug-associated gingival enlargement
- Gingival enlargement in leukaemia
- Mouth-breathing gingivitis

5.13.7   Diagnosis

- History
- Clinical examination

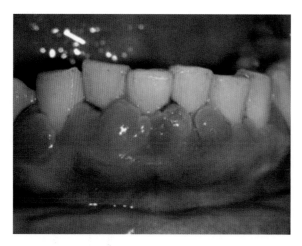

Figure 5.11   Inflammatory gingival hyperplasia induced by plaque in an otherwise healthy individual. Interdental papillae appear diffusely red, oedematous and enlarged with a tendency to bleed (*source:* by kind permission of Amit Arvind Agrawal, MGV's KBH Dental College and Hospital, Nashik, Maharashtra, India).

5.13.8   Management

- Elimination of causative factors
- Maintenance of oral hygiene
- Antiseptic mouth rinses
- In severe cases with fibrous enlargement, surgery may be necessary

5.13.9   Prognosis

- Good

5.14   Generalized Gingival Hyperplasia in Pregnancy

5.14.1   Definition/Description

- Inflammatory gingival hyperplasia is initiated by microbial dental plaque and exacerbated by higher levels of endogenous estrogen and progesterone in pregnancy

5.14.2   Frequency

- Common
- Nearly 60–75% of pregnant women have gingivitis
- Up to 5% of women with pregnancy gingivitis may sometimes develop localized gingival enlargements (pregnancy epulis/pregnancy tumours)

5.14.3   Aetiology/Risk Factors

- Dental plaque accumulation as in non-pregnant individuals
- Increased levels of estrogen and progesterone accentuate gingival response to plaque
- There is an increase in gingival inflammation between the 14th and 30th weeks of pregnancy
- Changes in the subgingival microbiota such as an increase in the proportion of *Prevotella intermedia* in bacterial plaque

5.14.4   Clinical Features

- Generalized maxillary and mandibular gingival swelling with oedema, erythema, and gingival bleeding (Figure 5.12)
- Common in the second trimester
- Aesthetic problems
- Sometimes seen as localized gingival enlargements (pregnancy epulis/pregnancy tumour)

5.14.5   Microscopic Features

- Hyperplastic stratified squamous epithelium
- Increased collagen fibres in the connective tissue
- Intense and diffuse inflammatory cell infiltrate

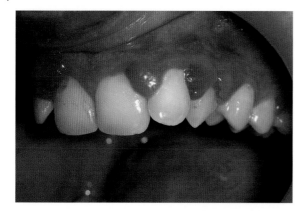

Figure 5.12   Generalized gingival enlargement with erythema and oedema in a pregnant woman (*source:* by kind permission of Amit Arvind Agrawal, MGV's KBH Dental College and Hospital, Nashik, Maharashtra, India).

5.14.6   Differential Diagnosis

- Inflammatory (plaque-induced) gingival hyperplasia
- Drug-associated gingival enlargement
- Gingival enlargement in leukaemia
- Mouth-breathing gingivitis

5.14.7   Diagnosis

- History
- Clinical examination
- Microscopic examination if excision is carried out

5.14.8   Management

- Full mouth scaling and root planning
- In severe enlargement, surgical intervention may be necessary

5.14.9   Prognosis

- Good
- Gingival enlargement regresses after pregnancy

5.15   Drug-Induced Gingival Hyperplasia

5.15.1   Definition/Description

- An abnormal proliferation of gingival tissue in response to the use of anticonvulsants, immuno-suppressive drugs, and anti-hypertensive agents

5.15.2   Frequency

- Available estimates:

– Anticonvulsants: phenytoin-induced gingival hyperplasia 25–50%
– Immunosuppressive agents: cyclosporine-induced gingival hyperplasia 27%
– Antihypertensive agents: calcium channel blocker-induced gingival hyperplasia 10–20%

5.15.3   Aetiology/Risk Factors

- Common medications that cause gingival hyperplasia include:
  – Anticonvulsants (phenytoin)
  – Immunosuppressant (cyclosporine)
  – Calcium channel blockers (nifedipine, diltiazem, amlodipine, and verapamil)

5.15.4   Clinical Features

- Gingival enlargement within a few months of starting medication
- Painless gingival enlargement starts in the interdental papillae and progresses in all directions
- Enlarged gingiva is lobulated, firm, and fibrotic (Figure 5.13)
- Anterior gingiva is frequently involved
- Enlargement causes pseudopockets
- Enlargement covers the crown of teeth resulting in difficulty in oral hygiene maintenance and eating
- Non-inflamed gingiva are pink in colour
- When inflamed, colour is dark red and oedematous and bleeds readily
- Aesthetically unpleasant
- Edentulous areas usually not involved

5.15.5   Microscopic Features

- Epithelium shows elongation of rete ridges
- Increased amount of fibrous tissue in lamina propria
- Relative lack of vasculature
- In inflamed gingiva, increased vasculature and lymphocytic and plasma cell infiltration

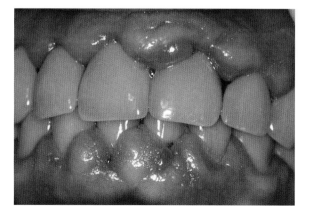

Figure 5.13   Gingival enlargement caused by nifedipine, an antihypertensive drug (*source:* by kind permission of Adj. Associate Professor John Highfield, University of Sydney, Australia).

5.15.6 Differential Diagnosis

- Gingival enlargement in pregnancy
- Gingival fibromatosis
- Leukaemic gingival enlargement
- Idiopathic gingival enlargement
- Gingival enlargement in granulomatosis with polyangiitis (Wegener's granulomatosis)
- Chronic inflammatory gingival enlargement

5.15.7 Diagnosis

- History (medical history)
- Clinical examination
- Histopathology to rule out gingival enlargement due to leukaemia and other causes

5.15.8 Management

- When possible, consult the patient's physician to replace the medication (e.g. cyclosporin, calcium channel blockers)
- Test for serum folate level and supplement folic acid if necessary
- Plaque control is important
- Home oral hygiene care and folic acid oral rinse or chlorhexidine gluconate 0.12% oral rinse
- Surgical resection of the fibrous gingival enlargement (gingivectomy or gingivoplasty) after oral hygiene is optimal
- Regular check up

5.15.9 Prognosis

- Good

5.16 Familial Gingival Hyperplasia

5.16.1 Definition/Description

- A rare, slowly progressive familial or idiopathic gingival enlargement characterized by a collagenous overgrowth of gingival fibrous connective tissue
- Also known as hereditary gingival fibromatosis

5.16.2 Frequency

- Rare
- Estimated prevalence: 1 in 750 000

5.16.3 Aetiology/Risk Factors

- Familial/idiopathic
- Familial: autosomal dominant pattern of inheritance in most cases

5.16.4 Clinical Features

- Gingival enlargement begins before the age of 20 years in most cases
- May cause delay or failure in tooth eruption
- Interferes with lip closure
- Teeth are covered
- Aesthetically unpleasant
- All four quadrants may be involved
- In the maxilla, palatal surfaces are predominantly enlarged
- Affected gingiva is firm, stippled and normal in colour (Figure 5.14)
- Other findings in some patients may include:
  - Hypertrichosis
  - Epilepsy
  - Intellectual disability
  - Deafness
  - Hypothyroidism

5.16.5 Microscopic Features

- Hypocellular, hypovascular fibrous connective tissue arranged in interlacing bundles
- Long epithelial rete ridges
- Lack of inflammation

5.16.6 Differential Diagnosis

- Gingival enlargement in pregnancy
- Drug-induced gingival enlargement
- Leukaemic gingival enlargement

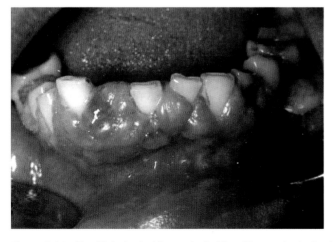

Figure 5.14 Familial gingival hyperplasia. Firm fibrous gingival enlargement in a patient with a history of familial gingival enlargement in the family (*source:* reproduced with permission from Ramdas, K., Lucas, E., Thomas, G et al. (2008). *A Digital Manual for the Early Diagnosis of Oral Neoplasia.* Lyon: IARC. Available from http://screening.iarc.fr/atlasoral.php?lang=1).

- Idiopathic gingival enlargement
- Gingival enlargement in Wegener's granulomatosis
- Chronic inflammatory gingival enlargement

5.16.7 Diagnosis

- History
- Clinical examination
- Histopathology to rule out gingival enlargement due to leukaemia and other causes

5.16.8 Management

- Scaling and root planning for mild cases
- Surgical removal of enlarged tissue for more advanced cases
- Follow up

5.16.9 Prognosis

- Fair to good

5.17 Gingival and Periodontal Abscesses

5.17.1 Definition/Description

- Gingival abscess is a localized purulent infection that involves the marginal gingiva or interdental papilla without involving the periodontal ligament or alveolar bone
- Periodontal abscess is the result of acute inflammation of periodontal pocket resulting in collection of pus alongside a vital tooth

5.17.2 Frequency

- Gingival and periodontal abscesses are common
- Periodontal abscess is the third most frequent dental emergency, representing 7–14% of all the dental emergencies

5.17.3 Aetiology/Risk Factors

- Gingival abscess:
  - Plaque or foreign body entrapped in the gingival sulcus
- Periodontal abscess:
  - Acute exacerbation of untreated chronic periodontitis
  - The consequence of the treatment of chronic periodontitis
  - Foreign body (such as toothbrush bristle or fish bone) in the periodontal pocket
  - Food impaction between the teeth with poor contact points
  - Pericoronitis

- Role of microbes:
  - Gingival abscess: a wide variety of microbes to colonize, including Porphyromonas, streptococci and Actinomyces
  - Periodontal abscess: Gram-negative anaerobic rods are predominantly found in periodontal abscesses. Organisms include *Porphyromonas gingivalis*, *Prevotella intermedia*, *Fusobacterium nucleatum*, *Campylobacter rectus, and Capnocytophaga* spp.

5.17.4 Clinical Features

- Gingival abscess:
  - Localized gingival erythematous swelling (Figure 5.15a)
  - Pain
  - Feeling of malaise
- Periodontal abscess:
  - Rapid onset
  - Mild discomfort to severe throbbing pain
  - Vital tooth
  - Sensitivity on palpation and/or percussion on the affected tooth
  - Fever and/or malaise
  - Superficial abscess shows swollen red fluctuating tender gingiva along the lateral aspect of the root. (Figure 5.15b)
  - A deep periodontal abscess might be less obvious.
  - Pus, either spontaneous or provoked, through a fistula or from a periodontal pocket
  - Tooth mobility and/or tooth elevation
  - Foul taste
  - Regional lymphadenopathy

(a)   (b)

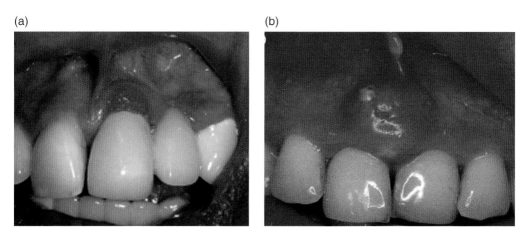

Figure 5.15 (a) Gingival abscess: acute gingival abscess showing an erythematous gingival swelling above the maxillary left central incisor (*source:* by kind permission of Amit Arvind Agrawal, MGV's KBH Dental College and Hospital, Nashik, Maharashtra, India). (b) Acute periodontal abscess with a history of sudden onset of painful gingival swelling. Note a well-circumscribed swelling on the attached gingiva with points of fluctuation (*source:* by kind permission of Adj. Associate Professor John Highfield, University of Sydney, NSW, Australia).

5.17.5 Microscopic Features

- Gingival abscess:
  - Acute inflammatory cell infiltrate in the connective tissues
  - Evidence of pus
- Periodontal abscess:
  - Osteoclasts along the bony wall
  - Dense infiltration of neutrophils
  - Destruction of periodontal fibres
  - Evidence of pus

5.17.6 Differential Diagnosis

- Periapical abscess
- Periodontal abscess for gingival abscess
- Gingival abscess for periodontal abscess
- Lateral periodontal cyst
- Periodontic–endodontic lesion

5.17.7 Diagnosis

- History of onset and duration of symptoms and recent dental/periodontal interventions and trauma
- Clinical examination: determination of the existence of a periodontal pocket in periodontal abscess (absent in gingival abscess)
- Confirmation of the presence of purulent exudate
- Radiographical evidence of bone loss alongside the tooth in periodontal abscess (seen for periodontal abscesses of more than a week's duration)
- Gingival abscesses do not cause alveolar bone loss

5.17.8 Management

5.17.8.1 Gingival Abscess
- Drainage of pus
- Subgingival curettage
- Analgesics for pain

5.17.8.2 Periodontal Abscess
- Abscess to be drained (through the pocket or by incision)
- Subgingival curettage and root surface debridement
- Analgesics for pain
- If periodontal involvement is severe, tooth extraction is required
- Antibiotic is prescribed if fever is present

5.17.9 Prognosis

- Good

5.18 Pericoronitis/Pericoronal Abscess

5.18.1 Definition/Description

- An inflammatory process that arises within the tissues surrounding the crown of a partially erupted or impacted tooth
- Based on symptoms, three types are recognized: acute, subacute, and chronic (recurrent) pericoronitis

5.18.2 Frequency

- Estimated prevalence of pericoronitis: 4.92%

5.18.3 Aetiology/Risk Factors

5.18.3.1 Aetiology
- Entrapment of plaque and food debris between crown of tooth and overlying gingival flap or operculum
- Oral streptococci and various anaerobic species

5.18.3.2 Risk Factors
- Presence of unerupted/partially erupted tooth
- Mandibular third molar impaction (placed vertical or distoangular)
- Presence of periodontal pocket adjacent to unerupted/partially erupted teeth
- Opposing tooth/teeth in relation to pericoronal tissues surrounding unerupted/partially erupted tooth. When an opposing tooth bites into the operculum, it can initiate or exacerbate pericoronitis resulting in a spiralling cycle of inflammation and trauma
- Previous history of pericoronitis
- Poor oral hygiene
- Respiratory tract infections and tonsillitis

5.18.3.3 Microbial Association
- Bacterial species which are predominant in pericoronitis are *Streptococcus* species, Actinomyces spp., and *Propionibacterium* spp. but microbial flora become predominantly anaerobic

5.18.3.4 Clinical Features
- Common in teens and young adults
- Can present as asymptomatic gingival flaps around the partially erupted tooth (usually the lower third molar)
- Long periods of chronic inflammation present minimal symptoms
- Food debris and bacteria are trapped in the inflamed tissues and trauma from occlusal forces may exacerbate the inflammatory process causing an abscess
- Other features include:
  – Continuous dull or severe pain, extra oral swelling, and tenderness
  – Difficulty in mouth opening, closing, and discomfort in swallowing
  – Lymphadenitis of the associated lymph nodes
  – Fever and malaise

   – Unpleasant breath/taste

   – Purulent exudate (expressed on palpation) from the inflamed/abscessed tissue (operculum) surrounding the partially erupted tooth (Figure 5.16)

   – Loss of appetite

- Complications: this infection can spread to the cheeks, orbits or periorbital tissues, and other parts of the face or neck, and occasionally can lead to airway compromise (e.g. Ludwig's angina) requiring emergency hospital treatment

5.18.4 Microscopic Features

- Hyperplastic epithelial lining of pericoronal flap
- Connective tissue underneath epithelium shows oedema increased vascularity, dense diffused infiltration with lymphocytes, plasma cells and polymorphonuclear leukocytes

5.18.5 Differential Diagnosis

- Tonsillar infections
- Lymphoma
- Paradental cyst

5.18.6 Diagnosis

- History (onset, duration, symptoms, etc.)
- Clinical examination
- Radiography (to evaluate type of tooth impaction)

5.18.7 Management

- Non-surgical:
  - Irrigation of the pericoronal space with warm saline
  - Gentle curettage and swabbing the underneath surface of flap with antiseptic

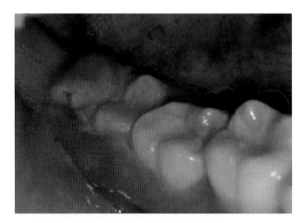

Figure 5.16 Pericoronal abscess. Note a pus-filled swelling partially covering the occlusal surface of the erupting third molar and erythematous area of the buccal gingival tissue (*source:* by kind permission of Amit Arvind Agrawal, MGV's KBH Dental College and Hospital, Nashik, Maharashtra, India).

- If an opposing tooth is traumatizing with the pericoronal flap, then occlusal adjustment is required
- Establishing the drainage of pus if abscess has formed
- Application of caustic agents such as chromic acid, trichloroacetic acid or Howe's ammoniacal solution
- In severe cases of pericoronitis or if systemic symptoms are present, antibiotics and appropriate analgesics:
- Antibiotic of choice is amoxicillin 500 mg three times a day for five days in combination with metronidazole 400 mg three times a day for five days
- Surgical:
  - Operculectomy
  - Extraction

5.18.8   Prognosis

- Favourable

5.19   Gingival Enlargement in Granulomatosis with Polyangiitis (Wegener's granulomatosis)

5.19.1   Definition/Description

- Granulomatosis with polyangiitis (Wegener's granulomatosis) is a potentially immunologically mediated fatal form of vasculitis

5.19.2   Frequency

- Uncommon
- A prevalence of 3 in 100 000 cases
- Majority of cases are in white populations

5.19.3   Aetiology/Risk Factors

- Believed to be an autoimmune disorder
- Abnormal immune response to an inhaled environmental antigen or infectious agent
- Hereditary predisposition is possible for some cases

5.19.4   Clinical Features

- Wide age range
- Both sexes are equally affected
- Weight loss
- Nasal congestion, chronic sinus pain, epistaxis and fever are common
- Respiratory tract involvement includes dry cough, haemoptysis, and dyspnoea
- Kidney involvement results in glomerulonephritis (haematuria is common)
- Gingival enlargement: granular and red bulbous projections (strawberry gingivitis) (Figure 5.17)

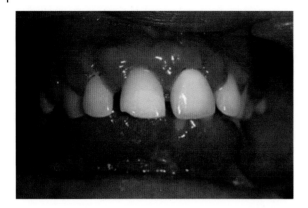

Figure 5.17 Gingival enlargement in granulomatosis with polyangiitis (Wegener's granulomatosis), presents as reddish purple, exophytic gingival overgrowth often referred to as 'strawberry gingivitis' (*source: by kind permission of Amit Arvind Agrawal, MGV's KBH Dental College and Hospital, Nashik, Maharashtra, India*).

- Oral non-specific ulcerations, temporomandibular joint pain, and facial paralysis are other manifestations
- Saddle-nose deformity

5.19.5 Microscopic Features

- Microscopic features of oral lesions:
  - Epithelium shows pseudoepitheliomatous hyperplasia
  - Connective tissue: mixed inflammatory cell infiltrate around blood vessels (neutrophils, histiocytes, lymphocytes, eosinophils, and multinucleated giant cells)

5.19.6 Differential Diagnosis

- All gingival enlargements due to local and systemic causes
- All non-specific oral ulceration from other causes

5.19.7 Diagnosis

- History
- Clinical examination
- Complete blood count (CBC):
  - Raised white cell count (leucocytosis)
  - Reduced haemoglobin (normocytic normochromic anaemia)
  - Raised platelet count (thrombocytosis)
  - Raised erythrocyte sedimentation rate (ESR)
- Detection of anti-neutrophil cytoplasm antibodies (ANCA)
- Detection of antibodies against proteinase-3 (PR3-ANCA), together with enzyme-linked immunosorbent assay, is diagnostic
- Positive rheumatoid factor occurs in 50–60% of cases

5.19.8   Management

- Specialist treatment required
- Oral prednisone and cyclophosphamide
- Low doses of methotrexate and corticosteroids
- Other useful drugs and treatment modalities: azathioprine, intravenous immunoglobulin, plasma exchange and rituximab
- Disease must be monitored regularly: periodic blood tests (CBC, differential, ESR, antibody tests)

5.19.9   Prognosis

- Oral lesions respond to systemic treatment
- Prognosis varies:
  - If PR3-ANCA levels disappear, the prognosis is good
  - Disease may recur if PR3-ANCA levels persist

5.20   Gingival Enlargement in Leukaemia

5.20.1   Definition/Description

- Leukaemia is a haematological disorder which is characterized by a marked increase in circulating immature or abnormal white blood cells. The disease begins with the malignant transformation of one of the haematopoietic stem cells in the bone marrow and released into the peripheral circulation
- Leukaemia is classified based on clinical behaviour (acute or chronic) and the primary haematopoietic cell line involved (myeloid or lymphoid)
- The four principal diagnostic categories are
  - acute myelogenous leukaemia
  - acute lymphocytic leukaemia
  - chronic myelogenous leukaemia
  - chronic lymphocytic leukaemia

5.20.2   Frequency

- All four forms of leukaemia put together, approximately 13 cases per 100 000 population per year
- Slight preponderance for males

5.20.3   Aetiology/Risk Factors

- The causes of leukaemia are unknown
- Increased risk factors include large doses of ionizing radiation, certain chemicals (benzene), and infection with specific viruses (e.g. Epstein–Barr virus, human lymphotropic virus)
- Cigarette smoking and exposure to electromagnetic fields have also been implicated

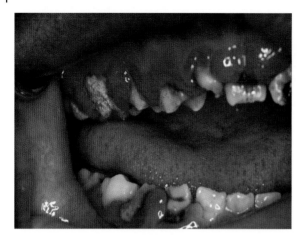

Figure 5.18 Gingival enlargement in a patient with acute lymphocytic leukaemia. The free and attached gingival tissues are swollen and erythematous. Note the gingival bleeding. (*Source:* by kind permission of Professor Newell Johnson, Brisbane, Australia)

5.20.4 Clinical Features

- Chronic leukaemia may last several years
- Acute cases may involve malaise, cervical lymphadenopathy, laryngeal pain, fever, enlarged tonsils, and pharyngitis
- 65% of patients have oral manifestations. These include:
  - Gingival bleeding, petechiae, ecchymosis
  - Gingival enlargement: gingiva appear swollen, devoid of stippling and pale red to deep purple in colour; more common in acute leukaemia (Figure 5.18)
  - Gingival ulceration and oral infection (herpetic infections and candidosis) are common

5.20.5 Microscopic Features

- Gingival tissue shows:
  - Destruction of tissue
  - Infiltration with poorly differentiated leukaemic cells

5.20.6 Differential Diagnosis

- Agranulocytosis
- Cyclic neutropenia
- Thrombocytopenic purpura
- Gingival fibromatosis
- Drug-induced gingival enlargement

5.20.7 Diagnosis

- History
- Clinical examination
- Laboratory investigations:

- CBC count: reduction in the number of normal circulating blood cells
- Identification of abnormal (poorly differentiated) leukaemic cells in the peripheral blood
- Bone marrow biopsy
- Cytochemical staining (myeloperoxidase), immunophenotyping (cell surface markers), and cytogenetic analysis of chromosomal abnormalities

5.20.8 Management

- Chemotherapy for leukaemia by oncologists
- Allogeneic haematopoietic cell transplantation by oncologists
- Supportive care
- Oral hygiene
- Antiviral and antifungal treatment if oral herpetic or candidal infections exist

5.20.9 Prognosis

- The average five-year survival rate for all types of leukaemia is 62.7%

5.21 Gingival Enlargement in Ascorbic Acid Deficiency

5.21.1 Definition

- A rare nutritional disorder due to deficiency of ascorbic acid (vitamin C)

5.21.2 Frequency

- Uncommon/rare

5.21.3 Aetiology/Risk Factors

- Severe vitamin C deficiency

5.21.4 Clinical Features

- Symptoms of scurvy develop after at least three months of severe or total vitamin C deficiency
- Systemic manifestations:
  - Patients initially complain of weakness, fatigue, and aching limbs in the legs
  - If left untreated, reddish/bluish bruise-like spots surrounding hair follicles occur
  - The papules may join to form large areas of palpable ecchymoses (bruises)
  - Bleeding in the joints causing swollen and tender joints
  - Dry eyes, irritation, light intolerance, transient visual blurring, and conjunctival bleeding
  - Anaemia
  - Shortness of breath
- Oral manifestations:
  - Red, soft, spongy, swollen gingiva (Figure 5.19)
  - Spontaneous gingival bleeding

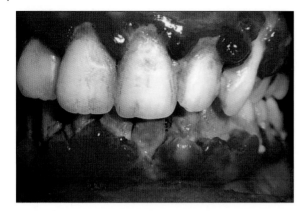

Figure 5.19 Shiny, soft, bulbous, spongy gingival enlargement in a patient with severe vitamin C deficiency (scurvy) mimicking acute necrotizing ulcerative gingivitis (*source:* by kind permission of Sharanabasappa R. Japatti, Annasaheb Chudaman Patil Memorial Dental College and Hospital, Dhule, Maharashtra, India).

– Tooth mobility in severe cases
– Gingival features may mimic those of acute necrotizing ulcerative gingivitis

5.21.5   Microscopic Features

- Presence of intra-epidermal vesicles and spongiosis in the squamous epithelium
- The deeper connective tissue reveals marked vascularity and acute or chronic inflammatory infiltrate
- Subepithelial haemorrhages and capillaries reveal fibrin thrombi

5.21.6   Differential Diagnosis

- Gingival enlargements due to local and systemic causes
- Necrotizing ulcerative gingivitis
- Agranulocytosis
- Thrombocytopenic purpura

5.21.7   Diagnosis

- History (dietary history to be included)
- Clinical examination
- CBC
- Blood test for ascorbic acid: plasma vitamin C concentration < 11 mmol/l (0.2 mg/dl) is said to be indicative of scurvy

5.21.8   Management

- Vitamin C 60–100 mg/day is effective
- Prevention: recommended daily intake of vitamin C is 30–60 mg/day
- Treatment of other vitamin deficiencies that may occur in conjunction with vitamin C deficiency

- Consuming five servings of fruits and vegetables/day offers recommended daily intake of vitamin C
- Scaling and root planning
- Oral hygiene instructions

5.21.9 Prognosis

- Good

Recommended Reading

Agrawal, A.A. (2015). Gingival enlargements: differential diagnosis and review of literature. *World Journal of Clinical Cases* 3 (9): 779–788.

Amberkar, V.S., Mohan Kumar, K.P., Chawla, S.K., and Madhushankari, G.S. (2017). Peripheral ossifying fibroma: revisited. *International Journal of Oral Health Sciences* 7: 35–40.

Brierley, D.J., Crane, H., and Hunter, K.D. (2019). Lumps and bumps of the gingiva: a pathological miscellany. *Head and Neck Pathology* 13: 103–113.

Demirer, S., Özdemir, H., Şencan, M. et al. (2007). Gingival hyperplasia as an early diagnostic oral manifestation in acute monocytic leukaemia: a case report. *European Journal of Dentistry* 1 (2): 111–114.

Highfield, J. (2009). Diagnosis and classification of periodontal disease. *Australian Dental Journal* 54 (1 Suppl): S11–S26.

Japatti, S.R., Bhatsange, A., Reddy, M. et al. (2013). Scurvy-scorbutic siderosis of gingiva: a diagnostic challenge - a rare case report. *Dental Research Journal (Isfahan)* 10: 394–400.

Neville, B.W., Damm, D.D., Allen, C.M., and Chi, C.A. (2016). Periodontal diseases. In: *Oral and Maxillofacial Pathology 4e*, 14–159. St Louis MO: Elsevier.

Odell, E.W. (2017). Gingival and periodontal disorders. In: *Cawson's Essentials of Oral Pathology and Oral Medicine*, vol. 9e, 95–115. Edinburgh: Elsevier.

Prabhu, S.R. (2019). Benign mucosal swellings. In: *Clinical Diagnosis in Oral Medicine: A case based approach*, 205–239. New Delhi: Jaypee Brothers Medical Publishers.

Prabhu, S.R. and Wilson, D.F. (2016). Gingival and oral soft tissue lumps and swellings. In: *Handbook of Oral Diseases for Medical Practice* (ed. S.R. Prabhu), 107–122. New Delhi: Oxford University Press.

Ranjan, A., Sharma, R., Arora, M. et al. (2018). Pyogenic granuloma of oral cavity: case series and clinicopathologic correlation. *International Dental and Medical Journal of Advanced Research* 4: 1–4.

Savage, N.W. and Daly, C.G. (2010). Gingival enlargements and localized gingival overgrowths. *Australian Dental Journal* 55 (1 Suppl): 55–60.

Shaw, L., Harjunmaa, U., Doyle, R. et al. (2016). Distinguishing the signals of gingivitis and periodontitis in supragingival plaque: a cross-sectional cohort study in Malawi. *Applied and Environmental Microbiology* 82 (19): 6057–6067.

Shivalingu, M.M., Rathnakara, S.H., Khanum, N., and Basappa, S. (2016). Plasma cell gingivitis: a rare and perplexing entity. *Journal of Indian Academy of Oral Medicine and Radiology* 28: 94–97.

Part II

Pathology of Jaw Bones

6

Infections and Necrosis of the Jaw

CHAPTER MENU

6.1 Acute Suppurative Osteomyelitis
6.2 Chronic Suppurative Osteomyelitis
6.3 Sclerosing Osteomyelitis
6.4 Proliferative Periostitis (Garre's Osteomyelitis)
6.5 Actinomycosis of the Jaw
6.6 Cervicofacial Cellulitis (Cervicofacial Fascial Space Infection)
6.7 Osteoradionecrosis of the Jaw
6.8 Medication-Related Osteonecrosis of the Jaw

6.1 Acute Suppurative Osteomyelitis

6.1.1 Definition/Description

- An acute inflammatory process caused by an infection that involves the bone marrow of the jaw bones
- Infection usually lasts for less than one month

6.1.2 Frequency

- Uncommon in recent years

6.1.3 Aetiology/Risk Factors

- Causative microbes: predominantly anaerobes: *Bacteroides*, *Porphyromonas*, *Prevotella* species, and staphylococci in early stages
- Predisposing factors include diabetes mellitus, malnutrition, and immunosuppression
- Sources of infection: periapical infections, infected periodontal pocket, acute necrotizing ulcerative gingivitis or pericoronitis, bone fracture, radiation damage, etc.

6.1.4 Clinical Features

- Predominantly adult males are affected
- Commonly involves mandible
- Pain is severe, throbbing, and deep seated
- External (facial) swelling and redness due to inflammatory oedema
- Trismus
- Dysphagia
- Paraesthesia or anaesthesia of the lower lip (for mandibular osteomyelitis)
- Cervical lymphadenopathy
- Fever and malaise
- Teeth involved are tender to percussion
- Pus may be visible, which exudes from around the necks of teeth, from an open socket, or from other sites within the mouth or on the skin over the involved bone
- Sinuses open on the skin or oral mucosa
- Foetid odour

6.1.5 Radiographical Features

- Radiographical changes are not evident until after 10 days of infection
- Possible initial findings include widening of the periodontal ligament and loss of the lamina dura
- As disease progresses, loss of trabecular pattern is followed by irregular areas of radiolucency ('motheaten' appearance due to bone destruction; Figure 6.1)
- Area of dead bone (sequestrum)
- Untreated acute osteomyelitis of the mandible may proceed to chronic stage showing subperiosteal new bone formation below the lower border (seen on lateral radiographic views)
- Additional imaging modalities include computed tomography, magnetic resonance imaging, and scintigraphy

6.1.6 Microscopic Features

- Predominant acute inflammation and fibrin
- Loss of osteocytes from the lacunae
- Presence of necrotic bone with signs of peripheral resorption
- Bacterial colonization surrounding the inflammatory infiltrate

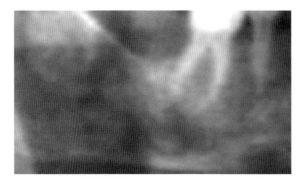

Figure 6.1 Cropped orthopantomogram of acute suppurative osteomyelitis of the mandible. Note motheaten appearance (*source:* by kind permission of ProProfs.com).

6.1.7 Differential Diagnosis

- Exacerbation of osteoradionecrosis
- Exacerbation of bisphosphonate-related osteonecrosis of the jaw
- Langerhans cell histiocytosis
- Metastatic neoplasms to the jaws with abscess formation
- Periapical granuloma or infected cyst

6.1.8 Diagnosis

- History
- Clinical examination
- Radiography and other imaging modalities
- Bacterial sampling and culture (from pus or a swab from the lesion)
- Blood investigations (complete blood count with differential in cases of active bacterial infection)

6.1.9 Management

- Antibiotics
- Empirical treatment initially
- Specific antibiotics should be started on the basis of culture and sensitivity reports:
  - The recommended antibiotic is penicillin V potassium 500 mg (one tablet four times daily for seven days) *or*
  - Amoxicillin 500 mg (one tablet three times daily for 7 days) or clindamycin 150 mg or 300 mg (one capsule four times daily for seven days)
  - For severe infections: amoxicillin/clavulanate potassium (co-amoxiclav) 500 mg (one tablet three times daily for seven days)
  - Intravenous antibiotics (penicillin G potassium, 12–24 million units/day, depending on the infection and its severity, administered in equal doses four to six times daily)
  - For anaerobic infections: amoxicillin 500 mg with metronidazole 250 mg three times daily
  - For pain: acetaminophen, 325 mg, six times daily; the maximum cumulative dose of acetaminophen is 4 g in 24 hours).
  - For severe pain: oxycodone 5 mg with acetaminophen 325 mg, 1 tablet four to six times daily)
  - If anaerobes are of periodontal in origin, a combination of amoxicillin 500 mg with metronidazole 250 mg three times daily is effective
- Hospitalization if there are signs and symptoms of sepsis or airway compromise
- Elimination of the source of infection (e.g. extraction or root canal treatment on the offending tooth)
- Sequestrectomy
- Use of hyperbaric oxygen (for radiation induced osteomyelitis)

6.1.10 Prognosis

- Generally good

6.2 Chronic Suppurative Osteomyelitis

6.2.1 Definition/Description

- A disease of the (jaw) bone characterized by chronic inflammatory processes that causes necrosis of mineralized and marrow tissues, suppuration, resorption, sclerosis, and hyperplasia
- Chronic osteomyelitis refers to a condition that has lasted over one month

6.2.2 Frequency

- Common (compared with the acute form)

6.2.3 Aetiology/Risk Factors

- Low-grade infection with *Staphylococcus aureus* and aerobic Gram-negative bacilli
- Odontogenic infection (most common)
- Post-extraction complication
- Infected periodontal pocket
- Inadequate removal of necrotic bone
- Early termination of antibiotic therapy
- Inappropriate selection of antibiotics for odontogenic infections
- Diagnostic failure
- Trauma to the jaw
- Inadequate treatment for fracture
- Irradiation to the mandible
- Actinomycosis
- Tuberculosis
- Underlying malignancy and associated osteomyelitis

6.2.4 Clinical Features

- Low-grade pain
- Mandible commonly involved
- Bone exposure
- Pus, fistula, and sequestration
- Low-grade fever in some cases

6.2.5 Radiographical Features

- Radiographical features include:
  - Radiolucent areas
  - Bony destruction
  - Sequestrum formation (Figure 6.2)

6.2.6 Microscopic Features

- Inflammatory cell infiltrate predominantly with lymphocytes and plasma cells
- Scanty polymorphonuclear cell infiltrate

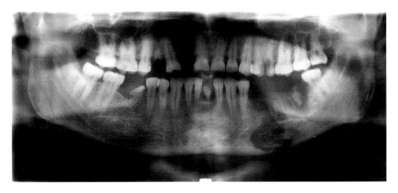

Figure 6.2 Chronic suppurative osteomyelitis. Orthopantogram showing radiolucent areas extending between left mandibular first premolar and third molar (*source:* by kind permission of Dr Hemant Mehra, Babu Banarasi Das College of Dental Surgery, Lucknow, Uttar Pradesh India).

- Marrow fibrosis, reactive woven bone formation, minimal marrow adipose tissue
- Periosteum still contains osteogenic potential in most cases, which contributes to formation of a bony shell (involucrum) covering the necrotic bone (sequestrum)

6.2.7 Differential Diagnosis

- Paget's disease
- Hypercementosis
- Fibrous dysplasia
- Early stage of bone malignancy
- Osteosarcoma
- Osteoradionecrosis
- Medication-related osteoradionecrosis

6.2.8 Diagnosis

- History
- Clinical examination
- Radiography and other imaging modalities
- Bacterial sampling and culture (from pus or a swab from the lesion)
- Blood investigations (complete blood count with differential in cases of active bacterial infection)

6.2.9 Management

- Aggressive antibiotic therapy (see section 6.1.9, treatment protocol for acute suppurative osteomyelitis)
- Removal of sequestrum (non-viable bone)

6.2.10 Prognosis

- Good

6.3   Sclerosing Osteomyelitis

6.3.1   Definition/Description

- Sclerosing osteomyelitis is characterized by the process of sclerosis of bone due to low grade non-suppurative inflammation
- Sclerosing osteomyelitis is of two types: focal and diffuse
- Focal sclerosing osteomyelitis, also known as condensing (or sclerosing) osteitis refers to a relatively common, focal, well-circumscribed radiopaque condensation of bone surrounding the apex of a root which is often inflamed or is associated with necrotic dental pulp
- Diffuse sclerosing osteomyelitis refers to a condition affecting a large portion of the bone, usually the mandible, and is associated with mandibular expansion remodelling and clinical symptoms

6.3.2   Frequency

- Focal sclerosing osteomyelitis: common as a sequel to low-grade odontogenic infection
- Diffuse sclerosing osteomyelitis: less common compared with focal sclerosing osteitis

6.3.3   Aetiology/Risk Factors

- Focal sclerosing osteomyelitis: low-grade periapical infection in an individual with strong host defensive response
- Diffuse sclerosing osteomyelitis: periapical or periodontal chronic infection around the bone

6.3.4   Clinical Features

- Focal sclerosing osteomyelitis (condensing osteitis):
  - Children and adolescents are usually affected
  - Premolar and molar regions are predominantly involved in sclerotic change
  - Associated tooth is usually non-vital or with chronic pulpitis
  - No jaw expansion

- Diffuse sclerosing osteomyelitis:
  - Usually affects adults
  - Both sexes are equally affected
  - Persistent dull pain but no jaw expansion is seen

6.3.5   Radiographical Features

- Focal sclerosing osteomyelitis:
  - Focal zone of sclerosis in the jaw is associated with periapical tissues (Figure 6.3a)
  - Widened periodontal space
  - Usually the mandibular premolar/molar region
- Diffuse sclerosing osteomyelitis:
  - Extensive cortical and medullary sclerosis in the jaw sometimes combined with subperiosteal bone formation (Figure 6.3b)

(a)

(b)

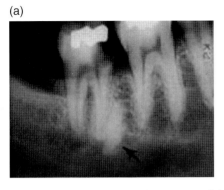 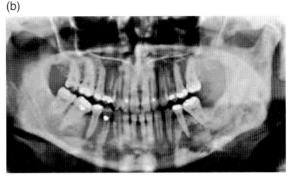

Figure 6.3 (a) Focal sclerosing osteomyelitis: an intraoral radiograph showing focal sclerosing osteomyelitis (condensing osteitis) around the decayed second molar root (black arrow). (*Source:* by kind permission from Professor Charles Dunlap, Kansas City, USA). (b) Diffuse sclerosing osteomyelitis: an orthopantogram showing diffuse sclerosing osteomyelitis of the mandible. *Source:* DOI:https://doi. org/10.1016/S1042-3699(02)00073-0

6.3.6 Microscopic Features

- Focal sclerosing osteomyelitis:
  - Appears as replacement of cancellous bone with compact bone and, in some cases, shows chronic inflammatory infiltrate and areas of fibrosis
- Diffuse sclerosing osteomyelitis:
  - Sclerosis and remodelling of bone are predominant features
  - Little marrow tissue
  - Necrotic bone tissue separates from the adjacent vital tissue and becomes surrounded by granulation tissue
  - Bacterial colonization is often present

6.3.7 Differential Diagnosis

- For focal sclerosing osteomyelitis:
  - Cemento-osseous dysplasia
- For diffuse sclerosing osteomyelitis:
  - Florid cemento-osseous dysplasia
  - Osteoradionecrosis
  - Medication-related osteoradionecrosis

6.3.8 Diagnosis

- History
- Clinical examination
- Radiographical findings:
  - Sclerosis and remodelling of bone are predominant features
  - Little marrow tissue
  - Necrotic bone tissue separates from the adjacent vital tissue and becomes surrounded by granulation tissue
  - Bacterial colonization is often present

6.3.9 Management

- Elimination of the focus of odontogenic infection (endodontic treatment or extraction of the offending tooth) for both forms

6.3.10 Prognosis

- Generally good

6.4 Proliferative Periostitis (Garre's Osteomyelitis)

6.4.1 Definition/Description

- Proliferative periostitis (also known as Garre's osteomyelitis) is the proliferation of new bone formation, resulting in the expansion of the mandibular cortex as a periosteal reaction to low-grade inflammation in children and adolescents

6.4.2 Frequency

- Uncommon

6.4.3 Aetiology/Risk Factors

- Periapical/dentoalveolar low-grade chronic infection

6.4.4 Clinical Features

- Usually children and adolescents are affected
- Unilateral asymptomatic hard swelling of the lower border of the mandible

6.4.5 Radiographical Features

- Medullary radiolucent and radio-opaque appearance with ill-defined margins
- Periosteal–cortical expansion is seen
- Concentric or parallel layering of cortex ('onion-skin' appearance) seen on occlusal radiography (Figure 6.4a)

6.4.6 Microscopic Features

- Formation of new bone or osteoid tissue in a fibrous connective tissue stroma
- Osteoblasts bordering osteoid tissue
- Some areas of bone show resorption and reversal lines
- Lymphocytes and plasma cells in marrow spaces (Figure 6.4b)

6.4.7 Differential Diagnosis

- Ewing's sarcoma
- Langerhans cell disease (histiocytosis X)

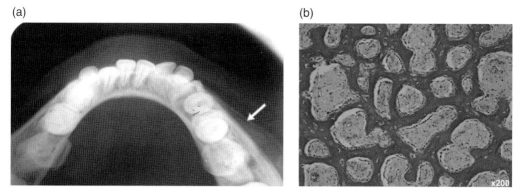

Figure 6.4 (a) Proliferative periostitis of the mandible: preoperative mandibular occlusal radiograph showing the peripheral sub-periosteal bone deposition on right side (white arrow). (b) Photomicrograph showing the mixture of woven bone, mature bone, osteoblastic rimming, mild fibrotic changes in the marrow space and mild inflammatory cell infiltrate.

- Osteosarcoma
- Fibro-osseous lesion
- Metastatic tumours

6.4.8 Diagnosis

- History
- Clinical examination
- Radiography

6.4.9 Management

- Elimination of the focus of odontogenic infection (endodontic treatment or extraction of the offending tooth)
- In some cases, antibiotics may be required

6.4.10 Prognosis

- Good

6.5 Actinomycosis of the Jaw

6.5.1 Definition

- A chronic suppurative infection of the jaw caused by Gram-positive anaerobic, microaerophilic filamentous bacteria *Actinomyces israelii*

6.5.2 Frequency

- Actinomycosis of the jaws (actinomycosis osteomyelitis) is relatively uncommon

6.5.3   Aetiology/Risk Factors

- Filamentous bacteria *A. israelii* (a commensal organism in the mouth)
- Preceding trauma from tooth extractions/jaw fracture (predisposing factors)
- Poor oral hygiene, and immunocompromised status (risk factors)

6.5.4   Clinical Features

- Men 30–60 years of age are predominantly affected
- Trismus and minimal pain
- Subcutaneous collection of pus
- Multiple abscesses and discharging sinuses
- Sulphur granules from the pus
- Jawbone involvement is uncommon
- Majority of reported cases are in the mandible
- Low-grade fever
- Regional lymphadenopathy is uncommon

6.5.5   Microscopic Features

- Rounded masses of filaments with peripheral radially arranged club shaped thickenings
- Neutrophils
- Chronic inflammatory cell infiltrate
- Fibrous connective tissue wall of the abscess

6.5.6   Differential Diagnosis

- Dentoalveolar abscess
- Osteomyelitis
- Malignancy
- Other chronic granulomatous lesion (tuberculosis or fungal infections such as coccidioidomycosis)

6.5.7   Diagnosis

- History
- Clinical findings
- Culture: microscopy of pus reveals colonies of actinomyces: Gram staining reveals Gram-positive long-branching filaments
- computed tomography
- nucleic acid probes and polymerase chain reaction methods have been developed for rapid and accurate identification of the bacteria

6.5.8   Management

- Antibiotics are the cornerstone of treatment
- To be treated with high doses of intravenous penicillin G over two to six weeks, followed by oral penicillin V

- If there is extensive necrotic tissue, or sinus tracts, fistulas, or if patients do not respond to medical treatment, surgical treatment may be necessary
- Two to six weeks of antibiotics with surgical drainage are adequate for most patients

6.5.9 Prognosis

- Good, if treated adequately

6.6 Cervicofacial Cellulitis (Cervicofacial Fascial Space Infection)

6.6.1 Definition

- Acute inflammation of the soft tissue spaces of the facial and cervical region due to spreading odontogenic infection

6.6.2 Frequency

- Common in less developed countries; uncommon in the developed regions

6.6.3 Aetiology/Risk Factors

- Anaerobic bacteria from odontogenic sources (mandibular molars in particular)

6.6.4 Clinical Features

- Severe pain
- Swelling (oedematous, red, and shiny) of the facial spaces with board-like firmness (Figure 6.5)
- Sublingual and submandibular spaces usually involved
- If swelling is bilateral and involves parapharyngeal space, the condition is called Ludwig's angina (life threatening)
- Fever

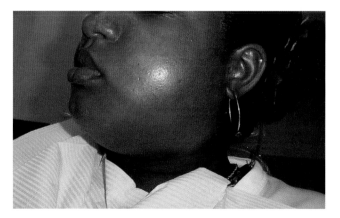

Figure 6.5 Cervicofacial cellulitis from odontogenic infection. Note diffuse inflammatory swelling of the face and submandibular region.

6.6.5 Diagnosis

- History
- Clinical findings
- Haematology

6.6.6 Management

- Immediate hospitalization
- Securing airway
- Obtaining sample for culture and sensitivity testing
- Aggressive empirical antibiotic treatment: specific antibiotic administration to be based on the sensitivity results
- Spreading odontogenic infection:
  - Empirical antibiotics in the form of amoxicillin 500 mg orally every eight hours for adults and metronidazole 400 mg orally every eight hours are recommended
  - For those with penicillin allergy, clindamycin should be considered
  - Severely ill patients need intravenous cefotaxime 1 g every 12 hours and intravenous metronidazole 500 mg every eight hours.
  - Drainage of the swelling to reduce the pressure

6.6.7 Prognosis

- If treated early and adequately, prognosis is good
- Complications include glottic oedema and spread of the infection into the mediastinum

6.7 Osteoradionecrosis of the Jaw

6.7.1 Definition/Description

- Osteoradionecrosis of the jaw is a complication of irradiated jawbone resulting in sequestrum formation

6.7.2 Frequency

- Uncommon due to improved radiation techniques

6.7.3 Aetiology/Risk Factors

- Radiation usually greater than 60 Gy to the head and neck region
- Radiation causes damage to the microvasculature (vascular endarteritis). This leads to hypoxia, which, in turn causes hypocellularity and necrosis in the jawbone

6.7.4 Clinical Features

- The mandible is usually affected
- Exposed necrotic bone with or without formation of external fistula (Figure 6.6a)

(a) (b)

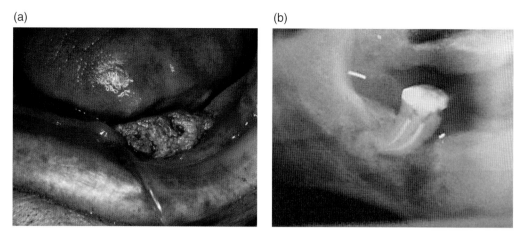

Figure 6.6 (a) Osteoradionecrosis of the mandible. (a) Note the exposed bone. (b) Radiographical appearance of an early case of osteoradionecrosis of the mandible in a patient who was treated with radiation for a tumour of the right cheek. Note the irregular areas of radiolucency and radiopacity of bone around the endodontically treated molar. (*source:* Cesar A. Migliorati. 2014. The cancer patient/oral complications of cancer therapy and management. In: *Diagnosis and Management of Oral Lesions and Conditions: A resource handbook for the clinician*, ed. Cesar A. Migliorati and Fotinos S. Panagakos. IntechOpen. doi: 10.5772/57597.

- Pain is common
- Pathological fracture is a possibility

6.7.5 Radiographical Features

- Irregular areas of mixed radiolucency and radiopacity (Figure 6.6b)
- Presence of sequestrum

6.7.6 Microscopic Features

- Presence of necrotic bone
- Lack or absence of inflammation
- Hypovascularity
- Absence of osteoclasts
- Aggregates of microorganisms

6.7.7 Differential Diagnosis

- Locally recurrent tumour
- Metastatic tumour
- Osteomyelitis
- Osteosarcoma
- Radiation-induced sarcoma
- Medication-related osteonecrosis

6.7.8 Diagnosis

- History of radiation
- Clinical findings
- Radiography
- Biopsy is not mandatory but can confirm non-vital bony sequestrum

6.7.9 Management

- Elimination of infection at least three weeks prior to treatment is required
- After biopsy, sequestrectomy of non-vital bone
- Hyperbaric oxygen therapy before and after sequestrectomy
- Resection of the jaw (if required) to be followed by reconstruction
- Preventive care

6.7.10 Prognosis

- Variable

6.8 Medication-Related Osteonecrosis of the Jaw

6.8.1 Definition/Description

- Medication-related osteonecrosis of the jaw is a rare adverse event of antiresorptive drugs such as bisphosphonates and denosumab used for osteoporosis or antiangiogenic therapy for cancer with no history of radiotherapy

6.8.2 Frequency

- Rare
- The reported prevalence is less than 1 case in 1000 in patients receiving oral bisphosphonate therapy or denosumab

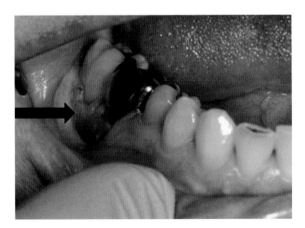

Figure 6.7 Medication-related osteonecrosis of the mandible (black arrow) in a patient who had been administered intravenous bisphosphonates (*source:* by kind permission of Dr Nagamani Narayana, UNMC Nebraska, USA).

6.8.3   Aetiology/Risk Factors

- Use of antiresorptive drugs in those exposed to trauma to the jaws, dental extractions, prolonged corticosteroids, smoking, anaemia, ill-fitting dentures, or poor oral hygiene
- More common in patients with cancer receiving antiresorptive drugs
- Note: intravenous bisphosphonates are used to treat breast and prostate cancer and hypercalcaemia. Oral bisphosphonates are used to treat osteoporosis, Paget's disease, and osteogenesis imperfecta

6.8.4   Clinical Features

- Presence of exposed bone in the maxillofacial region which does not heal within eight weeks after identification by a healthcare provider (Figure 6.7)
- No history of radiation therapy to the head and neck region
- Exposed bone but soft tissue inflammation in early cases can occur
- Pain, soft tissue swelling, infection, and external fistula in advanced cases
- Loose teeth
- Non-healing extraction socket
- Halitosis

6.8.5   Radiographical Features

- Thickening of the lamina dura
- Diffuse osteosclerosis
- Osteolysis, presence of bone sequestrum
- Disruption of medullary trabecular bone and alveoli with delayed remodelling

6.8.6   Microscopic Features

- Enlarged irregular osteoclasts containing intracytoplasmic vacuoles
- Trabeculae of sclerotic lamellar bone show loss of osteocytes
- Peripheral resorption of bone with bacterial colonization
- Variable amount of inflammation

6.8.7   Differential Diagnosis

- Locally recurrent tumour
- Metastatic tumour
- Osteomyelitis
- Osteosarcoma
- Radiation-induced sarcoma

6.8.8   Diagnosis

- History of taking antiresorptive drugs
- Trauma to the jaw (dental treatment, denture trauma, etc.)
- No history of radiation
- Clinical findings: exposed bone persisting for more than eight weeks

6.8.9 Management

- Antimicrobial mouth rinses
- Antibiotics and analgesics
- Resection of necrotic bone
- Hyperbaric oxygen therapy
- Prevention:
  - Invasive dental treatment to be carried out prior to commencing antiresorptive medication
  - Maintenance of good oral hygiene

Prognosis

- Fair to good

Recommended Reading

Ayekinam, K., Saliha, C., and Wafaa, E.W. (2017). Chronic suppurative osteomyelitis of mandible complicating molar extraction: a case report. *Journal of Medical and Surgical Research* 4 (2): 457–460.

Chronopoulos, A., Zarra, T., Ehrenfeld, M., and Otto, S. (2018). Osteoradionecrosis of the jaws: definition, epidemiology, staging and clinical and radiological findings: a concise review. *International Dental Journal* 68: 22–30.

Mehra, H., Gupta, S., Gupta, H. et al. (2013). Chronic suppurative osteomyelitis o*f mandible: a case report. Craniomaxillofacial Trauma & Reconstruction* 6 (3): 197–200.

Migliorati, C.A. (2014). The cancer patient/oral complications of cancer therapy and management. In: *Diagnosis and Management of Oral Lesions and Conditions: A resource handbook for the clinician* (eds. C.A. Migliorati and F.S. Panagakos). London: IntechOpen https://doi.org/10.5772/57597.

Montonen, M. and Lindqvist, C. (2013). Diagnosis and treatment of diffuse sclerosing osteomyelitis of the jaws. *Oral and Maxillofacial Surgery Clinics of North America* 15: 69–78.

Neville, B.W., Damm, D.D., Allen, C.M., and Chi, C.A. (2016). Physical and chemical injuries. In: *In: Oral and Maxillofacial Pathology*, 4ee, 111–136. St Louis, MO: Elsevier.

Odell, E.W. (2017). Infections of the jaws. In: *Cawson's Essentials of Oral Pthology and Oral Medicine*, vol. 9e, 117–128. Edinburgh: Elsevier.

Pazianas, M. (2011). Osteonecrosis of the jaw and the role of macrophages. *Journal of the National Cancer Institute* 103: 232–240.

Prabhu, S.R. (2019). Miscellaneous disorders. In: *Clinical Diagnosis in Oral Medicine: A case based approach*, 285–310. New Delhi: Jaypee Brothers Medical Publishers.

Ruggiero, S.L. (2013). Emerging concepts in the management and treatment of osteonecrosis of the jaw. *Oral and Maxillofacial Surgery Clinics of North America* 25: 11–20.

Suma, R., Vinay, C., Shashikanth, M.C., and Subba Reddy, V.V. (2007). Garre's sclerosing osteomyelitis. *Journal of the Indian Society of Pedodontics and Preventive Dentistry* 25 (Suppl S1): 30–33.

7

Cysts of the Jaw

7.1   Radicular, Lateral Radicular, and Residual Radicular Cysts

7.1.1   Definition/Description

- Cyst is defined as a fluid filled pathological cavity lined by epithelium
- Odontogenic jaw cyst refers to a pathological cavity derived from and lined by odontogenic epithelium
- Odontogenic cysts can be inflammatory or developmental
- Radicular cyst: a common odontogenic inflammatory cyst located at the apex of a non-vital tooth; also known as a periapical cyst
- Lateral radicular cyst: a radicular type of cyst located at the lateral surface of a non-vital tooth
- Residual radicular cyst: a radicular cyst that has persisted after extraction of the causative non-vital tooth

7.1.2   Frequency

- Radicular cyst is the most common type of jaw cyst. They comprise about 52–68% of all the cysts affecting the jawbone
- Lateral radicular cyst: less common than the radicular type
- Residual radicular cyst: less common than the radicular type

Handbook of Oral Pathology and Oral Medicine, First Edition. S. R. Prabhu.
© 2022 John Wiley & Sons Ltd. Published 2022 by John Wiley & Sons Ltd.
Companion website: www.wiley.com/go/prabhu/oral_pathology

7.1.3 Aetiology/Risk Factors

- Radicular cyst: Caused by proliferation of odontogenic epithelium in a periapical granuloma due to stimulation derived from chronic inflammation from non-vital pulp
- Lateral radicular cyst is caused by the proliferation of odontogenic epithelium in the periodontal tissues at the lateral aspect of a non-vital tooth. Stimulation for chronic inflammation is derived from the non-vital tooth
- Residual radicular cyst is caused by proliferation of odontogenic epithelium in a radicular cyst that has persisted after extraction due to inadequate curettage
- Cystic expansion in all three types of cysts occurs because of the effects of osmotic gradient within the epithelial lining layers and mediators of inflammation

7.1.4 Clinical/Radiographical Features

- Radicular cyst:
  - Common in the 20–60 years age group
  - More common in males (male to female ratio 3 : 2)
  - Common in permanent teeth; rare in deciduous teeth
  - Asymptomatic in most cases (unless inflammatory exacerbation occurs)
  - The maxilla is affected more than three times as frequently as the mandible
  - Slowly progressive hard swelling of the jaw
  - Large cyst may cause cortical expansion and reduction in bone thickness causing eggshell thickness (crackling under palpating fingers)
  - Occasionally part of the wall of the cyst may be soft and fluctuant on palpation and seen as a bluish swelling beneath the mucous membrane
  - Associated tooth is non-vital
  - Asymptomatic small cysts are often detected on routine radiography
  - Round radiolucency with sharp outline (Figure 7.1a)
  - Associated tooth may show large carious lesion or restoration
  - Adjacent tooth may be displaced if the cyst is large
- Lateral radicular cyst:
  - Common in middle age
  - Usually asymptomatic
  - Associated tooth is non-vital
  - Often detected on radiography as an oval radiolucency along the lateral aspect of the root (often mistaken for periodontal cyst; Figure 7.1b)
  - Loss of lamina dura
- Residual radicular cyst:
  - Usually in older individuals
  - Asymptomatic in most cases
  - Radiographical features: seen as round to oval radiolucency in the alveolar ridge at the site of previous tooth extraction (Figure 7.1c)
  - Occasionally central radio-opaque deposits may be seen in the radiographs

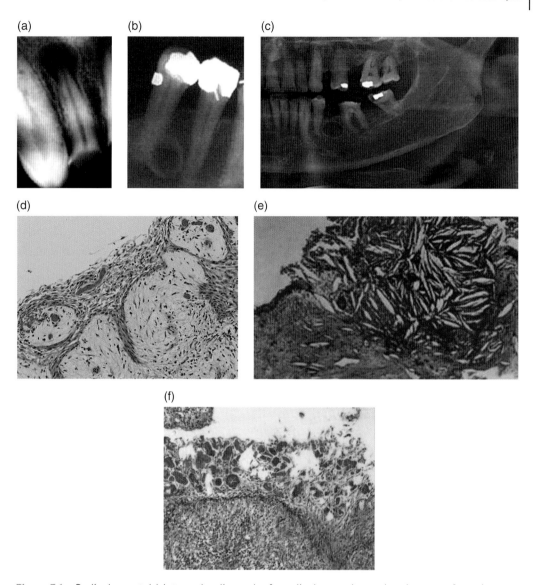

Figure 7.1   Radicular cyst. (a) Intraoral radiograph of a radicular cyst located at the apex of a carious non-vital maxillary lateral incisor. Note well-defined radiolucency with sharp outline. (b) Lateral radicular cyst arising from a non-vital mandibular second premolar. (c) Residual radicular cyst; cropped orthopantogram shows a well-defined oval-shaped residual radicular cyst located in the edentulous region of the mandible (*source:* by kind permission of Dr Amar Sholapurkar JCU School of Dentistry, Cairns, Australia). (d) Photomicrograph showing proliferating non-keratinizing epithelial cyst lining and chronic inflammatory cell infiltrate. (e) Photomicrograph showing numerous spindle shaped cholesterol cleft in the cyst lining and the fibrous wall. (f) Rushton bodies (hyaline bodies) seen as acellular, eosinophilic structures within the squamous lining (*source:* by kind permission of Dr Pereira, D Y Patil University, Mumbai, India).

7.1.5 Microscopic Features

- All three types:
  - Non-keratinizing stratified squamous cell epithelial lining (Figure 7.1d)
  - Neutrophils in the lumen
  - Cholesterol clefts in the cyst lining and cholesterol crystals in the cyst fluid (Figure 7.1e)
  - Hyaline or Rushton bodies in the epithelium (Figure 7.1f)
  - Fibrous wall with collagenous connective tissue with chronic inflammatory cell infiltrate

7.1.6 Differential Diagnosis

- Periapical granuloma
- Central giant cell granuloma
- Odontogenic tumours
- Lateral periodontal cyst
- Solitary bone cyst

7.1.7 Diagnosis

- History
- Clinical findings
- Radiography
- Microscopy

7.1.8 Management

- For radicular and lateral radicular cysts:
  - Root canal therapy
  - Periapical surgery
  - Tooth extraction and curettage
- Enucleation and curettage for residual radicular cyst

7.1.9 Prognosis

- Good
- No recurrences if treated adequately

7.2 Dentigerous Cyst

7.2.1 Definition/Description

- An odontogenic developmental cyst that surrounds the crown of an unerupted tooth, with the epithelial lining attached around the cemento-enamel junction
- Also known as a follicular cyst because of its origin from the dental follicle

7.2.2 Frequency

- Common; 20% of all epithelial lined jaw cysts

7.2.3 Aetiology/Risk Factors

- Expansion of the dental follicle caused by the separation of the reduced enamel epithelium from the enamel and accumulation of fluid between the crown and the reduced enamel epithelium

7.2.4 Clinical Features

- More common in males (male to female ratio 2 : 1)
- Common between 10 and 30 years of age
- More common in the mandibular third molars, followed by maxillary canines and mandibular premolars
- Asymptomatic in the early stages
- Often detected as chance finding on radiography
- Jaw expansion causes facial asymmetry and becomes symptomatic in later stages

7.2.5 Radiographical Findings

- Unilocular round radiolucency containing the crown of an unerupted tooth (Figure 7.2a)
- Radiolucent cavity shows corticated outline
- Large cyst may occasionally show multilocular appearance (pseudoloculation)
- The affected tooth may be displaced
- Enclosed tooth may show signs of resorption in some cases

7.2.6 Microscopic Features

- Thin cuboidal, non-keratinizing epithelial cyst lining (Figure 7.2b)
- Lack of epithelial rete ridges
- Loose collagen bundles with scattered epithelial islands
- Variable amount of chronic inflammatory cells and proliferating rete ridges appear if cyst is secondarily infected

(a) (b)

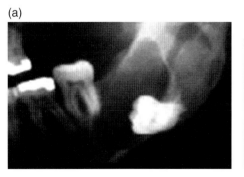 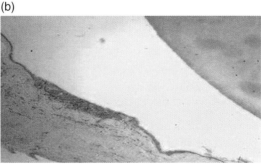

Figure 7.2 Dentigerous cyst. (a) Cropped orthopantogram showing a dentigerous cyst with the crown of an impacted third molar enclosed in the cyst cavity (*source:* by kind permission of Professor Charles Dunlap, Kansas City, USA). (b) Photomicrograph of dentigerous cyst showing an epithelial cyst lining and a fibrous connective tissue wall devoid of inflammation. The top right hand corner of the image shows dentine. Decalcification process has removed enamel leaving a clear space in between dentine and the cyst.

7.2.7 Differential Diagnosis

- Unilocular ameloblastoma
- Odontogenic keratocyst
- Adenomatoid odontogenic tumour
- Calcifying odontogenic cyst

7.2.8 Diagnosis

- History
- Clinical findings
- Radiography
- Microscopy

7.2.9 Management

- Enucleation of the cyst and extraction of the impacted tooth
- Marsupialization if the cyst is large

7.2.10 Prognosis

- Good
- Note that large lesions may cause pathological fractures
- Dentigerous cyst lining may transform into ameloblastoma or rarely into intraosseous squamous cell carcinoma

7.3 Eruption Cyst

7.3.1 Definition

- An odontogenic developmental cyst surrounding the crown of a permanent or deciduous tooth during and close to eruption
- It is clinically seen as a soft swelling on the alveolus
- This is a soft tissue analogue of dentigerous cyst

7.3.2 Frequency

- Eruption cyst: less common compared with dentigerous cyst

7.3.3 Aetiology/Risk Factors

- Separation of dental follicle from the reduced enamel epithelium and accumulation of fluid between the enamel and floor of the cyst

7.3.4 Clinical Features

- Common in children younger than 10 years of age
- Mandibular central incisors followed by the first permanent molars and deciduous maxillary incisors are commonly involved

Figure 7.3 Eruption cyst associated with tooth 11. Bluish surface of the swelling is due to eruption haematoma (*source:* by kind permission of Nagaveni N B, College of Dental Sciences, Davangere, Karnataka, India).

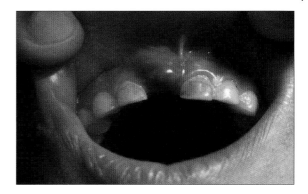

- Seen as a soft, rounded swelling on the alveolus with blue or purple colour (eruption haematoma; Figure 7.3)
- Most burst spontaneously

7.3.5 Microscopic Features

- Surface oral epithelium on the superior aspect of the cyst
- Underlying lamina propria shows inflammatory cell infiltrate
- Deeper layer (roof of the cyst) shows thin layer of non-keratinizing squamous epithelium

7.3.6 Differential Diagnosis

- Haemangioma
- Gingival cyst

7.3.7 Diagnosis

- History
- Clinical findings
- Radiographical identification of an erupting tooth
- Microscopy

7.3.8 Management

- Usually not required
- Large lesions may require incision of the roof of the cyst

7.3.9 Prognosis

- Excellent

7.4 Odontogenic Keratocyst (Keratocystic Odontogenic Tumour)

7.4.1 Definition

- Also known as keratocystic odontogenic tumour, the odontogenic keratocyst is a benign aggressive developmental cyst arising from cell rests of dental lamina

7.4.2 Frequency

- 5–15% of odontogenic jaw cysts

7.4.3 Aetiology/Risk Factors

- Mutation, deletion, or inactivation of the tumour suppressor gene (called patched gene [*PTCH*] on chromosome 9q)

7.4.4 Clinical Features

- Peak incidence is 20–30 years of age (60% of cases)
- Slight male predilection
- Posterior mandible is the site of predilection; 50% in the lower ramus
- Symptomless in early stages
- Slow growth mostly in the anteroposterior direction
- Pain, swelling in larger lesions
- Multiple odontogenic keratocysts can occur in patients with nevoid basal cell carcinoma syndrome (Gorlin's syndrome)
- Rarely occurs in extraosseous location, only in the gingival tissues

7.4.5 Radiographical Features

- Well-defined radiolucent area with corticated or scalloped margins (Figure 7.4a)
- Often multilocular radiolucency
- Cortical expansion is minimal, growth in anteroposterior direction
- In 25–40% of cases an unerupted tooth is enclosed in the cavity
- Association with the tooth may be apical, lateral, or periodontal in location
- Resorption of roots or displacement of adjacent teeth uncommon and minimal
- Occasionally third molar maybe absent (formerly called primordial cyst)

7.4.6 Microscopic Features

- Epithelium of uniform thickness (Figure 7.4b)
- Flat basal cell layer with reversed polarity
- Corrugated parakeratinized surface layer
- Lack of attachment of the epithelial layer to the fibrous connective tissue wall
- Satellite cysts in the fibrous wall (Figure 7.4c)
- Absence of inflammatory cells

7.4.7 Other Features

- Cyst content includes viscoid keratin
- Electrophoresis reveals low protein content, which is mostly albumin
- Total protein is found to be below 4 g/100 ml

7.4.8 Differential Diagnosis

- Dentigerous cyst
- Ameloblastoma

(a)

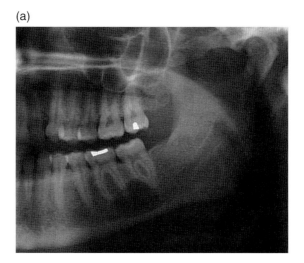

(b)   (c)

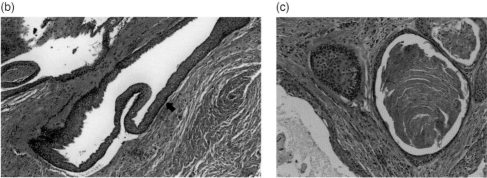

Figure 7.4   Odontogenic keratocyst. (a) Cropped Panoramic radiograph demonstrating an isolated radiolucent lesion in the posterior left mandible. (b) Stratified squamous epithelial lining shows uniform thickness and with a hyperchromatic, palisaded basal layer (black arrow). (*Source:* (a,b) by kind permission of Associate Professor Kelly Magliocca, Department of Pathology and Laboratory Medicine, Winship Cancer Institute at Emory University, Atlanta, GA, USA). (c) Satellite cysts in the fibrous connective tissue wall.

- Myxoma
- Radicular cyst
- Lateral periodontal cyst

7.4.9   Diagnosis

- History
- Clinical findings
- Radiography
- Microscopy (confirmatory)

7.4.10   Management

- Enucleation and curettage
- Peripheral osteotomy of the cavity or chemical cauterization with Carnoy's solution after the tumour removal (Carnoy's solution is a fixative composed of 60% ethanol, 30% chloroform, 10% glacial acetic acid, and 1 g of ferric chloride)

- Recurrence (range 5–62%). Greatest in those with Gorlin's syndrome
- Follow up

7.4.11 Prognosis

- Good, if adequately treated

7.5 Lateral Periodontal Cyst

7.5.1 Definition/Description

- A unilocular odontogenic developmental cyst that arises from the dental lamina situated in the periodontal ligament beside the mid-portion of the lateral aspect of the root of a vital tooth
- Botryoid odontogenic cyst is a rare multilocular variant of lateral periodontal cyst

7.5.2 Frequency

- Uncommon
- Less than 2% of all epithelium-lined jaw cysts

7.5.3 Origin/Aetiology/Risk Factors

- Proliferation of cell rests of Malassez, stimulus unknown

7.5.4 Clinical Features

- Middle-aged to elderly individuals commonly affected
- Asymptomatic
- Often detected during routine radiographical examination
- Usually seen in the mandibular canine/premolar region (65%)
- Displaces the adjacent teeth

7.5.5 Radiographical Features

- Well-circumscribed radiolucent area lateral to the root (of a vital tooth; Figure 7.5a)
- May show corticated outline
- Polycystic appearance in botryoid odontogenic cyst
- Rarely multilocular (botryoid odontogenic cyst)

7.5.6 Microscopic Features

- Thin (one to three cell layers thick) cuboidal non-keratinized squamous cell epithelium (Figure 7.5b)
- Foci of glycogen-rich clear cells in the epithelial lining
- Occasional nodular thickenings in the lining
- Lack of inflammatory cell infiltrate

(a) (b)

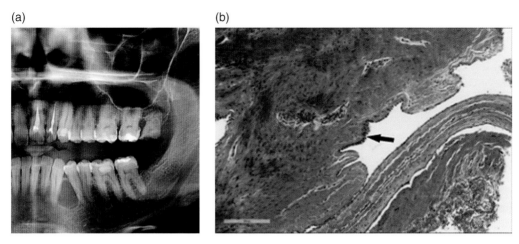

Figure 7.5 (a) Lateral periodontal cyst. Cropped orthopantogram showing well-circumscribed radiolucency with a sclerotic border in between roots of vital teeth 33 and 34. Note displacement of the roots. (b) Photomicrograph shows cystic lesion composed of reduced enamel epithelium-like lining comprising single or double layer(s) of flattened squamous or cuboidal cells and subtly thickened areas with more closely packed cells (arrow). (*Source:* by kind permission of Dr Sundar Ramalingam, King Saud University College of Dentistry, Riyadh, Saudi Arabia).

7.5.7 Differential Diagnosis

- Lateral radicular cyst
- Odontogenic keratocyst
- Ameloblastoma
- Glandular odontogenic cyst

7.5.8 Diagnosis

- Radiography
- Microscopy
- Enucleation

7.5.9 Prognosis

- Good.
- Recurrence unusual
- Increased rate of recurrence for botryoid odontogenic cyst
- Long-term follow-up recommended

7.6 Calcifying Odontogenic Cyst

7.6.1 Definition/Description

- Also known as cystic odontogenic tumour, gorlin cyst, and dentinogenic ghost cell tumour
- A benign cystic neoplasm of odontogenic origin, characterized by an ameloblastoma-like epithelium with ghost cells that may calcify

7.6.2 Frequency

- Rare; 6% of central odontogenic tumours

7.6.3 Origin/Aetiology/Risk Factors

- Odontogenic epithelial remnants trapped within the bones of the maxilla, mandible, or gingival tissues

7.6.4 Clinical Features

- Approximately 65–67.5% of cases occur in the anterior jaws
- No sex predilection
- Peak incidence: second decade of life
- Can occur as an intraosseous or extraosseous lesion
- Extraosseous lesion: gingival tissues: approximately 17% of cases
- 86–98% of cases demonstrate a cystic architecture while the solid (neoplastic) form comprises 2–16% of cases
- Most are asymptomatic; incidentally detected

7.6.5 Radiographical Features

- Well-delineated unilocular or multilocular radiolucency with calcifications (in one-third to one-half of cases)
- Root resorption and divergence common
- Impacted tooth occurs in approximately one-third of cases (Figure 7.6a)
- May be associated with odontomes

7.6.6 Microscopic Features

- Cyst lining composed of an outer layer of a columnar basaloid odontogenic epithelium
- Inner layer resembles stellate reticulum of the enamel organ.
- The presence of 'ghost cells' (loss of nuclei with basic cell outline intact and eosinophilic cytoplasm) and/or calcifications within the cyst lining or fibrous capsule are characteristic (Figure 7.6b)
- Ghost cell development may be due to coagulative necrosis, accumulation of enamel protein, aberrant keratinization of odontogenic epithelium
- Dentin/dentinoid may be laid down next to basal cells (Figure 7.6c)

7.6.7 Differential Diagnosis

- In earlier stages of intraosseous calcifying odontogenic cyst:
    - Dentigerous cyst
    - Odontogenic keratocyst
    - Unicystic ameloblastoma
- In later stages:
    - Adenomatoid odontogenic tumour
    - Partially mineralized odontoma

(a)

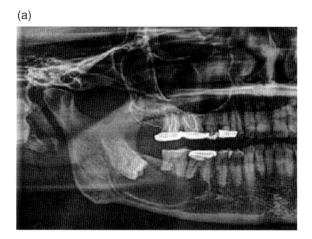

(b)   (c)

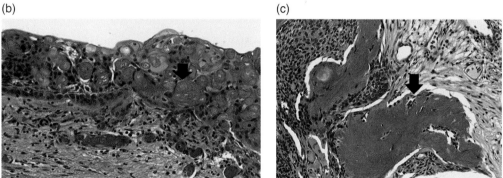

Figure 7.6 Calcifying odontogenic cyst. (a) Cropped orthopantogram showing a well-corticated unilocular radiolucent lesion containing crown of a molar tooth. Resorption of roots of adjacent molars is also evident. (b) Photomicrograph shows numerous ghost cells (black arrow) within the odontogenic epithelium lining. (c) Photomicrograph showing dentinoid (black arrow) and odontogenic epithelium present within the fibrous connective tissue cyst wall. (*Source:* images (b, c) by kind permission of Associate Professor Kelly Magliocca, Department of Pathology and Laboratory Medicine, Winship Cancer Institute at Emory University, Atlanta, GA, USA).

- – Calcifying epithelial odontogenic tumour
- – Ameloblastic fibro-odontoma
- The extraosseous calcifying odontogenic cyst:
  - – Gingival fibroma
  - – Gingival cyst
  - – Peripheral giant cell granuloma

7.6.8 Diagnosis

- History
- Clinical findings
- Radiography
- Microscopy (confirmatory)

7.6.9 Management

- Enucleation and curettage

7.6.10 Prognosis

- Prognosis excellent, few recurrences documented (less than 5%)
- Rarely malignant transformation reported

7.7 Orthokeratinized Odontogenic Cyst: Key Features

- A rare keratinizing odontogenic cyst with orthokeratinized epithelial lining
- Male predominance
- Frequent in mandible
- May be associated with unerupted third molars
- Usually seen radiographically as a unilocular radiolucent lesion, rarely multilocular
- Keratinizing odontogenic cyst with orthokeratinized epithelial lining with no palisading in the basal cells
- Treated with enucleation
- Recurrence is rare

7.8 Glandular Odontogenic Cyst: Key Features

- A rare odontogenic cyst with a histological appearance of small glands lined by mucous cells that secrete mucin located in the epithelial cyst lining
- Affects middle-aged adults
- The mandible is commonly affected
- Displaces the adjacent teeth
- Radiographically cyst is unilocular or multilocular
- Enucleation and curettage treatment of choice
- Recurrence common

7.9 Nasopalatine Duct Cyst (Incisive Canal Cyst)

7.9.1 Definition/Description

- Nasopalatine duct cyst is a common non-odontogenic cyst in the jaw located in the incisive canal

7.9.2 Frequency

- Common
- 5% of all jaw cysts

7.9.3 Aetiology/Risk Factors

- Arises from embryonic epithelial remnants of the nasopalatine duct
- Rarely, may develop within incisive papilla (cyst of incisive papilla, or cyst of palatine papilla)
- Irritation, trauma, or infection may trigger its development

7.9.4 Clinical Features

- Wide age range, most cases in the fourth through sixth decades of life
- Slight male predilection
- Asymptomatic, with the small lesion being detected on routine radiographs
- Superficial lesions may burst producing 'salty' discharge in the mouth
- Large lesion: swelling and pain (Figure 7.7a)
- Nearby teeth vital

(a)

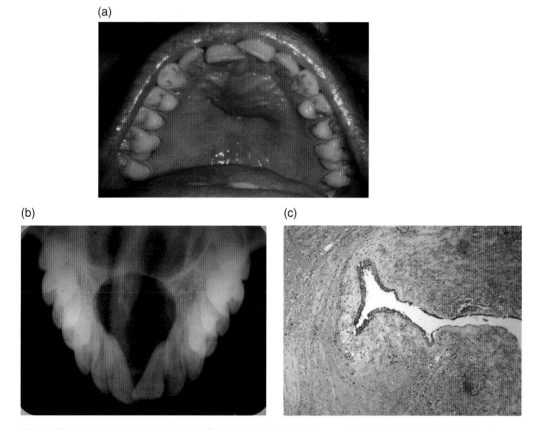

(b)   (c)

Figure 7.7 Nasopalatine duct cyst. (a) Clinical photograph shows a palatal swelling with evidence of displaced right central incisor. (b). Maxillary occlusal radiograph shows a round radiolucent lesion in the midline of the anterior palate with displaced roots of the central incisors and deviation of the nasal septum to the right side (c) Photomicrograph shows stratified squamous epithelium lining the cyst wall. (*Source:* Pratik Dedhia, Shely Dedhia, Amol Dhokar, and Ankit Desai. Nasopalatine duct cyst. *Case Reports in Dentistry* 2013: 869516. doi: 10.1155/2013/869516; reproduced under CC BY 3.0.)

7.9.5 Radiographical Features

- A rounded/heart-shaped radiolucent lesion at the site of the incisive canal apical to the roots of maxillary incisors (Figure 7.7b)
- Corticated outline seen

7.9.6 Microscopic Features

- Cyst lining: lined with stratified squamous epithelium alone (Figure 7.7c) or together with pseudostratified columnar epithelium (variable cilia and goblet cells), simple columnar epithelium or simple cuboidal epithelium
- Cyst wall: fibrous tissue with neurovascular bundles
- If infected, inflammatory cell infiltrate present

7.9.7 Differential Diagnosis

- Radicular cyst
- Ameloblastoma
- Central giant cell granuloma
- Odontogenic keratocyst

7.9.8 Diagnosis

- History
- Clinical findings
- Radiography
- Microscopy

7.9.9 Management

- Enucleation

7.9.10 Prognosis

- Excellent
- Does not recur

7.10 Pseudocysts of the Jaw: Solitary Bone Cyst, Aneurysmal Bone Cyst and Stafne's bone Cyst

- Pseudocysts are radiolucent cystic cavities with no epithelial lining

7.10.1 Definition/Description

- Solitary bone cyst is a single bone cavity filled with fluid or empty. Also known as haemorrhagic bone cyst, simple bone cyst and traumatic bone cyst

- Aneurysmal bone cyst is of two types: primary and secondary. The primary type is an example of benign neoplasm, whereas secondary type is an example of non-neoplastic lesion
- Stafne's bone cyst is a depression located on the lingual side of the mandible usually considered as a normal anatomical variation

7.10.2 Frequency

- All three are uncommon/rare

7.10.3 Aetiology

- Solitary bone cyst: aetiology inknown; bone injury followed by defective repair may be involved
- Aneurysmal cyst:
  - Primary: neoplastic proliferation of vascular tissue
  - Secondary: developmental malformation of vascular tissue
- Stafne's bone cyst (static bone cyst): possibly as the result of entrapment of embryonic salivary gland tissue within the bone

7.10.4 Clinical Features

- Solitary bone cyst:
  - Asymptomatic
  - Mostly occurs in teenagers
  - No sex predilection
  - Femur and humerus commonly involved
  - Mandibular alveolus and mandibular body are common sites in the jaws
  - Often detected on routine radiographs
  - Rarely cause bone expansion
  - Empty or fluid filled
  - Radiolucent lesion often extending between roots on radiography (Figure 7.8a)
- Aneurysmal bone cyst:
  - Both types expand the bone
  - Primary aneurysmal cyst is a benign neoplastic lesion
  - Long bones frequently affected
  - 1–2% occur in the jaws
  - Mandibular ramus and angle are preferred sites
  - Most patients are 10–20 years of age
  - Rapid painless growth
  - Adjacent teeth are displaced and vital
  - Multilocular radiolucency (soap-bubble appearance) or divided into multiple septa on radiography (Figure 7.8b)
- Stafne's bone cyst:
  - Asymptomatic
  - Usually discovered by chance during routine dental radiography
  - On radiography, shows a well-demarcated radiolucent defect located between the inferior dental canal and the inferior border of the posterior mandible between the molars and the angle of the jaw (Figure 7.8c)

(a)   (b)   (c)

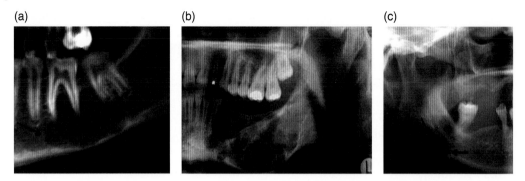

Figure 7.8 (a) Solitary bone cyst (simple bone cyst, black arrows). Note characteristic scalloped margins extending between the roots of the molars. (b) Aneurysmal bone cyst. Cropped orthopantogram showing multilocular radiolucency in the left mandible. (c) Stafne's bone cyst. Cropped orthopantogram of an asymptomatic individual showing well-circumscribed round/oval radiolucency near the angle of the mandible below the inferior dental canal (black arrows). (*Source:* From Werner Shintaku. 2014. Bony lesions. In: *Diagnosis and Management of Oral Lesions and Conditions: A resource handbook for the clinician* (ed. Cesar A. Migliorati and, Fotinos S. Panagakos), IntechOpen. doi: 10.5772/57597. Reproduced under CC BY 3.0).

    – Usually unilateral; rarely bilateral

7.10.5 Microscopic Features

- Solitary bone cyst:
  - Non-epithelialized (pseudocyst) cavity
  - Lined by fibrous tissue and bone
  - Lack of contents
- Aneurysmal bone cyst:
  - Highly cellular mass of blood-filled spaces with no endothelial lining
  - Occasional presence of giant cells
  - Spaces separated by fibrous septa
- Stafne's bone cyst:
  - Normal salivary gland tissue
  - Sometimes empty or presence of connective tissue, fat lymphoid tissue or blood vessels

7.10.6 Differential Diagnosis

- Solitary cyst:
  - Osteoporotic bone marrow defect
- Aneurysmal bone cyst: multilocular lesions such as:
  - Ameloblastoma
  - Odontogenic myxoma
  - Giant cell lesions
- Stafne's bone cyst
  - Unilocular ameloblastoma
  - Osteoporotic bone marrow defect
  - Intraosseous carcinoma

- Salivary gland tumours
- Lymph node

7.10.7 Diagnosis

- History
- Clinical findings
- Radiographic findings
- Microscopy (biopsy not required for Stafne's bone cyst)

7.10.8 Management

- Surgical curettage for solitary and aneurysmal cysts
- No recurrence in solitary cyst but aneurysmal cyst may recur
- Stafne's cyst does not require any treatment

7.10.9 Prognosis

- Good

7.11 Nasolabial Cyst: Key Features

- Develops outside the bone in the soft tissues deep to the nasolabial fold
- Uncommon
- Originates from the lower end of the nasolacrimal duct
- Middle-aged women commonly affected
- Painless swelling under the upper lip
- Nostril distorted
- No radiographical changes; occasionally pressure resorption of the underlying bone may be seen
- Pseudostratified epithelium lining is present
- Enucleation
- No recurrence

Recommended Reading

Dedhia, P., Dedhia, D., Dhokar, A., and Desai, A. (2013). Nasopalatine duct cyst. *Case Reports in Dentistry* 2013: 869516.

Manor, E., Kachko, L., Puterman, M.B. et al. (2012). Cystic lesions of the jaws: a clinicopathological study of 322 cases and review of the literature. *International Journal of Medical Sciences* 9 (1): 20–26.

Nagaveni, N.B., Umashankar, K.V., Radhika, N.B., and Maj Satisha, T.S. (2011). Eruption cyst: a literature review and four case reports. *Indian Journal of Dental Research* 22: 148–151.

Neville, B.W., Damm, D.D., Allen, C.M., and Chi, C.A. (2016). Odontogenic cysts and tumours. In: *In: Oral and Maxillofacial Pathology*, 4ee, 632–651. St Louis, MO: Elsevier.

Neville, B.W., Damm, D.D., Allen, C.M., and Chi, C.A. (2016). *Pulpal and periapical disease. In. Oral and Maxillofacial Pathology*, 4ee, 111–136. St Louis, MO: Elsevier.

Odell, E.W. (2017). Cysts in and around the jaws. In: *Cawson's Essentials of Oral Pathology and Oral Medicine*, vol. 9e, 139–162. Edinburgh: Elsevier.

Ramalingam, S., Alrayyes, Y.F., Almutairi, K.B., and Bello, I.A. (2019). Lateral periodontal cyst treated with Enucleation and guided bone regeneration: a report of a case and a review of pertinent literature. *Case Reports in Dentistry* 2019: 4591019.

Robinson, R. (2017). Diagnosing the most common odontogenic cystic and osseous lesions of the jaws for the practicing pathologist. *Modern Pathology* 30: S96–S103.

8

Odontogenic Tumours

CHAPTER MENU

8.1 World Health Organization Classification of Odontogenic Tumours (2017)

- Benign odontogenic tumours:
  - Epithelial origin:
  - Ameloblastoma:
    ○ Conventional type (solid/multicystic)
      ❑ Unicystic type
      ❑ Extraosseous, peripheral type
    ○ Squamous odontogenic tumour
    ○ Calcifying epithelial odontogenic tumour
    ○ Adenomatoid odontogenic tumour

- Mixed (epithelial and mesenchymal) origin
  - ○ Ameloblastic fibroma
  - ○ Primordial odontogenic tumour
  - ○ Odontoma
    - ❏ Complex type
    - ❏ Compound type
  - Dentinogenic ghost cell tumour
- Mesenchymal origin
  - Odontogenic fibroma
  - Odontogenic myxoma/myxofibroma
  - Cementoblastoma
  - Cemento-ossifying fibroma

- Malignant odontogenic tumours:
  - Ameloblastic carcinoma
  - Primary intraosseous carcinoma
  - Sclerosing odontogenic carcinoma
  - Clear cell odontogenic carcinoma
  - Ghost cell odontogenic carcinoma
  - Odontogenic carcinosarcoma
  - Odontogenic sarcoma

8.2 Ameloblastoma

8.2.1 Definition/Description

- A locally invasive slow-growing benign tumour derived from the odontogenic epithelium with solid, multicystic, or unicystic radiographical presentation
- Types: ameloblastomas present in four forms:
  - Conventional (solid/multicystic)
  - Unicystic (see section 8.3)
  - Peripheral (within gingival tissue)
  - Desmoplastic

- Origin: Odontogenic epithelium
  - Dental lamina
  - Developing enamel organ
  - Epithelial lining of dentigerous cyst

8.2.2 Frequency

- 1% of all oral tumours
- 9–11% of odontogenic tumours

8.2.3 Aetiology/Risk Factors

- Unknown
- V 600E mutation in the *BRAF* gene is detected in many cases
- Aetiological association of the gene has not been established

8.2.4 Clinical Features

- Conventional type:
  - Usually presents between 30 and 50 years
  - Mean age: 44 years
  - No sex predilection seen
  - 75–80% in the mandible mainly the third molar region
  - 15–20% in the posterior maxilla
  - Asymptomatic in early stages
  - Slow growing, locally invasive
  - Lingual and buccal cortical expansion
  - Large tumours may infiltrate medullary spaces
  - Crepitation or eggshell crackling on palpation in large tumours
  - Paraesthesia or pain are rare
  - Extraosseous or peripheral variant arises in gingival tissues of older adults (fifth to seventh decades)

8.2.5 Radiographical Features

- Small tumours are often detected on routine x-rays
- 'Soap-bubble' or 'honeycomb' multilocular appearance in most cases
- Occasionally 'spider-like', multilocular appearance
- Associated with unerupted tooth (commonly a mandibular third molar) in the radiolucent defect (Figure 8.1a)
- Unilocular radiolucency in minority of cases (Figure 8.1b)
- Margins of radiolucent defect show irregular scalloping
- Thinning and expansion of buccal and lingual cortical plates in large tumours
- Displaced and resorbed roots of adjacent teeth are common

8.2.6 Microscopic Features

- Follicular, plexiform types:
  - In follicular and ameloblastoma, islands of odontogenic epithelium are surrounded by mature fibrous connective tissue (Figure 8.1c)
  - In plexiform ameloblastoma, strands of odontogenic epithelium surrounds mature fibrous connective tissue (Figure 8.1d)
    - In both types, odontogenic epithelium resembles enamel organ epithelium (stellate reticulum -like cells surrounded by tall columnar ameloblast-like cells)
    - Ameloblast-like cells in both types show nuclei at the opposite pole to the basement membrane. This phenomena is called reverse polarity
    - Microcysts/cysts are common in the epithelial islands of the follicular type and in the stromal cells of the plexiform type
- Less common types include granular cell (Figure 8.1e), acanthomatous (Figure 8.1f) and basaloid types (Figure 8.1g). These types have no clinical relevance
- Desmoplastic type is characterized by sparse epithelial islands and predominance of dense collagenous (desmoplastic) tissue (Figure 8.1h)
- Ameloblastomas are keratin positive. The tumour cells express CK5 and CK14
- The stellate reticulum cells co-express CK8, CK18, and CK19

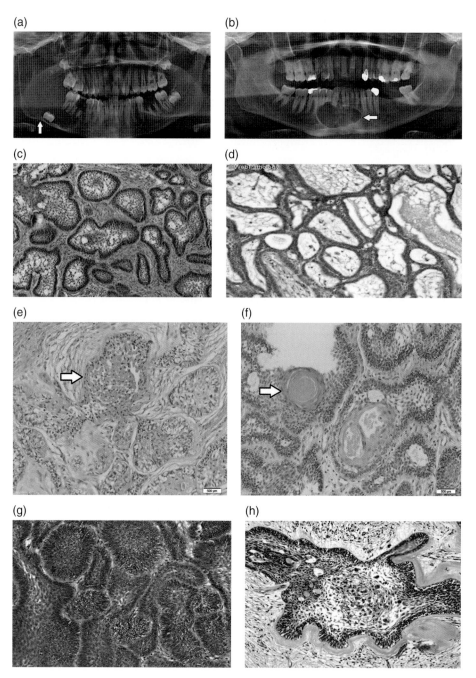

Figure 8.1 Ameloblastoma. (a) Pantomogram showing multilocular appearance of an ameloblastoma in the right mandible associated with an unerupted third molar (white arrow). (b) Pantomogram showing unilocular ameloblastoma in the anterior mandible with signs of root resorption (white arrow). (c) Follicular pattern: this pattern consists of round, oval, or irregular islands of epithelium. The nests and islands show peripheral palisading of columnar cells with reverse polarity. (d) Plexiform pattern. This pattern consists of interconnected thin lamina like strands or cords of basaloid cells, often without peripheral palisading and reverse nuclear polarity. The surrounding stroma is composed of loose connective tissue. Cyst formation is uncommon in plexiform type. (e) Granular pattern of follicular ameloblastoma. This pattern shows clusters of epithelial cells (arrow) with abundant granular eosinophilic cytoplasm due to lysosomal accumulation. (f) Acanthomatous pattern of follicular ameloblastoma -like cells showing extensive squamous metaplasia with keratin formation (arrow) within the stellate reticulum in the central portion of the epithelial islands. Such cases must be differentiated from squamous odontogenic tumour as well as squamous cell carcinoma. (g) The basaloid type consists of islands of uniform basaloid cells. (h) Desmoplastic variant shows cords or strands of odontogenic epithelium in a densely collagenized (desmoplastic) stroma. (*Source:* (a,b,e,f) by kind permission of Fadi Titinchi, University of the Western Cape, Cape Town, South Africa; (c,d,g,h) by kind permission of Dr Dharam Ramani, Webpathology, Richmond, Virginia, USA.)

8.2.7 Diagnosis

- History
- Clinical examination
- Radiography
- Biopsy and histology is mandatory
- Ameloblastomas are keratin positive; the ameloblast-like tumour cells express CK5 and CK14
- The stellate reticulum -like cells co-express CK8, CK18, and CK19
- Desmoplastic type is characterized by sparse epithelial islands and predominance of dense collagenous (desmoplastic) tissue

8.2.8 Differential Diagnosis

- Odontogenic keratocyst
- Odontogenic myxoma
- Calcifying epithelial odontogenic tumour
- Central giant cell granuloma
- Dentigerous cyst (if unerupted tooth is present in the radiolucent defect)
- Ossifying fibroma
- Intraosseous haemangioma
- Aneurysmal bone cyst
- Giant cell granuloma

8.2.9 Management

- Surgical excision (including approximately 10 mm of normal bone surrounding the tumour)
- Partial resection of the jaw for large tumours
- Regular radiographical follow-up

8.2.10 Prognosis

- Generally good
- Recurrence if not completely removed

8.3 Unicystic Ameloblastoma

8.3.1 Definition/Description

- An uncommon variant of ameloblastoma
- Predilection for younger individuals
- Shows a typically unilocular appearance on radiography
- Origin:
  - Odontogenic epithelium as for conventional ameloblastoma:
    - Developing enamel organ (reduced enamel epithelium)
    - Epithelial lining of dentigerous cyst

- Types: Unicystic ameloblastoma presents in three histological forms:
  o Luminal type (tumour epithelium limited to a single layer lining the lumen)
  o Intraluminal (plexiform) type (papillary projections of ameloblastoma into the lumen)
  o Mural type (showing tumour invading the connective tissue)

8.3.2 Frequency

- Account for 10–15% of all intraosseous ameloblastomas

8.3.3 Aetiology/Risk Factors

- Unknown
- Likely to be similar to that of conventional ameloblastoma (i.e. V 600E mutation in the *BRAF* gene; aetiological association has not been established

8.3.4 Clinical Signs and Symptoms

- Usually presents in the second or third decade (two decades earlier than conventional types)
- Male sex predilection seen
- 80–90% in the mandible mainly the third molar region
- Asymptomatic in early stages
- Slow growing
- Less aggressive than conventional ameloblastomas
- Often clinically unerupted molar detected

8.3.5 Radiographical Features

- Small tumours detected on routine radiography
- Unilocular radiographical appearance in most cases
- Associated with unerupted tooth (commonly a mandibular third molar) in the radiolucent defect (Figure 8.2a)
- Displaced and resorbed roots of adjacent teeth in large tumours

8.3.6 Microscopic Features

- Luminal type: ameloblastic epithelium lining seen with polarized basal cells; overlying cells resemble stellate reticulum like cells (Figure 8.2b)
- Intraluminal type: intraluminal plexiform ameloblastic cells projecting into the cystic lumen (Figure 8.2c)
- Mural type: follicular type of ameloblastic epithelium infiltrating the connective tissue

8.3.7 Differential Diagnosis

- Conventional type of ameloblastoma
- Odontogenic keratocyst
- Calcifying epithelial odontogenic tumour
- Central giant cell granuloma
- Dentigerous cyst (if unerupted tooth is present in the radiolucent defect)
- Ossifying fibroma

(a)

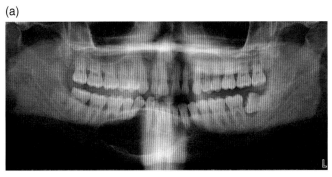

(b)   (c)

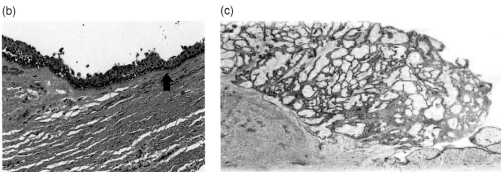

Figure 8.2 Unicystic ameloblastoma. (a) Panoramic radiograph demonstrating radiolucent lesion with corticated borders located in the anterior mandible. (b) Luminal type: epithelial lining exhibiting reverse polarity in the lining odontogenic epithelium (black arrow). (c) Intraluminal type: note plexiform ameloblastic epithelium projecting into the lumen. (*Source:* (a and b) by kind permission of Associate Professor Kelly Magliocca, Department of Pathology and Laboratory Medicine, Winship Cancer Institute at Emory University, Atlanta, GA, USA.)

8.3.8   Diagnosis

- History
- Clinical examination
- Radiography
- Biopsy and microscopy is mandatory

8.3.9   Management

- By enucleation
- Partial resection of the jaw for large tumours followed by reconstruction
- Regular radiography follow-up

8.3.10   Prognosis

- Good
- Better prognosis than conventional type of ameloblastoma
- Recurs if not completely removed

8.4 Squamous Odontogenic Tumour

8.4.1 Definition/Description

- A rare benign locally aggressive odontogenic tumour derived from odontogenic squamous epithelium
- Usually occupies the alveolar processes close to the roots of vital teeth
- Originates from:
  - Cell rests of Malassez
  - Remnants of the dental lamina
  - Gingival surface epithelium

8.4.2 Frequency

- Rare (50 plus cases reported to date)

8.4.3 Aetiology/Risk Factors

- Unknown

8.4.4 Clinical features

- Fourth decade of life
- Slight male predilection
- Painless or mildly painful swelling of the alveolar process
- Mobility and displacement of teeth seen
- Predilection for the anterior maxilla and the posterior mandible (equal distribution)

8.4.5 Radiographical Features

- Often detected on routine intraoral radiography
- A triangular-shaped unilocular radiolucency associated with the roots of erupted teeth
- Mimics interproximal bone loss due to periodontitis
- Rarely multilocular radiolucency, if located deeper

8.4.6 Microscopic Features

- Multiple islands of squamous epithelium surrounded by a mature connective tissue stroma (Figure 8.3)
- Occasionally cystic degeneration or calcification in the epithelial islands occur

8.4.7 Differential Diagnosis

- Periodontal pathology
- Lateral periodontal cyst
- Glandular odontogenic cyst.
- Lateral radicular and residual cyst

Figure 8.3 Squamous odontogenic tumour. Bland irregularly shaped odontogenic epithelium seen within dense fibrous connective tissue (*source:* by kind permission of Associate Professor Kelly Magliocca, Department of Pathology and Laboratory Medicine, Winship Cancer Institute at Emory University, Atlanta, GA, USA).

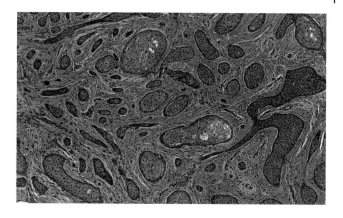

- Keratocystic odontogenic tumour (odontogenic keratocyst)
- Adenomatoid odontogenic tumour
- Central odontogenic fibroma
- Unicystic and multicystic ameloblastoma
- Langerhans's cell histiocytosis
- Multiple myeloma

8.4.8 Diagnosis

- History
- Clinical examination
- Radiography
- Biopsy and microscopy are mandatory

8.4.9 Management

- Curettage
- Extraction if teeth are involved

8.4.10 Prognosis

- Good
- Recurrence is uncommon

8.5 Calcifying Epithelial Odontogenic Tumour (Pindborg Tumour)

8.5.1 Definition/Description

- A rare locally aggressive benign odontogenic tumour composed of epithelial strands, deposits of amyloid and areas of calcification
- First reported by Pindborg in 1956
- Originates from:
  - Stratum intermedium
  - Primitive dental lamina

8.5.2 Frequency

- Rare tumour representing less than 1% of odontogenic tumours

8.5.3 Aetiology/Risk Factors

- Unknown

8.5.4 Clinical Features

- Fourth to sixth decade of life
- No sex predilection
- Painless or mildly painful swelling
- Mandible frequently involved (mandible : maxilla ratio 2 : 1)
- 52% are associated with unerupted tooth
- 6% as extra oral lesions

8.5.5 Radiographical Features

- Small lesions often detected on routine radiography
- A well-defined radiolucency in initial stages
- Mixed radiolucent/radiopaque appearance in later stages (Figure 8.4a)
- Adjacent teeth: displaced, roots resorbed

8.5.6 Microscopic Features

- Polyhedral neoplastic epithelial cells showing abundant eosinophilic finely granular cytoplasm with nuclear pleomorphism and prominent nucleoli
- Most cells are arranged in anastomosing sheet like masses
- An extracellular eosinophilic homogenous material staining like amyloid (characteristic) and concentric calcific deposits in the epithelial islands are predominant features (Figure 8.4b)

8.5.7 Differential Diagnosis

- Adenomatoid odontogenic tumour
- Calcifying odontogenic cyst
- Ameloblastic fibro odontoma
- Odontomes

8.5.8 Diagnosis

- History
- Clinical examination
- Radiography
- Biopsy and microscopy are mandatory

Figure 8.4 Calcifying epithelial odontogenic tumour. (a) Cropped panoramic radiograph demonstrating expansile mixed radiolucent and radiopaque lesion surrounding impacted mandibular third molar. (b) Photomicrograph showing amyloid like material (black arrow), calcifications (grey arrow) and cords of odontogenic epithelium (white arrows). (Images *source:* by kind permission of Associate Professor Kelly Magliocca, Department of Pathology and Laboratory Medicine, Winship Cancer Institute at Emory University, Atlanta, GA, USA.)

(a)

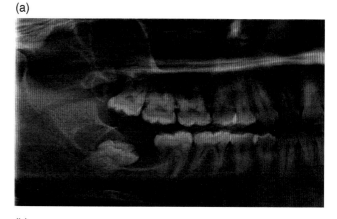

(b)

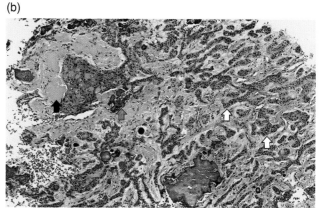

8.5.9 Management

- Small lesions: curettage/enucleation
- Large lesions: resection with removal of normal bone surrounding the tumour

8.5.10 Prognosis

- Fair to good
- Recurrence: 10–20%
- Malignant transformation is extremely rare

8.6 Adenomatoid Odontogenic Tumour

8.6.1 Definition/Description

- An uncommon hamartomatous odontogenic benign tumour characterized by duct-like histological structures
- Originates from:
  - Stratum intermedium
  - Primitive dental lamina

8.6.2 Frequency

- Uncommon tumour representing less than 3–7% of all odontogenic tumours

8.6.3 Aetiology/Risk Factors

- Unknown

8.6.4 Clinical features

- Common in late adolescence/young adulthood
- Female predilection
- Painless slow growing swelling
- Anterior maxilla frequently involved
- Associated with unerupted tooth

8.6.5 Radiographical Features

- Well-demarcated unilocular radiolucency
- May show unerupted tooth associated with the lesion
- Fine calcifications (snowflakes) may be seen, a feature that may be helpful in differentiating an adenomatoid odontogenic tumour from a dentigerous cyst (Figure 8.5a)
- Smooth cortical border
- Most lesions are pericoronal or juxta coronal
- Divergence of roots and displacement of teeth

8.6.6 Microscopic Features

- A well-defined capsule
- Duct-like structures lined by columnar epithelial cells (Figure 8.5b)
- Scanty connective tissue
- Epithelium may show rosettes, trabecular or cribriform patterns
- Homogeneous eosinophilic material in the duct-like structures
- Areas of dystrophic calcifications (Figure 8.5c)

8.6.7 Differential Diagnosis

- Dentigerous cyst
- Calcifying odontogenic cyst
- Calcifying epithelial odontogenic tumour
- Unicystic ameloblastoma
- Odontogenic keratocyst
- Ameloblastic fibro-odontoma

8.6.8 Diagnosis

- History
- Clinical examination
- Radiography
- Biopsy and microscopy are mandatory

(a)

(b)

(c)

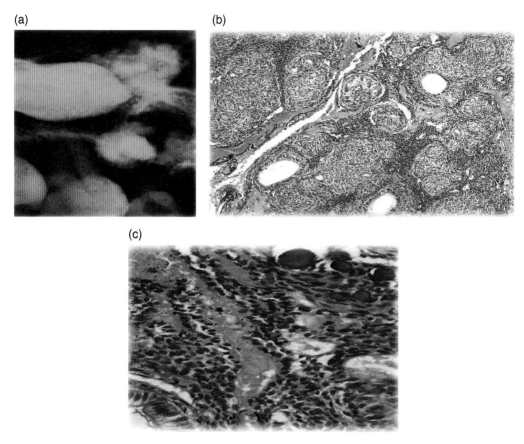

Figure 8.5   Adenomatoid odontogenic tumour. (a) Radiograph showing an unerupted maxillary canine surrounded by radiolucency and associated with radiopaque foci (snowflakes) of calcifications. (b) Photomicrograph showing duct-like structures lined by columnar epithelial cells. (c) Photomicrograph showing areas of dystrophic calcifications at the top right corner.

8.6.9   Management

- Enucleation
- Large lesions: resection with removal of normal bone surrounding the tumour

8.6.10   Prognosis

- Fair to good
- Recurrence: 10–20%
- Malignant transformation is extremely rare

8.7   Ameloblastic Fibroma

8.7.1   Definition/Description

- A mixed odontogenic benign tumour composed of strands of odontogenic epithelium in a cellular mesenchymal tissue resembling dental lamina
- Originates from epithelial and ectomesenchyme (mixed)

8.7.2 Frequency

- Rare tumour

8.7.3 Aetiology/Risk Factors

- Unknown

8.7.4 Clinical features

- Occur in childhood and adolescence
- Slight male predilection
- Painless slow-growing swelling
- Posterior mandible followed by posterior maxilla preferred sites
- 75% of cases associated with impacted tooth
- 20% detected on routine radiography

8.7.5 Radiographical Features

- Unilocular/multilocular radiolucency with well demarcated borders (Figure 8.6a)
- Tooth may be embedded in the radiolucency, in some cases mimicking a dentigerous cyst

8.7.6 Microscopic Features

- Strands or islands of odontogenic epithelium (resembling cap stage of tooth bud)
- Cellular mesenchyme resembling dental papilla (Figure 8.6b)

(a) (b)

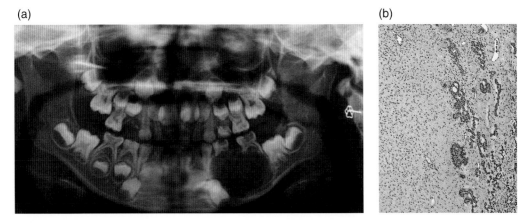

Figure 8.6 Ameloblastic fibroma. (a) Orthopantomogram showing a well-defined radiolucent lesion with a sclerotic border in the left body of the mandible. The second deciduous molar has been displaced distally and is supraerupted. (b) Photomicrograph shows cellular/fibroblastic fibromyxoid stroma resembling primitive mesenchyme or developing dental papilla. (*Images source:* Carroll. C., Gill, M., Bowden, E. et al. Ameloblastic fibroma of the mandible reconstructed with autogenous parietal bone: report of a case and literature review. *Case Reports in Dentistry* 2019: 5149219. doi: 10.1155/2019/5149219. Reproduced under Creative Commons Licence 3.0.)

8.7.7 Differential Diagnosis

- Dentigerous cyst
- Ameloblastoma
- Adenomatoid odontogenic tumour
- Ameloblastic fibro-odontome

8.7.8 Diagnosis

- History
- Clinical examination
- Radiography
- Biopsy and microscopy are mandatory

8.7.9 Management

- Enucleation/curettage
- Conservative resection

8.7.10 Prognosis

- Fair
- 33% recurrence
- Potential for malignant transformation exists

8.8 Ameloblastic Fibrodentinoma and Ameloblastic Fibro-Odontome

8.8.1 Definition/Description

- A mixed odontogenic benign tumour resembling ameloblastic fibroma showing dentine formation (ameloblastic fibrodentinoma) or with complex odontome (ameloblastic fibro-odontome)
- Originates from odontogenic epithelium and ectomesenchyme (mixed)

8.8.2 Frequency

- Rare tumour (1–3% of all odontogenic tumours)

8.8.3 Aetiology/Risk Factors

- Unknown

8.8.4 Clinical features

- Occurs in childhood (mean age 11.5 years)
- Slight male predilection
- Painless slow growing swelling

- Posterior mandible preferred site
- May be associated with impacted tooth
- Commonly detected on routine radiography

8.8.5 Radiographical Features

- Radiolucency and radiopacity
- Tooth embedded in the radiolucency in most cases (Figure 8.7a)

8.8.6 Microscopic Features

- Islands, cords, and strands of stellate reticulum like odontogenic epithelium
- Dental papilla like ectomesenchyme stroma
- Irregular dentine (ameloblastic fibrodentinoma)
- Enamel matrix and irregular dentine (ameloblastic fibro-odontome), and occasionally cementum (Figure 8.7b)

8.8.7 Differential Diagnosis

- Immature complex odontoma
- Odontoameloblastoma
- Ameloblastic fibrodentinoma
- Ameloblastic fibroma

8.8.8 Diagnosis

- History
- Clinical examination
- Radiography
- Biopsy and microscopy

(a)   (b)

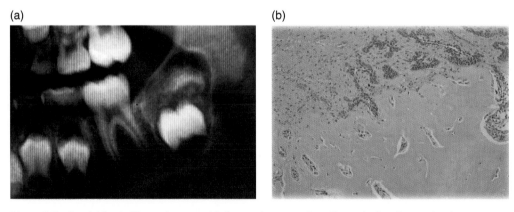

Figure 8.7 Ameloblastic fibro-odontome. (a). Cropped panoramic radiograph showing a mixed radiolucent–radiopaque lesion with an unerupted tooth in the left angle of the mandible. (b) Photomicrograph shows structures resembling ameloblastic fibroma in the upper half and calcified tissue matrix resembling dentine and cementum in the lower half of this section.

8.8.9 Management

- Enucleation

8.8.10 Prognosis

- Fair
- Little potential for recurrence

8.9 Odontome (Odontoma)

8.9.1 Definition/Description

- Odontome (odontoma) is a developmental malformation of odontogenic epithelial and mesen-chymal components of dental tissues and is not a neoplasm
- Origin dental lamina

8.9.2 Frequency

- Most common of the odontogenic tumours (malformations)
- Constitute 22% of all odontogenic tumours

8.9.3 Aetiology/Risk Factors

- Uncertain aetiology, but the following factors are suspected:
  - Trauma during primary dentition
  - Inflammatory and infectious processes
  - Family history
  - Anomalies which are hereditary in nature including
  - Hermann's syndrome and Gardner's syndrome
  - Hyperactivity of the odontoblast
  - Genetic alterations causing aberrations in signalling pathways controlling tooth development

8.9.4 Clinical Features

- Two types: complex and compound
- Complex odontome:
  - Common between the ages of 10 and 20 years
  - Male and females equally affected
  - Posterior mandibular region followed by anterior maxilla frequently involved
  - Occur on the right side of the jaw rather than the left
  - Commonly associated with permanent teeth; rare in deciduous teeth
  - Relative frequency among odontogenic tumours 5–30%
  - Painless, slow-growing, often associated with an unerupted permanent tooth
  - Often detected on routine radiography
  - Usually stops growing once mature

- Compound odontome:
  - Painless, slow-growing swelling
  - Slightly more common than the complex odontome
  - Occur on the right side of the jaw rather than the left
  - Common in anterior maxilla
  - Commonly associated with permanent teeth, rare in deciduous teeth
  - Seen between the ages of 10 and 20 years
  - Often associated with unerupted permanent tooth
  - Frequently detected on routine radiography
  - Relative frequency among odontogenic tumours 9–37%
  - Usually stops growing once mature

8.9.5 Radiographical Features

- Complex odontome:
  - An amorphous mass of calcified material with radio density of tooth structure surrounded by a radiolucent rim (Figure 8.8a)
- Compound odontome:
  - Multiple small radiopaque calcified structures (denticles; Figure 8.8b)
  - A radiolucent rim surrounding the calcified mass
  - Denticles are anatomically similar to normal teeth

8.9.6 Microscopic Features

- Complex odontome:
  - Dentine of the mature tubular form enclosing enamel (empty enamel spaces)
  - All dental tissues seen in a disorganized arrangement (Figure 8.8c)

- Compound odontome:
  - Tooth-like structures (denticles) embedded in a matrix composed of loose fibrous connective tissue
  - Denticles show an organized structure as in normal teeth (Figure 8.8d)

8.9.7 Differential Diagnosis

- Ameloblastic fibrodentinoma
- Ameloblastic fibro-odontoma
- Adenomatoid odontogenic tumour
- Pindborg's tumour

8.9.8 Diagnosis

- History
- Clinical examination
- Radiography
- Biopsy (surgically removed lesion)/microscopy

(a)

(b)

(c)

(d)

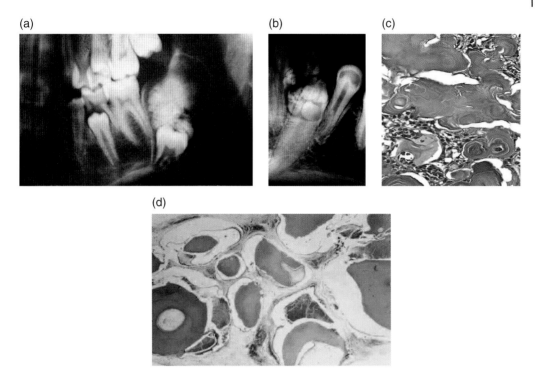

Figure 8.8 (a) Odontome: Radiograph of a complex odontome. Note dense radiopacity and a retained molar. (b) Radiograph of a compound odontome in the left canine region of the mandible. Tooth-like structures can be identified. The canine is impacted. (*Source:* (a,b) courtesy of Dr Ramadas. Reproduced with permission from Ramadas, K., Lucas, E., Thomas, G. et al., eds. 2008. *A Digital Manual for the Early Diagnosis of Oral Neoplasia.* Lyon: International Agency for Research on Cancer. Available from https://screening.iarc.fr/atlasoral.php. (c) Complex odontome. Photomicrograph shows a highly calcified tissue consisting of irregular masses of enamel (spaces), dentin-pulp, and cementum. (d) Compound odontome. Photomicrograph shows several small tooth-like structures are present with enamel (spaces) and dentin-pulp in their correct anatomical relationships.

8.9.9 Management

- Enucleation

8.9.10 Prognosis

- Good
- Extremely low recurrence

8.10 Dentinogenic Ghost Cell Tumour

8.10.1 Definition/Description

- Dentinogenic ghost cell tumour is characterized by an ameloblastomatous epithelium with areas of ghost cell formation and varying amounts of dentinoid
- It is a tumorous form of calcifying odontogenic cyst
- Origin: odontogenic epithelium

8.10.2   Frequency

- 6% of all odontogenic tumours
- The lesion accounts for 1% of all odontogenic jaw cysts

8.10.3   Aetiology/Risk Factors

- Uncertain

8.10.4   Clinical features

- Mean age 31 years
- No predilection for either sex
- 85% have cystic component
- 15% have solid pattern
- Usually anterior region of the jaws: incisor–cuspid region
- Slow growing, painless in initial stages
- May occur as an extraosseous lesion
- Solid lesions are more aggressive

8.10.5   Radiographical Features

- Round or ovoid shaped radiolucent lesion (unilocular; Figure 8.9a)
- Radiolucency surrounded by a narrow radio-opaque margin extending from the lamina dura of the tooth
- Rarely multilocular radiolucency
- Flecks of calcified masses in the radiolucent lesion
- Root resorption and displacement of adjacent teeth seen

8.10.6   Microscopic Features

- Epithelial lining of the cystic lesion is ameloblast-like
- Abnormal keratinization producing cluster of pale (ghost) cells are seen (Figure 8.9b)
- 'Ghost cells' calcify, and may induce a dentin-like matrix (dentinoid)

8.10.7   Differential Diagnosis

- Dentigerous cyst
- Radicular/residual cysts
- Odontogenic keratocyst
- Adenomatoid odontogenic tumour
- Odontoma
- Ameloblastic fibro-odontoma
- Calcifying epithelial odontogenic tumour
- Odontogenic fibroma

8.10.8   Diagnosis

- History
- Clinical examination

Figure 8.9 Dentinogenic ghost cell tumour. (a) An orthopantomogram showing a radiolucent lesion with areas of opacification and impacted right mandibular canine and first premolar teeth. (b) Photomicrograph shows epithelial lining of the cystic lesion, abnormal keratinization producing cluster of pale (ghost) cells and evidence of dentine like calcification of 'ghost cells'. (*Source:* by kind permission of Dr Yash Agrawal New Horizon Dental College and Research Institute, Bilaspur, Chhattisgarh, India.)

(a)

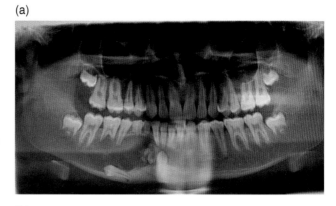

(b)

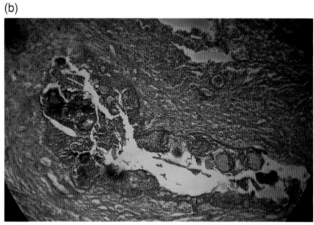

- Radiography
- Biopsy and microscopy

8.10.9   Management

Enucleation/curettage

8.10.10   Prognosis

- Good
- Solid lesions may recur

8.11   Odontogenic Myxoma

8.11.1   Definition/Description

- A benign odontogenic tumour of mesenchymal origin composed of loose myxoid ground substance and dispersed spindle shaped fibroblasts
- Origin: odontogenic mesenchyme: developing dental follicle and papilla

8.11.2 Frequency

- Third most common odontogenic tumour after odontomes and ameloblastoma

8.11.3 Aetiology/Risk Factors

- Uncertain

8.11.4 Clinical features

- Age: 10–30 years
- No predilection for either sex
- Posterior mandible commonly involved
- Asymptomatic swelling

8.11.5 Radiographical Features

- Radiolucent: multilocular/soap-bubble or honeycomb appearance (Figure 8.10a)
- Scalloped borders
- Adjacent teeth displaced

8.11.6 Microscopic Features

- Loose myxoid ground substance (Figure 8.10b)
- Dispersed fibroblasts with anastomosing processes
- Occasional collagen fibres and epithelial rests

8.11.7 Differential Diagnosis

- Ameloblastoma
- Central haemangioma
- Odontogenic keratocyst
- Glandular odontogenic cyst
- Central giant cell granuloma
- Odontogenic fibroma

8.11.8 Diagnosis

- History
- Clinical examination
- Radiography
- Biopsy/microscopy

8.11.9 Management

- Excision with bony curettage
- Bloc resection for large lesions

Figure 8.10 Odontogenic myxoma. (a) orthopantomogram showing a poorly defined multilocular radiolucency, extending from the midline to left ramus region causing cortical expansion and displacement of 34, 35 and 36 as well as root resorption of 34, 35, 36, 37 and 38. (b) Photomicrograph shows loosely arranged stellate-shaped cells with intermingled fibrillar processes in a homogenous mucoid ground substance. (Images *source:* by kind permission from Dr Suchitra Gupta Prasad, D J College of Dental Sciences, Ghaziabad, India.)

(a)

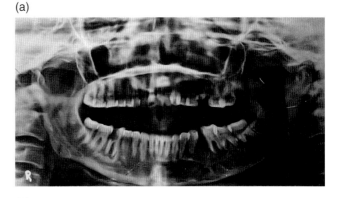

(b)

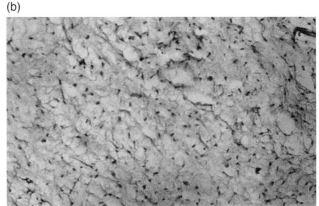

8.11.10   Prognosis

- Fair to good
- Occasionally recur

8.12   Odontogenic Fibroma (Central Odontogenic Fibroma)

8.12.1   Definition/description

- Odontogenic fibroma is a rare odontogenic tumour of mesodermal origin composed of mature fibrous tissue, with variable amounts of inactive-appearing odontogenic epithelium
- Two variants exist:
  - Central (intraosseous) odontogenic fibroma
  - Peripheral odontogenic fibroma (not discussed in this chapter)
- Origin: dental follicle, periodontal ligament, or dental papilla

8.12.2   Aetiology/Risk factors

- Unknown

8.12.3 Frequency

- Rare
- Different studies report high variability in the incidence rate, 3–23% of all odontogenic tumours
- Peak age of occurrence is 20–40 years

8.12.4 Clinical Features

- Common in the mandible posterior to the first molar
- In the maxilla, common anterior to the first molar
- Causes bony swelling by cortical expansion
- Related to the coronal or radicular portion of the teeth
- Root resorption and radiopaque flakes can be seen in some cases

8.12.5 Radiographical Features

- Unilocular or multilocular radiolucency with distinct borders
- Root resorption and radiopaque flakes can be seen in some cases

8.12.6 Microscopic Features

- Mature quite cellular fibrous connective tissue with islands of inactive odontogenic epithelium (Figure 8.11)
- Plump fibroblasts are common
- Calcification can be seen in association with odontogenic epithelium

8.12.7 Differential Diagnosis

- Cysts of odontogenic origin
- Ameloblastoma
- Adenomatoid odontogenic tumour
- Ameloblastic fibroma

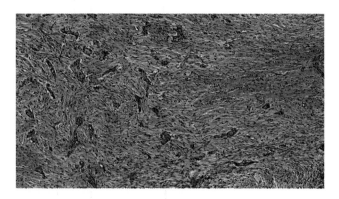

Figure 8.11 Odontogenic fibroma. Photomicrograph showing cellular fibrocollagenous tissue with scattered, small, inactive odontogenic epithelium in strands, cords, or nests (source: by kind permission of Associate Professor Kelly Magliocca, Department of Pathology and Laboratory Medicine, Winship Cancer Institute at Emory University, Atlanta, GA, USA.)

8.12.8 Diagnosis

- History
- Clinical examination
- Radiography
- Microscopic findings

8.12.9 Management

- The treatment of central odontogenic fibroma is conservative surgery by the enucleation of the lesion
- Recurrence is not common

8.13 Cementoblastoma

8.13.1 Definition/Description

- A benign odontogenic tumour of cementoblasts associated with the cementum
- Origin: odontogenic mesenchyme/ectomesenchyme

8.13.2 Frequency

- Less than 1% of all odontogenic tumours

8.13.3 Aetiology/Risk Factors

- Uncertain/unknown

8.13.4 Clinical Features

- Young adults (20–30 years of age)
- No predilection for either sex
- Slow growing painful swelling
- Bony expansion (lingual and buccal)
- Chance finding on radiography in early stages
- Mandibular first permanent molar roots commonly involved

8.13.5 Radiographical Features

- Typical: a well-circumscribed, radiopaque mass attached to the root of the involved tooth with a surrounding thin radiolucent zone (Figure 8.12a)
- Additional radiographical features:

  - Root resorption
  - Loss of the root outline
  - Invasion of the root canal

(a)

(b)

(c)

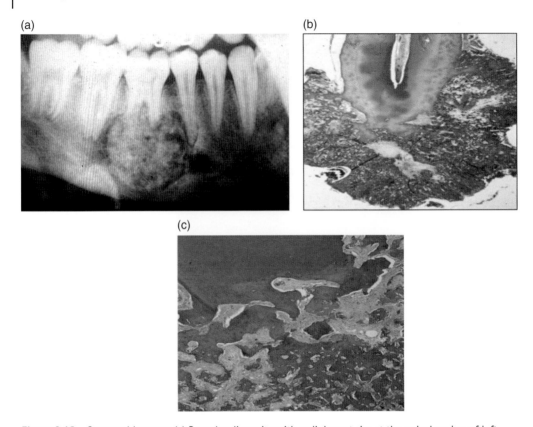

Figure 8.12 Cementoblastoma. (a) Round radiopacity with radiolucent rim at the apical region of left mandibular first molar tooth. (b) Note calcified mass fused to the root of a molar tooth. (c) Note cementum with basophilic reversal lines and intervening loose fibrovascular connective tissue stroma. (*source:* by kind permission of Dr Folk G S, Scripps Oral Pathology Service, San Diego, CA, USA).

- – Bony expansion
- – Displacement and involvement of adjacent teeth
- – Cortical erosion
- – Obliteration of the periodontal ligament space

8.13.6 Microscopic Features

- Calcified mass attached to the roots (Figure 8.12b)
- Masses of hypocellular cementum embedded in a fibrovascular stroma
- Prominent cementoblastic rimming
- Prominent reversal lines within the cementum (Figure 8.12c)
- Osteoclast-type multinucleated giant cells in fibrovascular stroma
- Plump osteoblasts in fibrovascular stroma
- Fibrous capsule at the periphery

8.13.7 Differential Diagnosis

- Osteoblastoma
- Osteosarcoma
- Osteoma
- Ossifying fibroma

8.13.8 Diagnosis

- History
- Clinical examination
- Radiography
- Microscopy (of surgically removed lesion)

8.13.9 Management

- Enucleation/curettage and extraction of the tooth involved

8.13.10 Prognosis

- Good
- Recurrence uncommon
- Regrowth possible if incompletely removed

Recommended Reading

Agrawal, Y., Naidu, G.S., Makkad, R.S. et al. (2017). Dentinogenic ghost cell tumour: a rare case report with review of literature. *Quantitative Imaging in Medicine and Surgery* 7 (5): 598–604.

Chang, H., Shimizu, M.S., and Precious, D.S. (2002). Ameloblastic fibro-odontoma: a case report. *Journal of the Canadian Dental Association* 68 (4): 243–246.

Dunlap, C. (2001). Odontogenic Tumors: The short version. University of Missouri-Kansas City School of Dentistry. https://dentistry.umkc.edu/dentistry-professionals/guides-manuals-documents (accessed 9 March 2021).

Gupta, S., Grover, N., Kadam, A. et al. (2013). Odontogenic myxoma. *National Journal of Maxillofacial Surgery* 4 (1): 81–83.

Huber, A.R. and Folk, G.S. (2009). Cementoblastoma. *Head and Neck Pathology* 3: 133–135.

Misra, S.R., Lenka, S., Sahoo, S., and Mishra, S. (2013). Giant Pindborg tumour (calcifying epithelial odontogenic tumour): an unusual case report with radiologic-pathologic correlation. *Journal of Clinical Imaging Science* 3 (Suppl 1): 11.

Neville, B.W., Damm, D.D., Allen, C.M., and Chi, C.A. (2016). Odontogenic cysts and tumours. In: *In: Oral and Maxillofacial Pathology,* 4ee, 632–681. St Louis, MO: Elsevier.

Odell, E.W. (2017). Odontogenic tumours and related jaw lesions. In: *Cawson's Essentials of Oral Pthology and Oral Medicine,* 9ee, 165–183. Edinburgh: Elsevier.

Ranchod, F.T., Behardien, N., and Morkel, J. (2020). Ameloblastoma of the mandible: analysis of radiographic and histopathological features. *Journal of Oral Medicine and Oral Surgery* 27: 6. https://doi.org/10.1051/mbcb/2020051.

Regezi, J. (2002). Odontogenic cysts, odontogenic tumors, fibroosseous, and giant cell lesions of the jaws. *Modern Pathology* 15: 331–341.

Speight, P.M. and Takata, T. (2018). New tumour entities in the 4th edition of the World Health Organization Classification of head and neck tumours: odontogenic and maxillofacial bone tumours. *Virchows Archiv* 472: 331–339.

9

Non-odontogenic Benign and Malignant Tumours of the Jaw

9.1   Osteoma

9.1.1   Definition/Description

- A benign tumour composed of mature compact and/or cancellous bone
- Two types: peripheral or periosteal and central or endosteal osteoma

9.1.2   Frequency

- Rare in the jaw

9.1.3   Aetiology

- Cause is unknown but injury or muscle traction may be contributing factors

9.1.4   Clinical Features

- Mandibular body (lingual to premolars) and the condyle are the sites of predilection
- Solitary and asymptomatic (Figure 9.1a)
- Slow growing, occasionally deformity of the face
- Limitation and deviation of mouth opening in condylar osteoma

Handbook of Oral Pathology and Oral Medicine, First Edition. S. R. Prabhu.
© 2022 John Wiley & Sons Ltd. Published 2022 by John Wiley & Sons Ltd.
Companion website: www.wiley.com/go/prabhu/oral_pathology

- Multifocal osteoma in Gardner's syndrome
- Paranasal sinus osteoma is common

9.1.5 Radiographical Features

- Round sclerotic mass (peripheral and central types. (Figure 9.1b)
- Dense sclerotic mass at the periphery and central trabeculation (periosteal osteoma)

9.1.6 Microscopic Features

- Compact osteoma: normal bone with minimal marrow (Figure 9.1c)
- Cancellous osteoma: bony trabeculae, fibrous/fatty tissue, and prominent osteoblastic activity

9.1.7 Differential Diagnosis

- Condensing osteitis (central type)
- Focal chronic sclerosing osteomyelitis (central type)

9.1.8 Diagnosis

- History
- Clinical findings

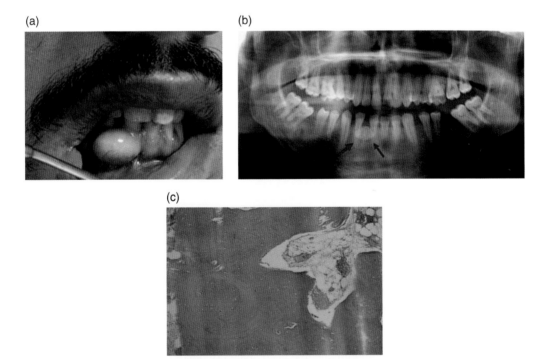

(a) (b)

(c)

Figure 9.1 Osteoma. (a). Clinical photograph of a 21 year old male with a slow growing hard painless lesion of over two years duration. Note a round nodule on the right anterior surface of the mandible adjacent to teeth number 41 and 42. (b) Panoramic radiograph of osteoma revealing a radiopaque lesion (red arrows). (c) Photomicrograph showing mature lamellar bone and minimal fatty bone marrow. *Source:* images a and b: Gumusok, M et al. (2015). Peripheral osteoma of the mandible: a case report. Journal of Istanbul University Faculty of Dentistry, 49, 47–50.

- Radiography
- Microscopy

9.1.9 Management

- Small asymptomatic osteoma needs no treatment
- Large and symptomatic osteoma should be removed surgically

9.2 Multiple Osteomas in Gardner's Syndrome

9.2.1 Definition

- A rare inherited disorder characterized by multiple intestinal polyps, osteomas of the cranium or mandible, epidermal cysts and fibromas, and abnormalities of the teeth
- Intestinal polyps tend to progress to colorectal cancer

9.2.2 Frequency

- Rare; 2–3 cases per 100 000 population

9.2.3 Aetiology

- Mutations in adenomatous polyposis coli gene

9.2.4 Clinical Features

- Colonic polyps
- Multiple bony swellings of the craniofacial bones (Figure 9.2a)
- Multiple epidermoid cysts
- Impacted/supernumerary teeth
- Odontomas
- Fibrous neoplasms (desmoid tumours)
- Congenital hypertrophy of the retinal epithelium (brown retinal maculae)
- Any of the above four findings suggest Gardner's syndrome

9.2.5 Radiographical Features

- Presence of dense bony masses (osteomas), odontomas, supernumerary teeth and other dental anomalies (Figure 9.2b)

9.2.6 Microscopic Features

- Presence of compact lamellar bone with haversian canals and lacunae (Figure 9.2c)
- Histiocytes and reversal and resting lines are other features present

(a)

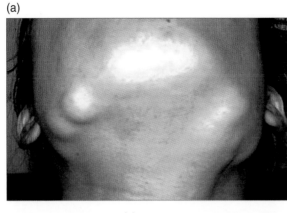

(b)   (c)

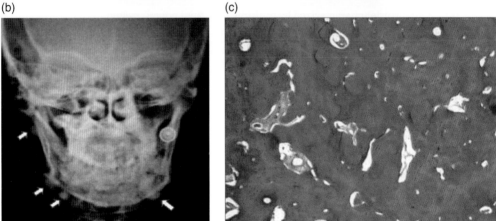

Figure 9.2 Gardner's syndrome. (a) Extraoral osteomas: multiple diffuse bilateral swellings along the mandibular border. (b) Posteroanterior radiograph shows extra-oral osteomas along the mandible (white arrows). (c) Photomicrograph shows the presence of compact lamellar bone with haversian canal, lacunae, histiocytes and reversal and resting lines suggestive of osteoma. (*Source:* by kind permission of Dr Sapna Panjwani, Institute of Dental Studies and Technologies, Modinagar, Ghaziabad, Uttar Pradesh, India.)

9.2.7   Differential Diagnosis

- Other familial intestinal polyposis syndromes
- Isolated forms of osteomas with other dental anomalies

9.2.8   Diagnosis

- History
- Clinical findings
- Radiography
- Endoscopy for intestinal polyposis

9.2.9   Management

- Surgery for intestinal polyps, skin tumours and jaw lesions

9.2.10   Prognosis

- Good prognosis for surgical removal of osteomas, odontomas, supernumerary teeth and other dental anomalies.

9.3   Central Haemangioma (Intraosseous Haemangioma)

9.3.1   Definition/Description

- Central (intraosseous) haemangioma is a true benign neoplasm of vascular origin

9.3.2   Frequency

- Rare in the maxillofacial bones
- Other bones: vertebral column and skull bones

9.3.3   Aetiology

- Endothelial proliferation which differentiates into blood vessels

9.3.4   Clinical Features

- Bone involvement is usually of cavernous type; it is congenital
- Mandibular ramus is mostly affected (premolar/molar area)
- Female sex predilection (female to male ratio 2 : 1)
- Peak incidence: second and fifth decade
- Asymptomatic in early stages
- More aggressive lesions are symptomatic: painless swelling, loose teeth and bleed from the gingival margins
- When overlying cortex is resorbed it appears as a bluish, pulsatile, soft lesion
- Supra eruption, premature exfoliation of primary teeth, and early eruption of permanent teeth are rarely reported

9.3.5   Radiographical Features

- Cyst-like radiolucency; often with soap-bubble appearance
- Formation of reactive spicula produced by the lesion is a classic radiographical feature of intrabony haemangioma (Figure 9.3a)

9.3.6   Microscopic Features

- Plexiform pattern of vascular spaces
- Spaces lined by a single layer of endothelial cells interspersed among bony trabeculae (Figure 9.3b)

(a) (b)

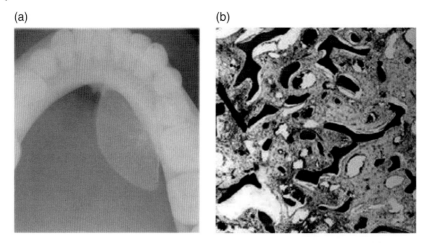

Figure 9.3 Central haemangioma. (a) Occlusal radiograph revealing a well-defined lesion surrounded by a sclerotic margin, containing reactive bone spicules which are characteristic for intraosseous cavernous hemangioma. (b) Photomicrograph shows blood-filled vascular space between the bone trabeculae. (*Source:* images © 2017 Medicina Oral S.L; from Elif, B., Derya, Y., Gulperi, K., Sevgi, B. 2017. Intraosseous cavernous hemangioma in the mandible: a case report. *Journal of Clinical and Experimental Dentistry* 9 (1): e153–e156. doi: 10.4317/jced.52864.)

9.3.7 Differential Diagnosis

- Ameloblastoma
- Odontogenic myxoma
- Fibrous dysplasia
- Aneurysmal bone cyst
- Central giant cell granuloma

9.3.8 Diagnosis

- History
- Clinical findings
- Radiography: orthopantomogram (OPG), computed tomography (CT), and magnetic resonance imaging (MRI), useful
- Angiography

9.3.9 Management

- Non-invasive radiotherapy
- Intralesional injection of sclerosing agents and selective arterial embolization
- Curettage and radiation
- Resection followed by osseous reconstruction
- Note: lesion should not be opened, or associated tooth extracted; these procedures may be fatal due to excessive haemorrhage

9.3.10 Prognosis

- Favourable

9.4 Melanotic Neuroectodermal Tumour of Infancy

9.4.1 Definition/Description

- Melanotic neuroectodermal tumour of infancy is a rare, destructive, benign, pigmented neoplasm of neural crest origin seen in early infancy

9.4.2 Frequency

- Rare; 90% are in infants
- Median age five months
- Slightly more common in males

9.4.3 Aetiology

- Unknown aetiology
- Tumour originates from neural crest

9.4.4 Clinical Features

- Occurs in the first few months of life
- Anterior maxilla commonly involved (60–80%), mandible (5.8%)
- Painless, non-ulcerative, locally aggressive, bluish black (pigmented) tumour mass (Figure 9.4a)
- Destroys underlying bone
- Prevents tooth development

9.4.5 Radiographical Features

- Destruction of the underlying bone
- Displacement of developing teeth

9.4.6 Microscopic Features

- Melanin containing epithelioid cells lining the slit like spaces and darkly stained small round cells in the cystic spaces and fibrous connective tissue (Figure 9.4b)
- Some degree of cellular atypia and mitotic figures

9.4.7 Differential Diagnosis

- Eruption cyst
- Congenital epulis

9.4.8 Diagnosis

- History from parent/guardian
- Clinical findings
- Radiography
- Microscopic findings

(a) (b)

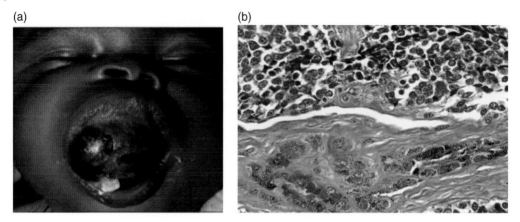

Figure 9.4 Melanotic neuroectodermal tumour of infancy. (a) Clinical photograph of a three-month-old female infant depicting a rapidly growing bluish mass on the anterior aspect of the maxilla. Growth involves the right upper vestibule, alveolar ridge, and anterior hard palate. Note an embedded tooth in the lesion (*source*: by kind permission of Dr Sachin Rai, Oral Health Sciences Centre, Postgraduate Institute of Medical Education and Research, Chandigarh, India). (b) Photomicrograph showing pigmented large epithelioid cells and smaller primitive cells (*source*: photo credit: Lestertheinvestor; https://en.wikipedia. org/wiki/Melanotic_neuroectodermal_tumor_of_infancy#/media/File:Oral_melanotic_neuroectodermal_ tumor_infancy_LDRT_369_13.tif; licensed under CC BY-SA 4.0).

9.4.9 Management

- Surgery

9.4.10 Prognosis

- Variable
- High recurrence rate: (10–60%); 15% in the first year of surgery
- Malignant transformation: 6.6%

9.5 Osteosarcoma

9.5.1 Definition/Description

- A malignant neoplasm of the bone that forms abnormal bone or osteoid

9.5.2 Frequency

- Rare; 5% of osteosarcomas arise in the jaw

9.5.3 Aetiology/Predisposing Factors

- 10% of jaw lesions are radiation induced
- Predisposing factors include:
  - Hereditary retinoblastoma
  - Paget's disease of the bone
  - A history of fibrous dysplasia or trauma

9.5.4   Clinical Features

- Median age is 30–40 years
- Maxilla and mandible are equally affected
- Local pain
- Numbness and facial dysesthesia
- Loose teeth
- Trismus and difficulty in mouth opening
- Nasal obstruction
- Bleeding
- Firm mass fixed to the underlying bone
- Systemic features: fever, headache, weight loss
- Very few cases with no symptoms (detected incidentally on radiography)

9.5.5   Radiographical Features

- Irregular bone destruction: a moth eaten appearance
- Periosteal elevation and new bone formation (Figure 9.5a)
- 'sun ray' appearance is often seen

9.5.6   Microscopic Features

- Histologically osteosarcoma can be classified according to the cellular differentiation as osteoblastic, chondroblastic, and fibroblastic
- Spindle-shaped atypical hyperchromatic neoplastic cells (osteoblasts/chondroblasts or fibroblasts; Figure 9.5b)
- Osteoid, disorganized woven bone or cartilage
- Mitotic bodies

(a)   (b)

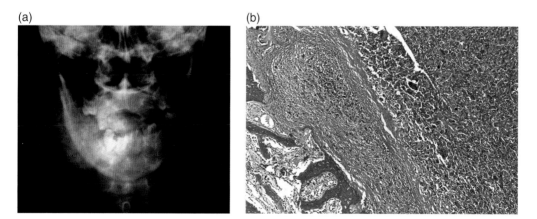

Figure 9.5   Osteosarcoma. (a) Radiographical findings in a case of chondroblastic osteosarcoma of the mandible. Note the bone forming mass in the right mandible with considerable displacement of teeth in the region (*source:* by kind permission of Dr Scott Riley Ong University of the Philippines, Manila, Philippines). (b). Photomicrograph showing osteosarcoma with poorly differentiated neoplasm (centre and right of image) adjacent to non-malignant bone (left bottom of image; *source:* Nephron; https://en.wikipedia.org/wiki/Osteosarcoma#/media/File:Osteosarcoma_-_intermed_mag.jpg. Licensed under CC BY-SA 3.0).

9.5.7 Differential Diagnosis

- Chondrosarcoma
- Fibrous dysplasia
- Osteomyelitis
- Osteoma
- Myositis ossificans
- Cemento-osseous dysplasia

9.5.8 Diagnosis

- History
- Clinical findings
- Radiography (OPG, CT, MRI)
- Microscopy
- Laboratory values: increased alkaline phosphatase or lactate dehydrogenase (LDH)

9.5.9 Management

- Radical surgery (hemi-mandibulectomy)

9.5.10 Prognosis

- Recurrence in 50% of cases
- Five-year survival is 70% for tumours of less than 5 cm in diameter and 0% for those greater than 15 cm

9.6 Chondrosarcoma: Key Features

- A malignant neoplasm of the chondrocytes that forms abnormal cartilage
- Rarer than osteosarcomas
- Affects adults
- Anterior maxilla is the site of predilection
- Painless swelling, loose teeth are common
- Radiography shows well or poorly demarcated radiolucent lesion with areas of calcification
- Radiography may show 'sun ray' appearance (Figure 9.6a), which is also a feature of osteosarcoma
- Microscopy shows new abnormal hyaline cartilage formation with atypia and mitosis in chondrocytes (Figure 9.6b)
- Management: surgery
- Radiotherapy or chemotherapy have no effect

9.6.1 Prognosis

- Five-year survival is 75%

(a) (b)

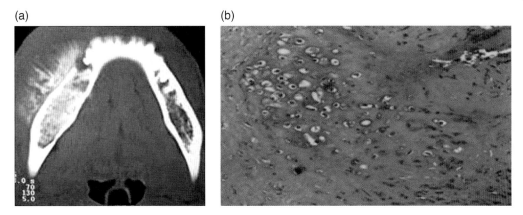

Figure 9.6 Chondrosarcoma. (a) Coronal computed tomography revealing the presence of a large osteolytic lesion involving the right body of mandible showing 'sun ray' appearance and expansion of the cortical plates (*source:* by kind permission of Dr Sanchita Kundu, Guru Nanak Institute of Dental Sciences and Research. Panihati, Kolkata, India). (b) Histology shows abnormal hyaline cartilage with atypia in chondrocytes (*source:* by kind permission of Bakyalakshmi, Tamil Nadu Dental College, Chennai India).

9.7 Ewing's Sarcoma

9.7.1 Definition/Description

- Ewing's sarcoma is an uncommon round cell malignant bone tumour with an aggressive course affecting mainly children and young adults

9.7.2 Frequency

- Approximately 4% in the bones of the head and neck, with 1% occurring in the jaws (predominantly mandible)
- Marked predilection for white populations
- Majority occur between the ages of 5 and 20 years
- Rare before 5 years and after 30 years of age

9.7.3 Aetiology/Risk Factors

- Unknown
- Genetically related to primitive peripheral neuroectodermal tumour via translocations
- Chromosomal translation, gene rearrangement and expression of the *MIC2* gene

9.7.4 Clinical Features

- Slight male preponderance
- Presenting signs and symptoms: swelling, pain, loose teeth, paraesthesia, ulceration, trismus and toothache
- Extraoral features: exophthalmos, ptosis, epistaxis, otitis media and sinusitis, fever, anaemia
- Rise in erythrocyte sedimentation rate, moderate leucocytosis and an increase in serum LDH are common

9.7.5 Radiographical Features

- Osteolysis (moth eaten appearance), cortical erosion, and periostitis (Figure 9.7a)

9.7.6 Microscopic Features

- Small, poorly differentiated cells with medium-size, round or oval nuclei exhibiting a fine chromatin pattern, small nucleoli, and scanty cytoplasm (Figure 9.7b)

9.7.7 Differential Diagnosis

- Osteosarcoma
- Eosinophilic granuloma
- Histiocytosis X
- Giant cell tumour
- Lymphoma
- Primitive rhabdomyosarcoma
- Neuroectodermal tumour of infancy
- Chondrosarcoma

(a)

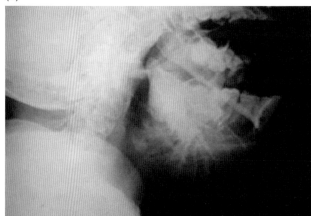

(b)

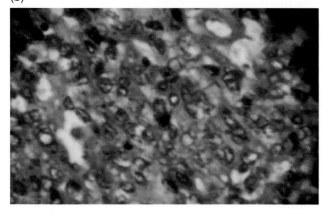

Figure 9.7 (a) Ewing's sarcoma. Cropped panoramic radiograph shows radiolucent ill-defined osteolytic lesion with bony spiculations, teeth displacement and missing 45. (b) Histopathology. Haematoxylin and eosin stain shows round cells with scanty cytoplasm and pleomorphic round or oval nuclei. (By kind permission of Dr. Sanki Reddy Shailaja, Panineeya Institute of Dental Sciences and Research Centre, Hyderabad, India)

9.7.8 Diagnosis

- History
- Clinical findings
- Radiography
- Microscopic findings

9.7.9 Management

- Radiotherapy
- Chemotherapy

9.7.10 Prognosis

- Five-year survival: 54–74%

9.8 Myeloma (Multiple Myeloma)

9.8.1 Definition/Description

- Multiple myeloma is a haematological malignancy characterized by the multicentric proliferation of a single clone of abnormal immunoglobulin-secreting plasma cells

9.8.2 Frequency

- About 1% of all malignancy and 10% of haematologic malignancy
- Common between 50 and 80 years of age
- Occurs twice as often in men as in women

9.8.3 Aetiology/Risk Factors

- Unknown

9.8.4 Clinical Features

- Early signs and symptoms: fatigue, bone pain, fever, anaemia, nephropathy and weight loss
- Posterior region of the mandible is the preferred site: molar region, ramus, angle, and occasionally condylar process
- Odontalgia, paraesthesia, tooth mobility, gingival haemorrhage and ulcerations in later stages of multiple myeloma

9.8.5 Radiographical Features

- Multiple radiolucent defects (punched out appearance) in the skull and the jaw with no sclerotic outline of the punched out radiolucent lesions (Figure 9.8a)

(a)

(b)

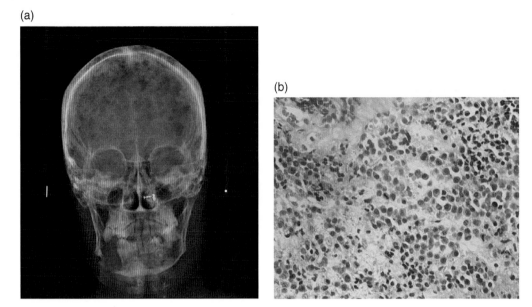

Figure 9.8 Multiple myeloma. (a) Radiograph shows multiple punched-out radiolucencies involving the skull bones, facial bones, and mandible. (b) Histopathology shows sheets of plasma cells with several atypical forms. (*Source:* images by kind permission of A.R. Subhashini, KLE Dental College, Bengaluru, India.)

9.8.6 Microscopic Features

- Diffuse sheets of neoplastic (monoclonal) plasma cells (Figure 9.8b)
- Deposition of amyloid
- Occasional mitotic bodies

9.8.7 Differential Diagnosis

- Plasmacytoma (solitary)
- Brown tumour
- Metastatic lesions
- Chronic osteomyelitis
- Arteriovenous malformations
- Langerhans' cell disease

9.8.8 Diagnosis

- History
- Clinical findings
- Radiography
- Laboratory test for Bence Jones proteins (positive)
- Microscopy

9.8.9 Management

- Incurable but life can be extended for many years
- Combination of chemotherapy, corticosteroids, proteasome inhibitors (bortezomib) and thalido-mide analogues
- Localized lesions may be treated with radiotherapy
- Bisphosphonates for those with a tendency for myeloma related bone fractures
- Bone marrow or stem cell transplants for some patients

9.8.10 Prognosis

- Fair
- Survival rate of six to seven years following diagnosis and treatment

9.9 Solitary Plasmacytoma

9.9.1 Definition/Description

- Plasmacytoma is a monoclonal, neoplastic proliferation of plasma cells that usually arises within bone marrow or soft tissue sites

9.9.2 Frequency

- Rare in the jaws
- 4.4% of the cases of solitary plasmacytoma of the bone occur in bone marrow-rich areas of posterior mandible

9.9.3 Aetiology/Risk Factors

- Aetiology is uncertain
- Proposed hypotheses include the role of radiation, chemical exposure, viruses, and genetic factors

9.9.4 Clinical Features

- May be the first manifestation of a subsequent multiple myeloma
- Mean age 55 years
- Predilection for males
- Often detected incidentally on radiography
- Bone paraesthesia or pain and swelling
- Pathological fracture
- Haemorrhage

9.9.5 Radiographical Features

- Well-defined solitary radiolucent lesion with no sclerotic outline (Figure 9.9a)
- Microscopically, sheets of neoplastic plasma cells with varying degree of differentiation

(a)

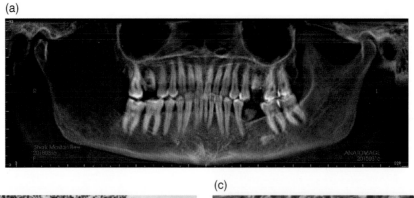

(b)   (c)

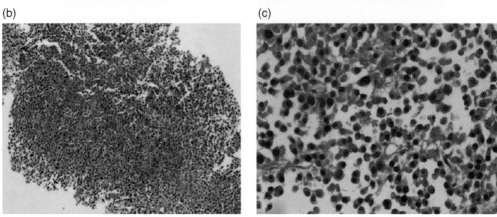

Figure 9.9 Plasmacytoma. (a) Orthopantomogram revealing ill-defined radiolucency involving the entire right side of the mandible. (b) Photomicrograph showing solid sheets of plasma cells. (c) Photomicrograph showing solid sheets of anaplastic cells with occasional binucleated forms. (*Source:* Chittemsetti, S., Guttikonda, V.R., Sravya, T., Manchikatta, P.K. 2019. Solitary plasmacytoma of mandible: a rare entity. *Journal of Oral and Maxillofacial Patholology* 23:136–139. doi: 10.4103/jomfp.JOMFP_175_18. © 2019 *Journal of Oral and Maxillofacial Pathology.*)

9.9.6 Microscopic Features

- Clusters or sheets of atypical plasma cells with varying degree of differentiation (Figure 9.9b)
- Sparse stroma
- Plasma cells are characterized by abundant cytoplasm with eccentrically placed nucleus with chromatin clumps typically arranged in cartwheel or clock-face pattern
- Occasionally binucleated cells (Figure 9.9c)
- Plasma cell differentiation may show mild, moderate or severe dysplasia

9.9.7 Differential Diagnosis

- Reactive inflammatory lesions such as plasma cell gingivitis
- Non-Hodgkin lymphoma
- Malignant melanoma
- Ameloblastoma
- Odontogenic myxoma
- Giant cell lesions
- Multiple myeloma

9.9.8 Diagnosis

- Skeletal radiological survey (to rule out multiple myeloma)
- Bone marrow aspiration
- Blood cell count
- Determination of calcium levels
- Detection of plasma protein M (or paraprotein) through electrophoresis of blood or urine samples (not diagnostic)
- Renal function

9.9.9 Management

- Radiotherapy (offers better result)
- Chemotherapy (alone has little effect)
- Surgery
- Combination of surgery and radiotherapy offer best results

9.9.10 Prognosis

- Course is relatively benign
- If recurrence is present, showing tendency toward multiple myeloma, the prognosis is worse
- Survival rate is 50–80% at 10 years
- If recurrence is present, survival rate drops to 16%

9.10 Burkitt's Lymphoma

9.10.1 Definition/Description

Burkitt's lymphoma is a most aggressive malignant solid tumour of B lymphocytes grouped under the umbrella of non-Hodgkin B-cell lymphoma

9.10.2 Frequency

- Burkitt's lymphoma is known to be endemic in Africa but can occur sporadically (non-endemic Burkitt's lymphoma) in other part of the world
- Accounts for 30-50% of all childhood cancers in equatorial Africa (predominantly children of four to seven years of age)
- The incidence rate of sporadic childhood Burkitt's lymphoma in the United States/Europe is around 10-fold lower than the incidence of endemic Burkitt's lymphoma (predominantly affects older individuals)
- Immunodeficiency-associated Burkitt lymphoma is associated with HIV infection (or those who received allografts) in older patients

9.10.3 Aetiology/Risk Factors

- Epstein–Barr virus is associated with 95% of the 'endemic' cases

- Infection of B cell lymphocytes with the virus causes the disease
- Malaria is a risk factor in endemic form of Burkitt's lymphoma
- Sporadic variant shows only a 20% association with Epstein–Barr virus and is seen mainly in Europe and North America
- Cytogenetic chromosomal translocations may be responsible for neoplastic transformation

9.10.4   Clinical Features

- 50–70% of endemic Burkitt's lymphoma affects the jawbone, but the sporadic form predominantly affects the abdomen (rarely in the jaw)
- Peak prevalence for endemic Burkitt's lymphoma is around seven years
- Greater predilection for males
- Predominantly affects posterior maxilla
- Facial swelling and severely mobile and displaced teeth are common presenting symptoms (Figure 9.10a)
- Premature exfoliation of teeth is common
- Lymphadenopathy is present

9.10.5   Radiographical Features

- Bone destruction with poorly defined and irregular margins

9.10.6   Microscopic Features

- Small, diffusely proliferated, monomorphic, immature, and undifferentiated lymphocytes interspaced by numerous macrophages within abundant cytoplasm giving a 'starry sky' microscopic appearance (Figure 9.10b)

(a)   (b)

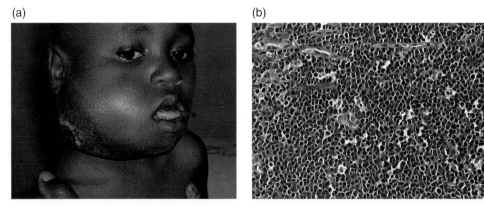

Figure 9.10   Burkitt's lymphoma. (a) Tumour in a seven-year-old Nigerian boy with a several-month history of jaw swelling, which had been treated with antibiotics. The tumour was ulcerated, infected and draining (*source:* Mike Blyth, https://commons.wikimedia.org/wiki/File:Large_facial_Burkitt%27s_Lymphoma.JPG#/media/File:Large_facial_Burkitt's_Lymphoma.JPG. Licensed under CC BY-SA 2.5). (b) Photomicrograph showing 'starry sky' appearance (*source:* CoRus13, https://en.wikipedia.org/wiki/Burkitt_lymphoma#/media/File:Burkitt's_lymphoma_in_a_kidney_biopsy,_very_high_mag.jpg. Licensed under CC BY-SA 4.0).

9.10.7 Differential Diagnosis

- Abscesses
- Apical lesion
- Ameloblastoma
- Other non-Hodgkin lymphoma
- Undifferentiated carcinomas
- Sarcoma

9.10.8 Management/Prognosis

- Fatal if not treated
- Burkitt's lymphoma is treated preferentially with intensive chemotherapy
- Five-year survival rates 75–95%, depending on the stage of the lesion at the time of diagnosis

Recommended Reading

Bakyalakshmi, K., Jayachandran, S., and Sureshkumar, M. (2015). Primary juxtacortical chondrosarcoma of mandibular symphysis: unique and rare case report. *Journal of Cancer Research and Therapeutics* 11: 1025.

Chittemsetti, S., Guttikonda, V.R., Sravya, T., and Manchikatta, P.K. (2019). Solitary Plasmacytoma of mandible: a rare entity. *Journal of Oral and Maxillofacial Pathology* 23: 136–139.

Kabukcuoglu, F., Ozagari, A., Tuncel, D., and Karsidag, S. (2015). Non-odontogenic tumors of the jaws. *Oral Surgery, Oral Pathology, Oral Medicine, Oral Radiology* 119 (3): E192.

Krishna, K.B.B., Thomas, V., Kattoor, J., and Kusumakaran, P. (2013). A radiological review of Ewing's sarcoma of the mandible: a case report with one year follow up. *International Journal of Clinical Pediatric Dentistry* 6: 109–111.

Kumar, D., Rattan, V., Rai, S. et al. (2015). Reconstruction of anterior maxillary defect with buccal pad fat after excision of melanotic neuroectodermal tumor of infancy. *Annals of Maxillofacial Surgery* 5 (2): 234–236.

Kundu, S., Pal, M., and Paul, R.R. (2011). Clinicopathologic correlation of chondrosarcoma of mandible with a case report. *Contemporary Clinical Dentistry* 2: 390–393.

Neville, B.W., Damm, D.D., Allen, C.M., and Chi, C.A. (2016). Fibro-osseous lesions of the jaws. In: *Oral and Maxillofacial Pathology*, 4ee, 592–622. St Louis, MO: Elsevier.

Odell, E.W. (2017). Non-odontogenic tumors of the jaws. In: *Cawson's Essentials of Oral Pthology and Oral Medicine*, vol. 9e, 187–200. Edinburgh: Elsevier.

Panjwani, S., Bagewadi, A., Keluskar, V., and Arora, S. (2011). Gardner's syndrome. *Journal of Clinical Imaging Science* 1: 65.

Raghavan, S.A., Nagaraj, P.B., Ramaswamy, B., and Nayak, D.S. (2014). Multiple myeloma of the jaw: a case report. *Journal of Indian Academy of Oral Medicine andRadiology* 26: 454–457.

10

Fibro-Osseous and Related Lesions of the Jaw

CHAPTER MENU

10.1 Ossifying Fibroma/Cemento-Ossifying Fibroma
10.2 Cemento-Osseous Dysplasias
10.3 Familial Gigantiform Cementoma: Key Features
10.4 Central Giant Cell Granuloma

10.1 Ossifying Fibroma/Cemento-Ossifying Fibroma

10.1.1 Definition/Description

- A benign bone tumour consisting of highly cellular, fibrous tissue that contains varying amounts of calcified tissue resembling bone, cementum, or both

10.1.2 Frequency

- Uncommon

10.1.3 Origin/Aetiology

- Origin: osteogenic
- Cause: unknown

10.1.4 Clinical/Radiographical Features

- Peak in the third to fourth decade
- Female predilection
- More common in mandible (premolar/molar area)
- Small lesions asymptomatic (detected incidentally on radiography)
- Large lesions: painless buccolingual swelling and facial asymmetry
- Unilocular radiolucency: mixed radiolucent radiopaque (Figure 10.1a)
- Thin radiolucent rim of mature lesions

(a)

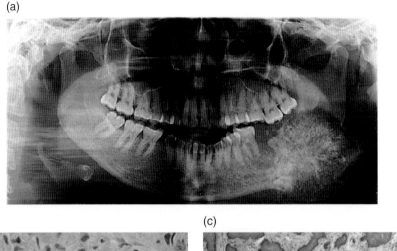

(b)   (c)

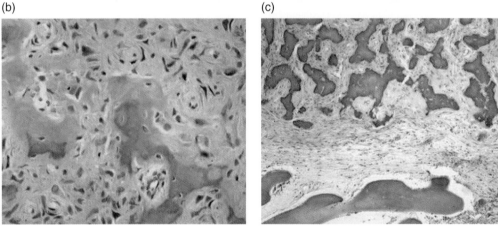

Figure 10.1 Ossifying fibroma. (a) Orthopantomograph showing a well-defined mixed radiopaque-radiolucent lesion causing bowing of the inferior border of the left side of the mandible (*source:* by kind permission of Karpal Singh Sohal. Muhimbili University of Health and Allied Sciences, Dar es Salaam, Tanzania). (b) Photomicrograph shows irregular islands of osteoid rimmed by osteoblasts and a fibrous stroma. (c) Photomicrograph showing the interface between normal bone (bottom) and ossifying fibroma (top). (*Source* (b, c): from Carvalho B., Pontes, M., Garcia, H. et al. (2012). Ossifying fibromas of the craniofacial skeleton. In: *Histopathology: Reviews and Recent Advances* (ed. E.P. Martinez), IntechOpen. doi: 10.5772/51030. Reproduced under CC BY 3.0.)

10.1.5 Microscopic Features

- Cellular fibrous tissue with mineralized component
- Mineralized product: islands of osteoid (Figure 10.1b) or cementum like spherules
- Bony trabeculae: woven and lamellar pattern (Figure 10.1c)

10.1.6 Differential Diagnosis

- Giant cell lesions
- Cementoblastoma
- Calcifying odontogenic cyst

10.1.7   Diagnosis

- History
- Clinical examination
- Radiography
- Microscopy

10.1.8   Management

- Conservative excision
- Enucleation with peripheral bony curettage

10.2   Cemento-Osseous Dysplasias

10.2.1   Definition/Description

- Cemento-osseous dysplasias are non-neoplastic disturbances of growth and remodelling of jaw-bone and cementum
- There are four subtypes:
  - Periapical cemento-osseous dysplasia
  - Focal cemento-osseous dysplasia
  - Florid cemento-osseous dysplasia
  - Familial gigantiform cementoma

10.2.2   Frequency

- Cemento-osseous dysplasias are the most common fibro-osseous lesions in the jaw

10.2.3   Aetiology

- Disturbances of growth and remodelling of bone and cementum

10.2.4   Clinical/Radiographical Features

- Periapical cemento-osseous dysplasia:
  - Predominantly involves periapical region at the anterior mandible with multiple foci
  - Marked female predilection
  - Incidentally diagnosed on radiography
  - Radiolucent and radiopaque mixed lesions (Figure 10.2a)
  - Periodontal ligament is intact
  - Associated teeth are vital
- Focal cemento-osseous dysplasia:
  - Involves a single site
  - 90% occur in females
  - Mean age 41 years
  - Ethnic predilection: African American, and East Asian

- Common in posterior mandible
- Incidental detection on radiography
- Asymptomatic
- Radiolucent and radiopaque single lesion with a peripheral radiolucent rim (Figure 10.2b)
- Florid cemento-osseous dysplasia:
    - Multiple teeth affected in one quadrant
    - Mandibular teeth commonly involved
    - Lesions seen around the roots
    - Lesions show central sclerosis being surrounded by a radiolucent rim (Figure 10.2c)
    - Teeth are vital

(a)   (b)

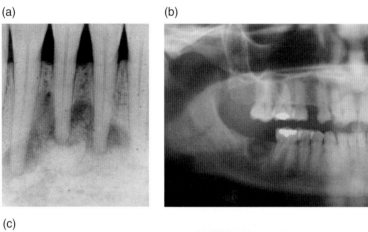

(c)

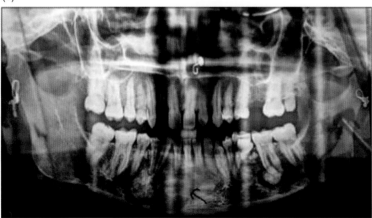

Figure 10.2 (a) Periapical cemental dysplasia; radiograph showing partly mineralized periapical lesion that merges with surrounding bone (*source:* courtesy of Dr K Ramadas. Reproduced with permission from IARC. 2008. *A Digital Manual for the Early Diagnosis of Oral Neoplasia.* Available from https://screening.iarc.fr/atlasoral.php). (b) Focal cemento-osseous dysplasia; panoramic radiograph showing isolated, mixed radio-opaque and radiolucent lesion with a 'bulls-eye' pattern (*source:* by kind permission of Associate Professor Kelly Magliocca, Department of Pathology and Laboratory Medicine, Winship Cancer Institute at Emory University, Atlanta, GA, USA). (c) Florid cemento-osseous dysplasia; orthopantomogram showing multiple bilateral radiopaque sclerotic lesions surrounded by peripheral radiolucent rim located apical to several mandibular teeth (*source:* by kind permission of Dr Sneha Choudhary, Theerthankar Mahaveer Dental College and Research Centre. Moradabad, UP India).

- Familial gigantiform cementoma:
  - Rare form of cemento-osseous dysplasia
  - Autosomal dominant condition
  - All quadrants are involved in childhood
  - Radiography: multiple radiolucencies in early stages, mixed (radiolucent and radiopaque) and completely radiopaque in later stages

10.2.5 Microscopic Features

- All four forms of cemento-osseous dysplasia show similar microscopic features:
  - Fibrovascular connective tissue in early stages
  - Variable mixture of woven and lamellar bone and cementum (Figure 10.3a, b and c)
  - Bony trabeculae may fuse in later stages of development

10.2.6 Differential Diagnosis

- Periapical cemento-osseous dysplasia:
  - Periapical abscess
  - Periapical granuloma

(a)   (b)

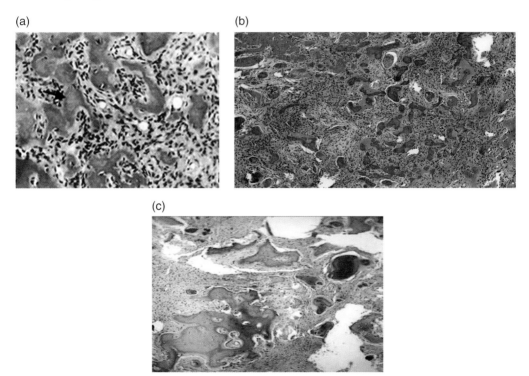

(c)

Figure 10.3   (a) Periapical cemental dysplasia; photomicrograph showing woven bone (black arrow) without osteoblastic rimming. (b) Focal cemento-osseous dysplasia; photomicrograph corresponding to the radiograph 2b above showing cemental droplets and immature bone within cellular fibroblastic stroma. Note the absence of osteoblastic or cementoblastic rimming (*source:* by kind permission of Associate Professor Kelly Magliocca, Department of Pathology and Laboratory Medicine, Winship Cancer Institute at Emory University, Atlanta, GA, USA). (c) Florid cemento-osseous dysplasia; photomicrograph showing numerous woven bony trabeculae in a fibrocellular stroma with multiple ossicles and a few cementicle-like areas (*source:* by kind permission of Dr Sneha Choudhary, Theerthankar Mahaveer Dental College and Research Centre. Moradabad, UP India).

    – Periapical cyst
    – Focal sclerosing osteomyelitis
- Focal cemento-osseous dysplasia:
    – Periapical cyst
    – Periapical granuloma
    – Stafne's cyst
    – Residual cyst
    – Ossifying fibroma
- Florid cemento-osseous dysplasia:
    – Gardener's syndrome
    – Paget's disease
    – Chronic diffuse sclerosing osteomyelitis
    – Cemento-ossifying fibroma
- Familial gigantiform cementoma:
    – Benign cementoblastoma
    – Osteoma
    – Ossifying fibroma

10.2.7 Diagnosis

- History
- Clinical findings
- Radiography
- Microscopy

10.2.8 Management

- Surgical procedures (extraction, biopsy, etc.) should be avoided in early stages
- Surgical exploration in later stages
- Osteomyelitis is a complication

10.2.9 Prognosis

- Good

10.3 Familial Gigantiform Cementoma: Key Features

- A rare benign fibro-osseous lesion
- Has an autosomal dominant mode of inheritance
- Usually starts in the first decade of life
- More common in white, African, and East-Asian populations
- Characterized by cemento-osseous proliferation involving multiple quadrants of the jaw
- Causes jaw expansion and facial deformity
- Painless, slow-growing lesion

- Radiographical features include a mixed radiolucent–radiopaque pattern
- Microscopic features are similar to those of florid cemento-osseous dysplasia
- Surgery is the treatment of choice

10.4 Central Giant Cell Granuloma

10.4.1 Definition/Description

- Central giant cell granuloma is an uncommon, benign, proliferative, intraosseous lesion

10.4.2 Frequency

- Represents less than 7% of all benign jaw lesions

10.4.3 Origin/Aetiology

- A reactive process, possibly secondary to trauma or inflammation

10.4.4 Clinical Features

- Predilection for females
- Common in second and third decades of life
- Slow-growing painless lesion in most cases
- Some grow rapidly causing pain and a purplish, soft tissue swelling through the alveolar ridge
- The mandible is commonly involved; anterior to the first molar is the preferred site

10.4.5 Radiographical Features

- The radiographical characteristics of central giant cell granuloma vary
- Most lesions are radiolucent while wispy opacification and trabeculation may be seen (Figure 10.4a)
- Occasionally soap-bubble appearance
- Roots of teeth displaced and resorbed

10.4.6 Microscopic Features

- Osteoclast-like multinucleated giant cells with a fibroblastic background (Figure 10.4b)
- Haemorrhage and haemosiderin, surrounded by giant cells
- Rich vascular connective tissue
- Osteoid may be seen in places

10.4.7 Differential Diagnosis

- Ewing's sarcoma
- Ameloblastoma
- Odontogenic myxoma
- Brown tumour of hyperparathyroidism

(a)   (b)

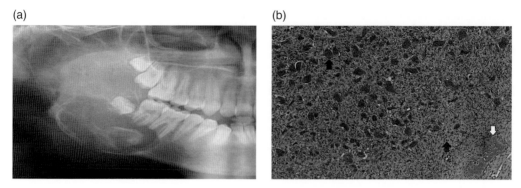

Figure 10.4 Central giant cell granuloma. (a) Cropped panoramic radiograph demonstrating expansile mixed radiolucent lesion near mandibular angle. (b) Photomicrograph shows Innumerable giant cells (black arrows) within a haemorrhagic fibroblastic background (grey arrow), with bone formation (white arrow). (*source:* by kind permission of Associate Professor Kelly Magliocca, Department of Pathology and Laboratory Medicine, Winship Cancer Institute at Emory University, Atlanta, GA, USA.)

10.4.8 Diagnosis

- History
- Clinical findings
- Radiography
- Microscopy

10.4.9 Management

- Curettage
- For rapidly growing aggressive lesions, additional treatment includes:
  - Intranasal calcitonin
  - Antiresorptive medications (e.g. bisphosphonates or denosumab)
  - Intralesional corticosteroid injections
  - Recurrence seen in 20% of cases
  - Second curettage is usually curative

10.4.10 Prognosis

- Good

Recommended Reading

Abramovitch, K. and Rice, D.D. (2016). Benign fibro-osseous lesions of the jaws. *Dental Clinics* 60: 167–193.

Carvalho, B., Pontes, M., Garcia, H. et al. (2012). Ossifying fibromas of the craniofacial skeleton. In: *Histopathology: Reviews and Recent Advances* (ed. E.P. Martinez). London: IntechOpen. doi: 10.5772/51030.

Choudhary, S.H., Supe, N.B., Singh, A.K., and Thakare, A. (2019). Florid cemento-osseous dysplasia in a young Indian female: a rare case report with review of literature. *Journal of Oral and Maxillofacial Pathology* 23 (3): 438–442.

Hall, G. (2017). Fibro-osseous lesions of the head and neck. *Diagnostic Histopathology* 23: 200–210.

Neville, B.W., Damm, D.D., Allen, C.M., and Chi, C.A. (2016). Fibro-osseous lesions of the jaws. In: *Oral and Maxillofacial Pathology*, 4ee, 592–622. St Louis, MO: Elsevier.

Odell, E.W. (2017). Odontogenic tumours and related jaw lesions. In: *Cawson's Essentials of Oral Pathology and Oral Medicine*, vol. 9e, 165–183. Edinburgh: Elsevier.

Potochny, E.M. and Huber, A.R. (2011). Focal osseous dysplasia. *Head and Neck Pathology* 5 (3): 265–267.

11

Genetic, Metabolic, and Other Non-neoplastic Bone Diseases

11.1   Osteogenesis Imperfecta

11.1.1   Definition/Description

- A group of genetic bone disorders characterized by low bone density (osteopenia) and increased bone fragility
- Also known as brittle bone disease

11.1.2   Frequency

- Affects about 1 in 15 000 people

11.1.3   Aetiology/Risk Factors

- Lack of type I collagen due to mutations in the *COL1A1* or *COL1A2* pro-collagen genes
- Often inherited from a person's parents in an autosomal dominant manner
- Over 12 types of osteogenesis imperfecta have been identified based on pattern of inheritance, genes affected and severity of clinical manifestations of the phenotype

11.1.4   Clinical Features

- Skeletal fragility with a tendency to fracture from minimal trauma
- Skeletal deformity, joint laxity, and scoliosis are common

Handbook of Oral Pathology and Oral Medicine, First Edition. S. R. Prabhu.
© 2022 John Wiley & Sons Ltd. Published 2022 by John Wiley & Sons Ltd.
Companion website: www.wiley.com/go/prabhu/oral_pathology

- Extra skeletal manifestations may include:
  - Hearing loss
  - Blue/grey sclera (Figure 11.1a)
  - Dentinogenesis imperfecta (Figure 11.1b)
  - Hypercalciuria
  - Aortic root dilatation
  - Macrocephaly
  - Hydrocephalus
- Disorder may be mild, moderate, or severe
- Children with severe osteogenesis imperfecta often exhibit anterolateral bowing of the femur and anterior bowing of the tibia
- Type II is the perinatal lethal form. Infants may be stillborn; if they survive birth, they usually die in the first two months of life
- Signs of dentinogenesis imperfecta are seen in types I (20%), III (80%), and IV (60%)
- Although rare, a tendency for fractures of the jaw has been reported

(a)

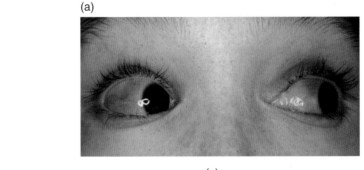

(b)   (c)

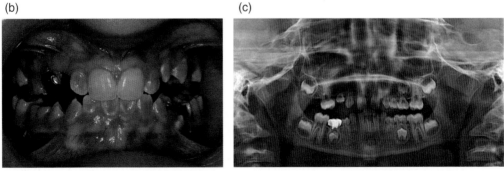

Figure 11.1 Osteogenesis imperfecta. (a) Characteristic blue sclera in a patient with osteogenesis imperfecta (Herbert L. Fred, MD, and Hendrik A. van Dijk, https://commons.wikimedia.org/wiki/File:Characteristically_blue_sclerae_of_patient_with_osteogenesis_imperfecta.jpg. Licensed under CC BY-SA 4.0). (b) Osteogenesis imperfecta showing features of dentinogenesis imperfecta. (c) Osteogenesis imperfecta. OPG showing bulbous crowns. Radiographical features are similar to those of dentinogenesis imperfecta. Note missing teeth. (*source*, images b and c: Rousseau, M., M, Retrouvey, J.M., Members of the Brittle Bone Diseases Consortium. 2018. Osteogenesis imperfecta: potential therapeutic approaches. *Peer J* 6: e5464. image a: https://doi.org/10.7717/peerj.5464/fig-1; image b: https://doi.org/10.7717/peerj.5464/fig-2).

11.1.5   Radiographical Features

- Dental radiographical features are identical to those of dentinogenesis imperfecta, such as bulbous crowns and short, slender roots (Figure 11.1c)

11.1.6   Diagnosis

- History
- Clinical findings
- Radiography
- DNA testing

11.1.7   Management

- Bisphosphonates
- Physical/rehabilitation therapy

11.2   Cleidocranial Dysplasia

11.2.1   Definition/Description

- Cleidocranial dysplasia is a rare skeletal dysplasia characterized by short stature, absent or defective clavicles, delayed closure of fontanelle and embedded supernumerary teeth

11.2.2   Frequency

- Rare
- Birth prevalence is approximately one in one million

11.2.3   Aetiology

- An autosomal dominant trait
- Mutation in the *RUNX2* gene that controls osteoblast and chondroblast differentiation
- Mutations in SH3-binding protein on chromosome 4p16.3

11.2.4   Clinical Features

- Hyperadduction of shoulders (Figure 11.2a)
- Delayed closure of fontanels
- Prominent forehead (frontal bossing)
- Short stature
- Absent or hypoplastic clavicles
- Maxillary hypoplasia
- Delayed tooth eruption of permanent teeth
- Retention of deciduous teeth
- Many unerupted supernumerary teeth
- Cysts around embedded teeth

(a)   (b)

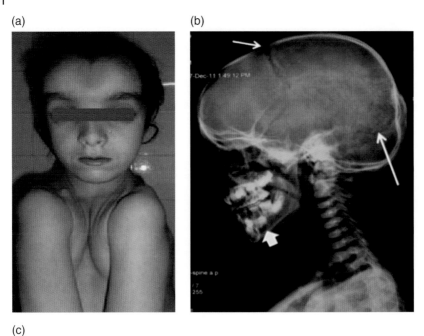

(c)

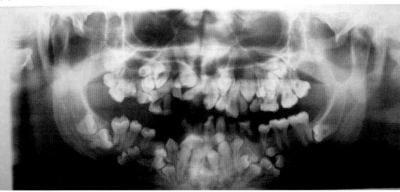

Figure 11.2   Cleidocranial dysplasia. (a) Extreme hyperadduction of shoulders almost approximated in midline. (b) X-ray skull lateral view showing open anterior fontanelle (short arrow), open cranial sutures (long arrow), frontal and parietal bossing and supernumerary teeth (arrowhead) (*Source:* By kind permission of Dr. Bashir Ahmad Laway, Sher-i-Kashmir Institute of Medical Sciences, Soura, Srinagar, J&K, India). (c) An OPG showing multiple supernumerary teeth in a patient with cleidocranial dysplasia. (*source:* courtesy of Charles Dunlap, UMKC Kansas City, USA.)

- Small paranasal sinuses
- High arched palate
- Ocular hypertelorism
- Pelvic bone deformities

11.2.5   Radiographical Features

- Open anterior fontanelle and cranial sutures (Figure 11.2b)
- Supernumerary teeth (Figure 11.2c)

- Maxillary hypoplasia
- Delayed tooth eruption of permanent teeth
- Cysts around the embedded teeth

11.2.6   Differential Diagnosis

- Achondroplasia
- Pyknodysostosis
- Hydrocephalus

11.2.7   Diagnosis

- History (family history)
- Clinical findings
- Radiography

11.2.8   Management

- Genetic counselling
- Surgical exposure of unerupted teeth and extraction of supernumerary teeth
- Early orthodontic intervention
- Dental reconstruction and correction of jaw deformities

11.3   Cherubism

11.3.1   Definition/Description

- An autosomal dominant developmental disorder characterized by plump cherubic face with bilateral symmetric expansion of the posterior mandible

11.3.2   Frequency

- Rare

11.3.3   Aetiology

- Dominant mutations in the *SH3BP2* gene on chromosome 4p16.3

11.3.4   Clinical Features

- Normal at birth, early signs in childhood (two to seven years of age)
- Cervical lymph node enlargement in early stages
- Bilateral, symmetrical, asymptomatic enlargement of mandible
- Maxillary involvement less common and less prominent
- Dental arch/occlusion discrepancies may be noted
- Permanent teeth may show hypodontia, rudimentary development of molars, abnormally shaped teeth, partially resorbed roots or delayed and ectopically erupting teeth

- Facial features include lower-third fullness and scleral exposure at a forward resting (heavenly) gaze
- Regresses spontaneously after puberty

11.3.5 Radiographical Findings

- Symmetric, multiloculated (soap bubble), expansile radiolucencies of mandibular body and ramus (Figure 11.3a)
- Impacted/displaced teeth
- Thinned cortices with scalloped medullary margins

11.3.6 Microscopic Features

- Loose fibrous tissue, endothelial cell proliferation and multinucleated giant cells (Figure 11.3b)
- Haemorrhagic areas
- Appearance is similar to central giant cell granuloma

(a)

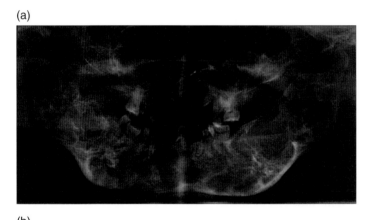

(b)

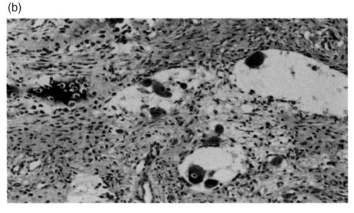

Figure 11.3 Cherubism. (a) An orthopantomogram showing multilocular appearance of the maxilla and mandible (excluding condyle) with numerous unerupted and displaced teeth. (b) Photomicrograph shows highly cellular mature fibrous connective tissue, numerous endothelial cell proliferations and multinucleated giant cells. (*source:* by kind permission of Dr Heena Mazhar, Chhattisgarh Dental College and Research Institute, Rajnandgaon, Chhattisgarh, India.)

11.3.7 Differential Diagnosis

- Brown tumour of hyperparathyroidism
- Central giant cell granuloma
- Noonan/multiple giant cell lesion syndrome
- Fibrous dysplasia
- Aneurysmal bone cyst
- Multiple odontogenic keratocysts

11.3.8 Diagnosis

- Clinical appearance
- Radiography
- Gene testing

11.3.9 Management

- Curettage of early lesion
- Cosmetic surgery until after puberty
- Stability is achieved by the end of skeletal growth

11.4 Gigantism and Acromegaly

11.4.1 Definition/Description

- Gigantism is characterized by overproduction of growth hormone by the anterior pituitary during skeletal growth in childhood resulting in overgrowth of the skeleton and course facial features
- Acromegaly is characterized by overproduction of growth hormone in middle age after the epiphyses have fused, which causes skeletal and soft tissue features

11.4.2 Frequency

- Uncommon/rare

11.4.3 Aetiology

- Pituitary adenoma in majority of cases for both forms of the disease
- McCune–Albright syndrome for about 20% of cases of gigantism

11.4.4 Clinical Features

- Gigantism:
  - Tall stature
  - Mild to moderate obesity (common)
  - Microcephaly

- Headaches
- Visual changes
- Exaggerated growth of the hands and feet, with thick fingers and toes
- Coarse facial features
- Prognathism
- Frontal bossing
- Peripheral neuropathies (e.g. carpel tunnel syndrome)
- Acromegaly:
  - Average age at diagnosis: 42 years
  - Enlargement of the lower lip and nose (the nose takes on a triangular configuration)
  - Enlarged swollen feet and hands
  - Doughy skin
  - Thick and hard nails
  - Swollen eye lids
  - Deepening of forehead creases and skin folds on the face
  - Wide spacing of the teeth (diastema)
  - Prognathism and bulging forehead (frontal bossing; Figure 11.4a)
  - Large tongue
  - Hypertrichosis
  - Hyperpigmentation (40% of patients) of the skin
  - Change in the voice

(a) (b)

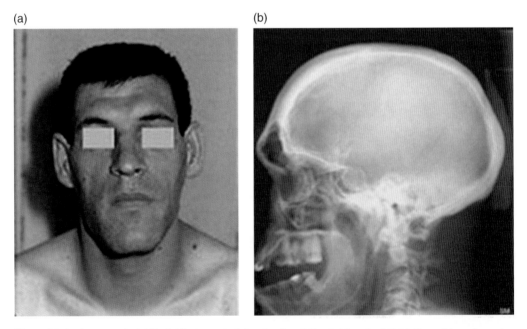

Figure 11.4 Acromegaly. (a) Facial features: bulging forehead (frontal bossing), thick lips, widened nasal bridge and prognathism. (b) Skull radiograph shows calvarial thickening, particularly of the inner table, frontal bossing, enlarged paranasal sinuses (especially frontal sinuses) and an enlarged sella turcica and mandibular prognathism. (*source:* by kind permission of Philippe Chanson, University of Paris, France.)

11.4.5   Radiographical Features

- Calvarial thickening, particularly of the inner table (Figure 11.4b)
- Frontal bossing
- Enlarged paranasal sinuses (especially frontal sinuses)
- Enlarged sella turcica
- The mandible also characteristically enlarges resulting in prognathism and gaps between the teeth

11.4.6   Diagnosis

- Blood tests can detect raised levels of growth hormone and insulin-like growth factor I.
- A pituitary adenoma can usually be seen on computed tomography (CT) or magnetic resonance imaging (MRI)
- Lateral skull radiography for prognathic mandible

11.4.7   Management

- Surgical removal of pituitary adenoma

11.5   Brown Tumour of Hyperparathyroidism

11.5.1   Definition/Description

- Hyperparathyroidism is a condition caused by excess production of parathyroid hormone
- Two types occur: primary and secondary

11.5.2   Frequency

- Uncommon to rare
- Primary hyperparathyroidism: 1–4 per 1000 in the general population

11.5.3   Aetiology

- Excessive parathyroid hormone due to:
  - Adenoma of the parathyroid gland (primary hyperparathyroidism)
  - Parathyroid hyperplasia (primary hyperparathyroidism)
  - Chronic low levels of serum calcium due to chronic renal failure (secondary hyperparathyroidism)

11.5.4   Clinical Features

- Common among people older than 60 years of age
- Female predilection
- Majority are asymptomatic
- Increased tendency for renal stones
- Subperiosteal resorption of phalanges

- Duodenal ulcers
- Confusion and dementia

11.5.5   Oral Manifestations

- Hyperparathyroidism can cause a non-neoplastic lesion in the jaws called brown tumour
- The reported prevalence of brown tumour is 0.1%
- Incidence of brown tumour in secondary hyperparathyroidism is 1.5–1.7%
- Common in females
- May be asymptomatic
- May present as a slow-growing soft to firm mass with varying degrees of tenderness
- Masticatory function is affected, facial deformities
- Generalized loss of lamina dura around roots of teeth

11.5.6   Radiographical Features

- Generalized loss of lamina dura around roots of teeth
- Well-demarcated unilocular or multilocular radiolucency (Figure 11.5a)

11.5.7   Microscopic Features

- Vascular granulation tissue
- Haemosiderin pigment (colouring the lesion brown, hence the name 'brown tumour')
- Multinucleated osteoclast-like giant cells (Figure 11.5b)
- Spicules of woven bone in a fibrovascular tissue

11.5.8   Differential Diagnosis

- Cherubism
- Paget's disease of bone
- Multiple odontogenic keratocysts
- Central giant cell granuloma

(a)

(b)

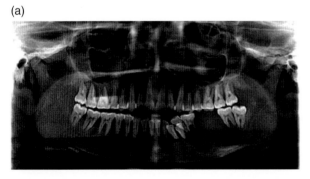
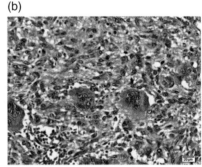

Figure 11.5   Brown tumour of hyperparathyroidism. (a) Orthopantomogram with large unilocular radiolucency on the left side, extending from mandibular first premolar to third molar. (b) Photomicrograph showing multinucleated giant cells deposition. (*Source:* (a) by kind permission of Dr Raquel Carvalho, Federal University of Mato Grosso do Sul, Campo Grande-MS, Brazil.)

11.5.9 Diagnosis

- History
- Clinical findings
- Radiography (radiolucency)
- Microscopy
- Serum calcium levels (high)
- Serum phosphorus levels (low)
- Serum alkaline phosphatase levels (raised)
- Plasma parathyroid hormone levels (high)

11.5.10 Management

- Surgery to remove the parathyroid gland (97% success)
- Treat the underlying cause (kidney failure for example)

11.5.11 Prognosis

- Good

11.6 Paget's Disease of Bone (Osteitis Deformans)

11.6.1 Definition/Description

- Paget's disease is characterized by disturbances in bone turnover causing irregular resorption, softening and sclerosis of bones

11.6.2 Frequency

- Most common bone disease after osteoporosis affecting 2–4% of adults over 55 years of age
- Uncommon in Scandinavia, Africa and Asia

11.6.3 Aetiology/Risk Factors

- Unknown
- Mutations in the sequestome-1 (*SQSTM1*) gene that controls development and activation of osteoclasts
- Family history

11.6.4 Clinical Features

- Common in the elderly
- Male predilection seen
- Common bones involved: sacrum, spine, femora, pelvis and skull
- Enlarged head, thickening of long bones
- Bone pain
- Increased tendency for fractures
- Deafness

- Deformity of skull
- Maxillary involvement causing symmetrical enlargement of alveolar process
- Development of diastema
- Ill-fitting dentures
- Hypertelorism
- Lion-like facial appearance (leontiasis ossea)
- Irregular hypercementosis
- Loss of lamina dura around roots resulting in ankylosis
- Obliteration of sinuses
- Neurological complications
- Occasionally development of osteosarcoma

11.6.5 Radiographical Features

- Lower bone density in early stages and sclerosis in later stages
- Patchy distribution of radiographical changes (cottonwool appearance; Figure 11.6a)
- Loss of lamina dura
- Pulpal radio-opacity
- Hypercementosis

11.6.6 Microscopic Features

- Irregular bone resorption and apposition (Figure 11.6b)
- Mosaic pattern of reversal lines

(a)

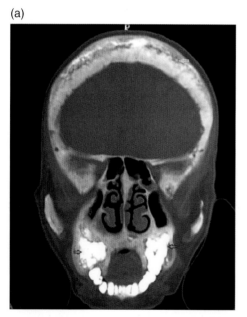

(b)

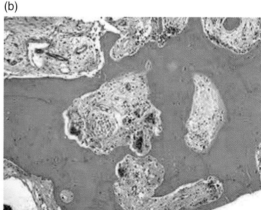

Figure 11.6 Paget's Disease of bone. (a) Computed tomography, coronal view, showing widened diploic space with sclerotic and lytic areas involving inner and outer tables of bony calvarium giving a cottonwool appearance (yellow arrow). Also note obliteration of the right maxillary antrum and osteosclerosis of maxillary alveoli (red arrows). (*Source:* by kind permission of Satya Ranjan Mishra Institute of Dental Sciences, Bhubaneswar, Odisha, India.) (b) Photomicrograph showing bone with irregular, scalloped edges, irregular cement lines, and numerous osteoclasts.

- Fibrovascular connective tissue
- Presence of osteoclasts and osteoblasts
- Osteoid rims around bone trabeculae

11.6.7 Differential Diagnosis of Jaw Lesions

- Fibrous dysplasia
- Fibro-osseous lesions
- Florid cemento-osseous dysplasia
- Chronic non-suppurative osteomyelitis
- Osteosarcoma

11.6.8 Diagnosis

- History
- Clinical findings
- Radiography of the affected bones
- Isotope bone scan
- Investigations:
  - Plasma total alkaline phosphatase levels (raised in most cases)
  - Liver function tests (to avoid diagnostic confusion since liver damage can also cause raised levels of plasma alkaline phosphatase levels)
  - Vitamin D levels (low)

11.6.9 Management

- Asymptomatic patients: no treatment is required
- For symptomatic patients:
  - Bisphosphonates
  - Vitamin D with ergocalciferol or cholecalciferol
  - Analgesics for pain
- Follow up

11.6.10 Prognosis

- Variable

11.7 Fibrous Dysplasia and McCune–Albright Syndrome

11.7.1 Definition/Description

- Fibrous dysplasia is characterized by focal replacement of normal bone by proliferation of cellular fibrous connective tissue. Three types occur:
  - Monostotic (single bone)
  - Polyostotic (multiple bones)
  - McCune–Albright syndrome (multiple bones plus endocrine abnormalities)

11.7.2 Frequency

- Uncommon to rare
- Represents about 2.5% of all bone tumours and over 7% of all benign tumours

11.7.3 Aetiology

- A growth disturbance of bone caused by mutation in the *GNAS1* gene
- Defect in osteoblastic differentiation and maturation

11.7.4 Clinical Features

- Monostotic fibrous dysplasia:
  - Most common form: 70–85% of patients with fibrous dysplasia are affected with monostotic type
  - Ribs, femur, tibia commonly involved
  - In 30% of patients, cranial or facial bones are affected
  - Maxilla is affected more often than mandible
  - Adjacent facial bones (zygoma, sphenoid, frontal, and ethmoid bones may be occasionally involved (craniofacial fibrous dysplasia)
  - Predilection in second and third decades of life
  - No sex predilection
  - Slow, unilateral painless growth
  - Adjacent teeth may be displaced
- Polyostotic fibrous dysplasia:
  - Two or more bones are involved in 25% of patients with fibrous dysplasia
  - 50% may affect craniofacial bones
  - Occurs usually under 10 years of age
  - Female predilection
  - Pain and fracture of long bones common
  - Facial asymmetry
- McCune–Albright syndrome:
  - Polyostotic fibrous dysplasia lesions with two or more bones involved
  - Cafe-au lait (colour of coffee with hot milk) skin pigmentation
  - Multiple endocrine abnormalities (sexual precocity, hyperthyroidism hyperparathyroidism, etc.)

11.7.5 Radiographical Features

- Monostotic fibrous dysplasia:
  - Lesion shows 'ground glass' appearance with poorly defined margins (Figure 11.7a)
  - Occasionally mixed (radiolucent and radiopaque) appearance
  - Large mandibular lesion: buccolingual expansion and superior displacement of the inferior alveolar canal
- Polyostotic fibrous dysplasia:
  - Multiple ground-glass appearances and radiolucencies of varying degree
- McCune–Albright syndrome:
  - Multiple ground-glass appearances and radiolucencies of varying degree

Figure 11.7 Fibrous dysplasia of the mandible. (a) Panoramic radiograph showing diffuse radio-opacity in the right maxilla with a ground glass appearance (*source:* reproduced with permission from Ramdas, K., Lucas, E., Thomas, G. et al. 2008) A Digital Manual for the Early Diagnosis of Oral Neoplasia. Lyon: IARC. Available from http://screening.iarc.fr/atlasoral.php?lang=1). (b) Photomicrograph showing irregular bone trabeculae in fibrous background. Note lack of osteoblastic rimming in the bony trabeculae. Spindle cells in the stroma are inactive. (*Source:* by kind permission of Dr Jose Mantilla, Department of Laboratory Medicine and Pathology University of Washington, USA).

(a)

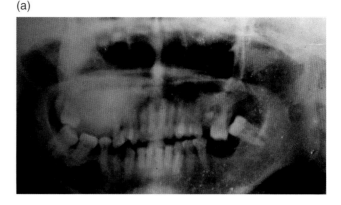

(b)

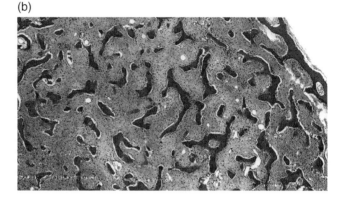

11.7.6   Microscopic features

- All three types:
  - Early stage:
    - Cell-rich fibrous connective tissue with area of slender trabecular woven bone (resembling Chinese characters; Figure 11.7b)
    - At the periphery, lesion fuses with normal bone without any capsule or demarcation
    - Osteoblastic activity is absent or minimal
  - Mature lesions:
    - Woven bone is replaced by lamellar bone

11.7.7   Differential Diagnosis

- Ossifying fibroma
- Cemento-ossifying fibroma
- Cemento-osseous dysplasia
- Central giant cell granuloma
- Giant cell tumour

11.7.8   Diagnosis

- History
- Clinical findings

- Radiography and CT
- Biochemistry: alkaline phosphatase levels (raised in polyostotic types)
- Microscopic findings (confirmatory)
- Genetic testing for *GNAS* mutation
- Correlation of clinical, imaging, biochemical investigation results microscopic findings are helpful

11.7.9 Management

- Stabilization upon skeletal maturation is often seen
- Bisphosphonates (relieve bone pain in fibrous dysplasia)
- Surgical shaving and debulking procedures
- In McCune–Albright syndrome, endocrinopathies should be detected and treated
- Osteosarcoma development in fibrous dysplasia lesions of McCune–Albright syndrome is a possibility

11.7.10 Prognosis

- Fair to good
- Regrowth often reported

11.8   Mandibular and Palatine Tori: Key Features

- Developmental localized swellings of the jawbone
- Very common
- May present denture problems
- Two types: torus mandibularis and torus palatinus
- Torus mandibularis:
  - Bony swelling lingual aspect of the mandible above the mylohyoid ridge usually lingual to the canine/premolar area
  - Small torus is single and smooth; may be seen as multiple hard nodules
  - Sometimes bilateral and symmetrical (Figure 11.8a)
- Torus palatinus:
  - Location: posterior of the midline of the hard palate
  - Sometimes lobular and symmetrical (Figure 11.8b)
- Tori may cause medication-related osteonecrosis if not prophylactically excised
- Other than tori, symmetrical bony exostoses are often found on the buccal aspect of the alveolar bone

11.9   Focal Osteoporotic Bone Marrow Defect: Key Features

- A radiolucent area in the bone of unknown aetiology probably a variation of normal bone
- Altered repair of a previously traumatized area of bone is implicated as the cause in some cases
- Shows female predilection
- Common in the fourth to the sixth decades

(a)

(b)

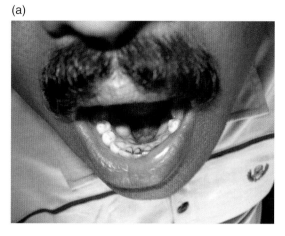

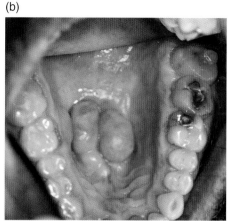

Figure 11.8 (a) Torus mandibularis. Note the bilaterally symmetrical nodular bony enlargement in the mandibular premolar region (*source:* reproduced with permission from Ramdas, K., Lucas, E., Thomas, G. et al. 2008) A Digital Manual for the Early Diagnosis of Oral Neoplasia. Lyon: IARC. Available from http:// screening.iarc.fr/atlasoral.php?lang=1). (b) Torus palatinus. Note the lobular bony swellings in the midline of the palate (*source:* by kind permission of Dr Anura Ariyawardana, JCU School of Dentistry, Cairns, Australia).

- Posterior mandible is the most common site, rare in maxilla
- Asymptomatic; detected on routine panoramic radiography
- Radiographically seen as a round to oval ill-defined radiolucency
- Often mistaken for cystic lesions or tumours
- Microscopic examination shows normal haematopoietic tissue with fat cells erythrocytes and leukocytes in various stages of maturation
- Usually no treatment required

Recommended Reading

Bhat, M.A., Laway, B.A., Mantoo, S. et al. (2012). Cleidocranial dysplasia: a rare cause of disproportionate severe short stature. *Oman Medical Journal* 27: 408–410.

Carvalho, R., Kurochka, V., Rocha, J., and Soares Fernandes, J. (2011). Brown tumor of the mandible: magnetic susceptibility demonstrated by MRI. *Radiology Case Reports* 7: 662.

Chandar, V.V. and Priya, A. (2010). Bilateral fibrous dysplasia of the mandible in a 7-year-old male patient-a rare case. *Journal of the Indian Society of Pedodontics and Preventive Dentistry* 28: 126–129.

Chanson, P. and Salenave, S. (2008). Acromegaly. *Orphanet Journal of Rare Diseases* 3: 17. https://doi. org/10.1186/1750-1172-3-17.

Dinkar, A.D., Sahai, S., and Sharma, M. (2014). Primary hyperparathyroidism presenting as an exophytic mandibular mass. *DFMR* 36 (6): 360–363.

Mazhar, H., Samudrawar, R., Gupta, R., and Kashyap, M.K. (2018). Cherubism in 12 year young female. *Annals of Maxillofacial Surgery* 8: 373–376.

Mir, S.A. (2012). Cleidocranial dysplasia: a rare cause of disproportionate severe short stature. *Oman Medical Journal* 27: 408–410.

Mundlos, S. (1999). Cleidocranial dysplasia: clinical and molecular genetics. *Journal of Medical Genetics* 36: 177–182.

Neville, B.W., Damm, D.D., Allen, C.M., and Chi, C.A. (2016). Bone pathology. In: *Oral and Maxillofacial Pathology*, e4, 572–591. St Louis, MO: Elsevier.

Odell, E.W. (2017). Genetic, metabolic and other non-neoplastic bone diseases. In: *Cawson's Essentials of Oral Pathology and Oral Medicine*, 9e, 205–221. Edinburgh: Elsevier.

Padbury, A.D. Jr., Tözüm, T.F., Taba, M. Jr. et al. (2006). The impact of primary hyperparathyroidism on the oral cavity. *Journal of Clinical Endocrinology and Metabolism* 91: 3439–3445.

Papdaki, M.E., Lietman, S.A., Levine, M.A. et al. (2012). Cherubism: best clinical practice. *Orphanet Journal of Rare Diseases* 7 (Suppl 1): S6.

Roberts, T., Stephen, L., and Beighton, P. (2013). Cleidocranial dysplasia: a review of the dental, historical, and practical implications with an overview of the South African experience. *Oral Surgery, Oral Medicine, Oral Pathology, Oral Radiology* 115: 46–55.

Rousseau, M., Retrouvey, J., and Members of the Brittle Bone Diseases Consortium (2018). Osteogenesis imperfecta: potential therapeutic approaches. *Peer J* 6: e5464. https://doi.org/10.7717/peerj.5464.

Shankar, Y.U., Misra, S.R., Vineet, D.A., and Baskaran, P. (2013). Paget disease of bone: a classic case report. *Contemporary Clinical Dentistry* 4 (2): 227–230.

Shetty, A.D., Namitha, J., and Jame, S.L. (2015). Brown tumour of mandible in association with primary hyperparathyroidism: a case report. *Journal of International Oral Health* 7 (2): 50–52.

Siddiqui, U.M., Nieves, C.A., Valencia-Guerrero, A.L., and Coyne, C. (2018). Paget disease of the mandible. *Clinical Case Reports* 4: e370–e374.

Part III

Pathology of the Oral Mucosa

12

Developmental Anomalies and Anatomical Variants of Oral Soft Tissues

---

CHAPTER MENU

12.1   Fordyce Granules: Key Features

- Sebaceous glands in the oral mucosa found in 80% of individuals
- Cannot be rubbed off with gauze
- Rarely spots fuse and seen as raised plaques
- Treatment is not required, reassurance is adequate
- For further information see Chapter 23 (section 23.6)

12.2   Double Lip: Key Features

- Fold of excess or redundant tissue on the mucosal side of the lip
- Upper lip affected more often than the lower lip
- Two types: congenital and acquired

Handbook of Oral Pathology and Oral Medicine, First Edition. S. R. Prabhu.
© 2022 John Wiley & Sons Ltd. Published 2022 by John Wiley & Sons Ltd.
Companion website: www.wiley.com/go/prabhu/oral_pathology

- Congenital form of double lip is thought to arise during the second or third month of gestation
- Acquired form of double lip may occur due to trauma or any oral habit
- Excess tissue interferes with mastication or speech or leads to habits as sucking or biting the redundant tissue
- Treatment for aesthetic purposes

12.3 Leukoedema: Key Features

- Diffuse, translucent, white, greyish thickening of the surface layers of mucosal epithelium (Figure 12.1)
- Common in people of African and Asian descent
- Common on labial and buccal mucosa
- Disappears on stretching, returns on releasing pressure
- Histological features:
  - Superficial layers show parakeratinization
  - Vacuolation of upper layers of prickle cell layers give 'basket weave' appearance
- Treatment is not required

12.4 Ankyloglossia: Key Features

- Ankyloglossia is also known as tongue-tie
- Two types: partial and complete ankyloglossia
- A congenital oral anomaly that may restrict the mobility of the tongue tip
- Caused by an unusually short, thick lingual frenulum (Figure 12.2)
- Prevalence of ankyloglossia reported in the literature varies from 0.1% to 10.7%
- Affects feeding, speech, chewing and oral hygiene
- Affected individuals may learn to compensate adequately for their decreased lingual mobility
- Surgery: frenectomy, frenuloplasty, or frenotomy

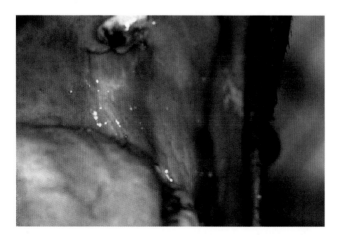

Figure 12.1 Leukoedema of the left buccal mucosa showing grey-white, diffuse, milky opalescent film. Usually, leukoedema is bilateral (*source:* reproduced with permission from Ramdas, K., Lucas, E., Thomas, G. et al. 2008. A Digital Manual for the Early Diagnosis of Oral Neoplasia. Lyon: IARC. Available from http://screening.iarc.fr/atlasoral.php?lang=1).

Figure 12.2 Ankyloglossia (*source:* Klaus D. Peter, Wiehl, Germany, https://da.wikipedia.org/wiki/ Fil:Frenulum_linguae.jpg. Licensed under CC BY-SA 3.0).

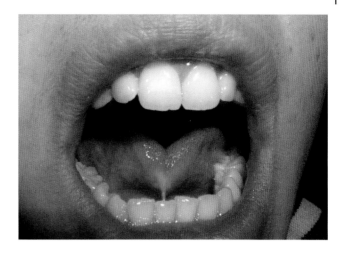

Figure 12.3 Geographic tongue.

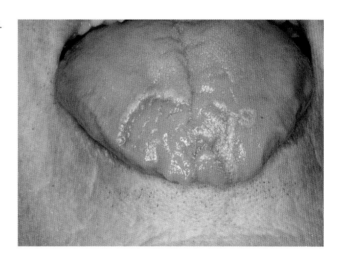

12.5 Geographic Tongue: Key Features

- Also known as erythema migrans and benign migratory glossitis
- Common condition: 2% of the population affected at any one time
- Dorsum of the tongue is the usual site
- Asymptomatic irregular smooth red map-like areas on the dorsum with a white raised margin (Figure 12.3)
- Lesions are migratory
- Thin epithelium; loss of filiform papillae
- Generally, no treatment is required for asymptomatic patients
- Reassurance that the condition is not serious and not contagious
- For symptomatic patients, treatment with antifungal agents combined with topical steroids are effective
- Treatment for symptomatic patients with nystatin–triamcinolone acetonide ointment to be applied after each meal and at bedtime

12.6   Hairy Tongue: Key Features

- Hair-like appearance on the dorsum of the tongue due to elongation of filiform papillae (Figure 12.4)
- Increased amount of keratin on the filiform papillae
- Common: affects 1% of the population
- Asymptomatic in most cases
- Common in smokers and patients with radiation and debilitating illness
- Gagging sensation or bad taste in some individuals
- Black hairy tongue in those on iron compounds, antibiotic lozenges, bismuth-containing antacids, chlorhexidine mouthwash and frequent consumption of coffee
- Not to be confused with hairy leukoplakia
- No treatment is required

12.7   Fissured Tongue: Key Features

- Presence of multiple grooves or fissures on the dorsum of the tongue (Figure 12.5)
- Unknown cause
- Often hereditary
- 2–5% prevalence in general population
- Usually asymptomatic; burning sensation in some patients
- May be associated with geographic tongue
- No specific treatment is required

12.8   Lingual Thyroid: Key Features

- Presence of ectopic thyroid between foramen caecum and the epiglottis (Figure 12.6a)
- Uncommon in general population
- Seen as a small asymptomatic nodule
- When symptomatic, patient complaints include dysphagia, dysphonia, and dyspnoea
- Hypothyroidism in 33% of patients with lingual thyroid
- Thyroid scan testing required for diagnosis

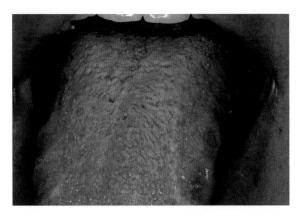

Figure 12.4   Hairy tongue (*source:* courtesy of Professor Azmi Darwazeh, Irbid, Jordan).

Figure 12.5 Fissured tongue (*source:* Laila, https://en.wikipedia.org/wiki/Fissured_tongue#/media/File:Fissured_Tongue.JPG. Licensed under CC BY-SA 3.0).

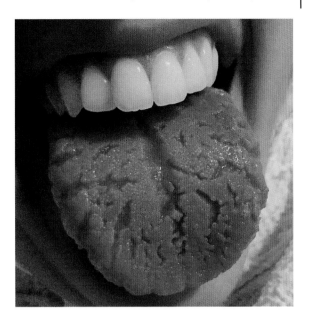

(a)

(b)

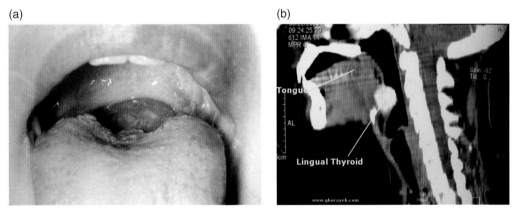

Figure 12.6 Lingual thyroid. (a) The dome shaped red fleshy mass at the base of the tongue was discovered on a routine examination of the pharynx. (b) Sagittal reconstruction of computed tomography of the neck, showing the lingual thyroid at the base of the tongue. (*Source:* images by kind permission of Bechara Y. Ghorayeb, Otolaryngology, Houston, USA.)

- CT, ultrasound, and MRI are helpful in determining the size and extent (Figure 12.6b)
- Asymptomatic patients need no treatment
- Supplemental thyroid hormone therapy for symptomatic patients
- Surgical removal of lingual thyroid for those who are not responsive for thyroid hormone therapy

12.9 Microglossia and Macroglossia: Key Features

- Uncommon developmental conditions characterized by abnormally small (Microglossia) or larger than normal (macroglossia) tongue size
- Microglossia may be associated with syndromes with hypogenesis of the mandible

- Noisy breathing, drooling, difficulty eating are common symptoms in macroglossia
- Macroglossia may cause crenations along the margins of the tongue (Figure 12.7)
- Causes of macroglossia include: lymphangioma, haemangioma, Down syndrome, neurofibromatosis, amyloidosis, myxoedema, acromegaly, and myasthenia gravis
- Reduction glossectomy is useful for symptomatic cases of macroglossia
- Asymptomatic cases do not require treatment
- Speech therapy is useful

12.10   Bifid Tongue: Key Features

- A congenital structural defect of the tongue in which its anterior part is divided
- longitudinally (Figure 12.8)
- Bifid tongue is a rare congenital anomaly usually associated with syndromes and infrequently associated with non-syndromic cases
- Most common condition in patients with orofacial–digital syndrome
- Abnormal or partial non-fusion of branchial arches may lead to congenital anomalies of tongue, including bifid tongue
- Presents feeding and speech difficulties
- Surgical correction is required

12.11   Bifid Uvula: Key Features

- Bifid uvula is usually found in infants; rare in adults
- Failure of the developmental process involved in the soft palate and uvula development can result in complete or partial clefts of the soft palate and uvula (Figure 12.9)
- Bifid uvula is often regarded as a marker for submucous cleft palate
- Bifid uvula can cause otitis media, speech problems, and regurgitation
- Bifid uvula is a feature of Loeys–Dietz syndrome
- Bifid uvula may be associated with increased risk of schizophrenia, mild mental retardation, and chromosomal disorder

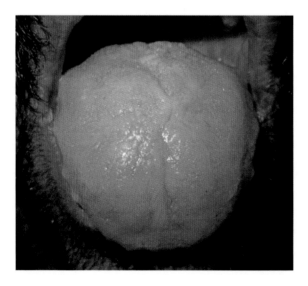

Figure 12.7   Macroglossia with crenations along the margins and loss of papillae on dorsum surface of the tongue (*Source:* Deshpande, P., Guledgud, M.V., Patil, K. et al., https://en.wikipedia.org/wiki/Crenated_tongue#/media/File:Macroglossia_with_crenations_along_the_margins_and_loss_of_papillae_on_dorsum_surface_of_the_tongue.png. Licensed under CC BY-SA 3.0).

Figure 12.8 Bifid tongue (*source:* by kind permission of Dr Aisha Siddiqua, Albadar Rural Dental College and Hospital, Gulbarga, Karnataka, India).

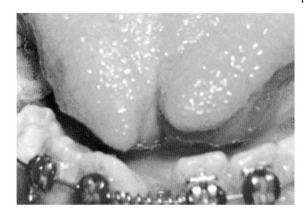

Figure 12.9 Bifid uvula.

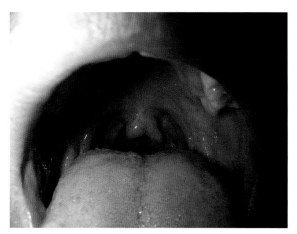

12.12 Cleft Lip: Key Features

- Cleft lip is caused by a failure of the normal orofacial development between 6 and 12 weeks of embryonic life
- Most common facial deformity. Most cases are associated with cleft palate
- Majority are idiopathic; however, a number of drugs during pregnancy have been implicated, including phenytoin, carbamazepine, steroids, and diazepam. Heavy smoking and folic acid deficiency during pregnancy are also risk factors
- It can be unilateral or bilateral and incomplete or complete (Figure 12.10 a, b and c)
- Cleft lip with cleft palate presents problems with feeding, speech, and hearing
- Corrective surgery is recommended

12.13 Calibre Persistent Labial Artery: Key Features

- A common vascular anomaly characterized by extension of main arterial branch into the superficial submucosal tissues without a reduction in its diameter
- Common among the elderly
- Lip is the most common site in the mouth; usually asymptomatic
- Seen as a raised linear or papular pink or blue coloured pulsatile elevation (Figure 12.11 a and b)

(a)   (b)   (c)

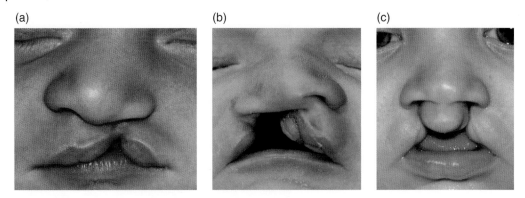

Figure 12.10   (a–c) Small, incomplete cleft lip (a), complete unilateral cleft lip (b) and bilateral cleft lip (c).

(a)   (b)

(c)

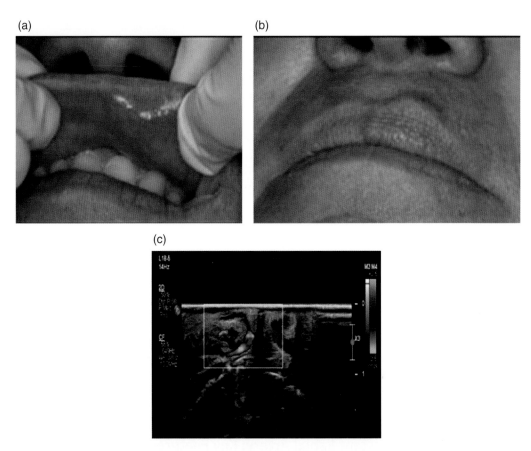

Figure 12.11   Calibre persistent labial artery. (a). Note a linear elevated pink submucosal mass on the left labial mucosa of the upper lip and (b) a linear swelling of the skin above the vermillion border corresponding to the mucosal lesion. (c). Ultrasonography of the lesion demonstrated a 6x6x10mm non-cystic lesion in the muscular layer of the upper lip with marked arterial flow, confirming the clinical diagnosis of a calibre persistent labial artery. (By kind permission of Dr. Jacinta Vu, UWA Dental School, Perth, Western Australia)

- Pulsation of the lesion is always felt with ungloved fingers
- Differential diagnosis includes mucocele, varicosities, venous lakes, haemangiomas and vascular malformations
- Ultrasound is confirmatory (Figure 12.11c)
- No treatment is required

12.14 Epstein's Pearl and Bohn's Nodules: Key Features

- Small developmental lesions of the newborn
- Common: 55–85% of the neonates
- Seen as small (1–3 mm) white or yellow-white papules in both instances but on different locations
- Epstein's pearl is a small, firm, white, keratin-filled cyst, located on the mid palatine raphe (Figure 12.12)
- Bohn's nodules: they occur on the alveolar ridge, more commonly on the maxillary than mandibular
- Microscopically keratin-filled cysts lined by stratified squamous epithelium
- No treatment is required, self-healing lesions

12.15 Dermoid and Epidermoid Cysts: Key Features

- Dermoid cyst: developmental cystic malformation characterized by dermal adnexal structures (hair follicles, sebaceous and sweat glands) in the epithelium lined cyst wall
- Epidermoid cyst: developmental cystic epithelium lined malformation without adnexal structures in the epithelium
- Dermoid/epidermoid cysts:
  - Common in the midline of the floor of the mouth (Figure 12.13a)
  - Size: a few millimetres to 12 cm in diameter
  - Common in children and young adults
  - 15% are congenital
  - Common symptoms: difficulty in eating, speaking
  - Slow-growing rubbery mass, pitting on pressure
  - Contents: cheesy keratinous material
  - If located above the geniohyoid muscle, tongue is elevated

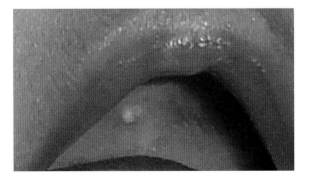

Figure 12.12   Epstein pearl in a five-week-old infant (*source:* Sghael).

(a)   (b)

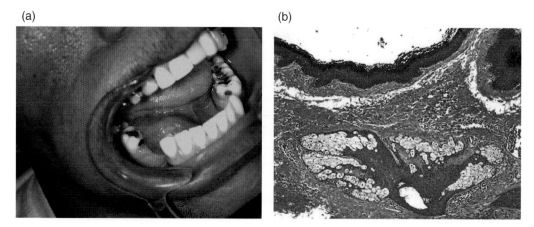

Figure 12.13 Oral dermoid cyst. (a) Presenting as a smooth-surfaced, soft tissue swelling on the floor of the mouth. (b) Histopathology shows a cystic lesion lined by hyperorthokeratinized stratified squamous epithelium with sebaceous glands and hair follicles. (*Source:* images from Vieira, E.M.M., Borges, A.H., Volpato, L.E.R. et al. (2014). Unusual dermoid cyst in oral cavity. *Case Reports in Pathology* 2014: 389752. doi: 10.1155/2014/389752. Reproduced under CC BY 3.0.)

- If located below the geniohyoid muscle, submental swelling results causing 'double chin'
- Differential diagnosis: ranula, unilateral or bilateral blockage of Wharton's ducts, lipoma, thyroglossal duct cyst, cystic hygroma, and branchial cleft cysts
- Diagnosis: history, clinical findings, fine needle aspiration, CT, and MRI
- Microscopy is confirmatory; histopathology of oral dermoid cyst shows cutaneous adnexal structures (Figure 12.13b). When cutaneous appendages are not found, the cyst is called an epidermoid cyst
- Treatment by surgical removal

12.16   Oral Varicosities: Key Features

- Varicosities are abnormally dilated veins
- Lingual varicosities are common on the ventral surface of the tongue (Figure 12.14)
- Labial and buccal mucosa may also be involved. On the lips they may resemble mucoceles
- Often found in the elderly
- Possibly caused by weakening of the vessel walls
- Clinically seen as purple, coloured dots, nodules, or tortuous veins
- Clinical appearance is diagnostic
- No treatment is required

12.17   Lymphoid Aggregates: Key Features

- Lymphoid aggregates are collection of normal or hyperplastic oral lymphoid tissue
- Common on the lateral surfaces of the tongue (Figure 12.15)
- Other sites: oropharynx and soft palate
- Usually asymptomatic
- Symptomatic when inflamed due to bacterial or viral infections

Figure 12.14 Lingual varicosities on the ventral tongue.

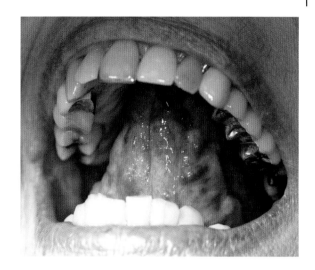

Figure 12.15 Lymphoid aggregate located at the posterolateral surface of the tongue. (*Source:* Molly S. Rosebush, K. Mark Anderson and Yeshwant B. Rawal (February 19th 2014). Normal Oral Cavity Findings and Variants of Normal, Diagnosis and Management of Oral Lesions and Conditions: A Resource Handbook for the Clinician, Cesar A. Migliorati and Fotinos S. Panagakos, IntechOpen, DOI: 10.5772/57597. Available from: https://www.intechopen.com/books/diagnosis-and-management-of-oral-lesions-and-conditions-a-resource-handbook-for-the-clinician/normal-oral-cavity-findings-and-variants-of-normal)

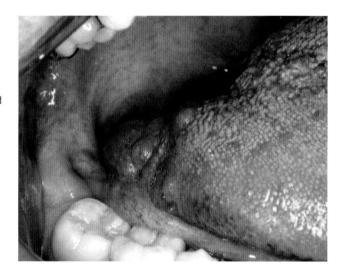

- Occasionally mistaken for oral squamous cell carcinoma or lymphoma
- Diagnosis on clinical grounds
- No treatment is required

12.18 Parotid Papilla: Key Features

- Parotid papilla is the projection seen at the oral opening of the duct of the parotid salivary gland (Figure 12.16)
- Located into the vestibule opposite the second upper left and right molar teeth
- This is a normal structure
- Diagnosed on clinical appearance
- No treatment is required

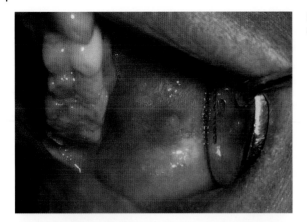

Figure 12.16 Parotid papilla appearing as a nodule on the buccal mucosa.

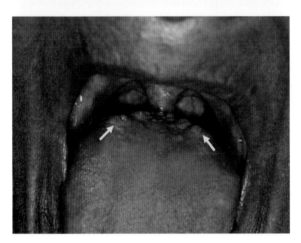

Figure 12.17 Prominent circumvallate papillae on the posterior tongue (yellow arrows) (*source:* reproduced with permission from Ramdas, K., Lucas, E., Thomas, G. et al. 2008. *A Digital Manual for the Early Diagnosis of Oral Neoplasia.* Lyon: IARC. Available from http://screening.iarc.fr/atlasoral. php?lang=1).

12.19   Circumvallate Papillae: Key Features

- The circumvallate papillae are 8–12 dome-shaped structures that are situated on the dorsum of the tongue immediately in front of the foramen caecum and sulcus terminalis
- These are normal structures
- Occasionally enlarged circumvallate papillae may be mistaken for pathology (Figure 12.17)
- Diagnosis on clinical appearance
- No treatment required

12.20   Physiological Pigmentation: Key Features

- Also known as racial pigmentation
- Commonly seen in individuals of African descent
- A normal physiological process
- Pigmented patches (brown to black) on the gingiva (Figure 12.18) or other oral mucosal sites
- Patches often mimic pigmentation of Addison's disease, smoker's melanosis, and drug related pigmentation

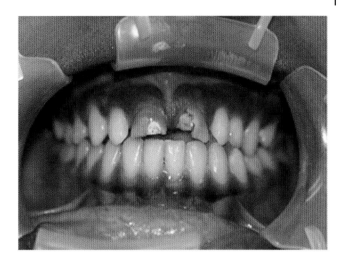

Figure 12.18 Generalized black-brown physiological melanin hyperpigmentation of the maxillary and mandibular gingiva, not transgressing the mucogingival junction. The patient's main concern was her carious incisors (*source:* reproduced with permission from Feller, L., Khammissa, R.A.G., Lemmer, J. et al. 2017. Oral mucosal melanosis. In: Melanin (ed. M. Blumenberg), doi: 10.5772/65567. IntechOpen. Available from: https://www.intechopen.com/books/melanin/oral-mucosal-melanosis).

- Pigmentation is usually diffuse and symmetrical
- Diagnosis on clinical grounds
- No treatment is required

Recommended Reading

Bakshi, P.S., Jindal, N., Kaushik, A., and Leekha, S. (2014). An appraisal of congenital maxillary lip with a case report. *European Journal of General Dentistry* 3: 199–201.

Neville, B.W., Damm, D.D., Allen, C.M., and Chi, C.A. (2016). Developmental defects of the oral and maxillofacial region. In: *Oral and Maxillofacial Pathology*, 4e, 1–22. St Louis, MO: Elsevier.

Odell, E.W. (2017). Disorders of development. In: *Cawson's Essentials of Oral Pathology and Oral Medicine*, 9e, 45–50. Edinburgh: Elsevier.

Pinna, P., Cocco, F., Campus, G. et al. (2019). Genetic and developmental disorders of the oral mucosa: epidemiology; molecular mechanisms; diagnostic criteria; management. *Periodontology 2000* 80: 12–27.

Vieira, E.M.M., Borges, A.H., Volpato, L.E.R. et al. (2014). Unusual dermoid cyst in oral cavity. *Case Reports in Pathology* 2014: 389752.

13

Bacterial Infections of the Oral Mucosa

13.1   Scarlet Fever: Key Features

- A systemic infection caused by group A *beta haemolytic streptococci*
- Common in children five to seven years
- Tonsils, pharynx and tongue become erythematous, oedematous (tonsillitis and pharyngitis)
- Tonsillar crypts fill with yellowish exudate
- Petechiae appear on the soft palate
- Skin rash appears due to the action of erythrogenic toxin produced by the organisms
- Tongue shows white coat through which red fungiform papillae are visible (white strawberry tongue
- White-coat desquamates and the tongue reveals an erythematous dorsal surface (red strawberry tongue) with hyperplastic fungiform papillae
- Fever, headache, malaise, and nausea are frequent
- Rash subsides in about six days
- Throat culture is diagnostic
- Penicillin V or amoxycillin are antibiotics of choice
- Ibuprofen for fever
- Prognosis is excellent with adequate treatment
- Complications may include pneumonia, otitis media, rheumatic fever, and hepatitis

13.2   Syphilis

13.2.1   Definition/Description

- Syphilis is an infectious venereal disease caused by the spirochete *Treponema pallidum*

Handbook of Oral Pathology and Oral Medicine, First Edition. S. R. Prabhu.
© 2022 John Wiley & Sons Ltd. Published 2022 by John Wiley & Sons Ltd.
Companion website: www.wiley.com/go/prabhu/oral_pathology

13.2.2 Frequency

- Syphilis remains prevalent in many developing countries
- Prevalent in some areas of North America, Asia, and Europe, especially Eastern Europe
- Syphilis acquisition increases the risk of HIV acquisition two- to five-fold

13.2.3 Aetiology/Risk Factors

- Spirochete *Treponema pallidum* is the causative agent
- Syphilis is transmissible by sexual contact
- Maternal infection is from mother to fetus in utero
- Infection via blood product transfusion is possible but rare
- Risk factors include:
  - Unprotected sex (genital, oral, anal)
  - Men having sex with men
  - HIV infection
  - Sex workers
  - Having a sexual partner who has tested positive for syphilis
- Humans are the only proven natural host

13.2.4 Clinical Features

- If untreated, acquired syphilis progresses through four stages: primary, secondary, latent, and tertiary
- Fetal infection causes congenital syphilis (not discussed in this chapter)
- Primary syphilis oral manifestations:
  - Chancre develops two to eight weeks after infection at the site of inoculation (Figure 13.1a)
  - Lips and tip of the tongue are commonly involved
  - Chancre progresses from a papule to an ulcer, which is typically painless, indurated, well circumscribed, round to oval with a clean base
  - Surface breaks and becomes an indurated raised ulcer after a few days
  - Regional lymph nodes are enlarged (rubbery consistency)
  - Chancres are highly infectious and heal spontaneously within one to six weeks
- Secondary syphilis oral manifestations:
  - Symptoms appear within one to four months after infection
  - A rash occurs in 75–100% of patients with secondary syphilis
  - Fever, malaise, and generalized lymphadenopathy are common
  - Pinkish symmetrically distributed macular skin lesions on the trunk
  - Ulcers on tongue, tonsils, and lips covered by greyish membrane (Figure 13.1b)
  - Mucosal 'snail's track' ulcers and mucous patches are characteristic
  - Papillary lesions called condyloma lata develop in some cases
  - Secondary syphilis is a highly infectious stage
- Latent syphilis:
  - Characterized by the persistence of *T. pallidum* organisms in the body without causing signs or symptoms
  - May last for several years
- Tertiary syphilis oral manifestations:
  - Nearly 30% of patients develop tertiary stage disease

(a)

(b)

(c)

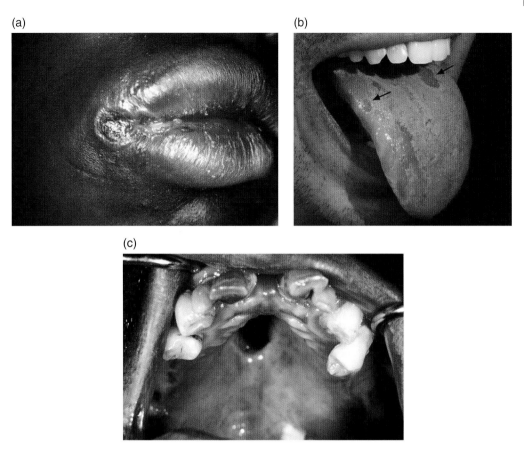

Figure 13.1 Syphilis. (a) Primary: oral chancre at the corner of the mouth. Syphilitic chancres are typically round, firm, and painless. (b) Secondary: shallow ulcers on the tongue (arrows). (c) Tertiary: palatal perforation (gumma). (*source:* a and c, Centers for Disease Control and Prevention Public Health Image Library (CDC/Robert E. Sumpter, 1967); b, reproduced with permission from National STD Curriculum. By Andrew W. Hahn, and Lindley A. Barbee, 24 February 2020; www.syphilis.uw.edu.)

- Oral lesions: interstitial glossitis, syphilitic leukoplakia and gumma (a necrotic lesion seen on the palate, tongue, or tonsils)
- Interstitial glossitis and leukoplakia seen on the dorsum of the tongue may carry malignant potential
- Palatal gumma may perforate the palate (Figure 13.1c)

13.2.5 Microscopic Features

- Non-specific chronic inflammation with plasma cells and lymphocytes
- Evidence of ulceration and endarteritis
- Granulomatous inflammation with giant cells and histiocytes in tertiary stage

13.2.6 Differential Diagnosis

- Ulcerative deep fungal infections
- Traumatic ulcer

- Squamous cell carcinoma presenting as an ulcer
- Tobacco-associated or idiopathic leukoplakia
- Midline granuloma
- Granulomatosis with polyangiitis (Wegener's granulomatosis)

13.2.7 Diagnosis

- History
- Clinical findings
- Serology and polymerase chain reaction results
- Dark ground illumination test of the smear from lesions
- Biopsy: immunohistochemical staining of tissue (to detect the organisms)
- Note: *T. pallidum* cannot be cultured

13.2.8 Management

- Parenteral penicillin is the antibiotic of choice (by specialists)
- Surgical and prosthetic interventions for palatal perforation (gumma)

13.2.9 Prognosis

- Prognosis is good for lesions of primary and secondary stage disease and fair for tertiary stage lesions

13.3   Gonorrhoea: Key Features

- A sexually transmitted bacterial disease caused by *Neisseria gonorrhoeae*
- Those at risk include injecting drug users, prostitutes, homosexual men, and those with low socioeconomic level
- Most lesions occur in the genital area with purulent discharge
- Often asymptomatic in women
- Symptomatic women complain of vaginal discharge, itching, and intermenstrual bleeding
- Uterus and ovaries can be affected, causing pelvic inflammatory disease
- In men, urethral discharge is common
- Disseminated disease results in about 3% of patients causing systemic bacteraemia
- Oropharyngeal/oral lesions may occur from oral sex or septicaemia
- Pharyngeal erythema and tonsillar inflammation with punctate pustules are common pharyngeal manifestations
- Oral mucosa is inflamed with erythematous, pustular, erosive, or ulcerated lesions (gonococcal stomatitis) (Figure 13.2)
- In males, purulent material from urethra stained with Gram stain is useful to demonstrate organisms
- Culture of organisms from endocervical swabs is diagnostic in women
- Cephalosporins are effective against gonorrhoea

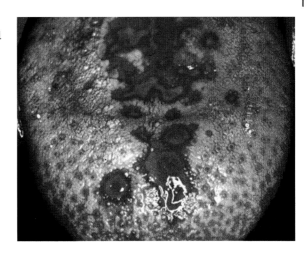

Figure 13.2 Gonococcal stomatitis. Note inflamed erythematous lesions on the dorsal surface of the tongue. (*Source:* Center for Disease Control and Prevention. USA)

13.4 Tuberculosis

13.4.1 Definition/Description

- Tuberculosis (TB) is a chronic granulomatous specific infection caused by *Mycobacterium tuberculosis*

13.4.2 Frequency

- Global estimates: two billion people infected

13.4.3 Aetiology/Risk Factors

- Causative agent: Acid fast bacillus *M. tuberculosis*
- Less common agent *M. avium intracellulare*
- At risk individuals include those with:
  - HIV infection
  - Substance abuse
  - Silicosis
  - Diabetes mellitus
  - Severe kidney disease
  - Low body weight
  - Organ transplants
  - Head and neck cancer
  - Crowded living conditions
  - Medical treatments such as corticosteroids or organ transplant
  - Specialized treatment for rheumatoid arthritis or Crohn's disease
- Types: primary and secondary:
  - Primary: usually involves lungs (pulmonary TB) of previously unexposed people
  - Secondary: usually infects people who have been previously infected or immunocompromised/immunosuppressed. This causes miliary TB (widespread dissemination by haematogenous spread)

13.4.4 Clinical and Radiological Features

- Pulmonary TB general symptoms:
  - Low-grade fever
  - Anorexia
  - Malaise
  - Night sweats
  - Weight loss
  - Productive cough
  - Haemoptysis
  - Chest pain
- Extra pulmonary TB includes:
  - Skin lesions (lupus vulgaris), bone, kidneys, central nervous system, and gastrointestinal tract
  - Head and neck sites: lymph nodes, larynx, pharynx, sinuses, nasal cavity, oesophagus, cervical spine, and oral cavity
  - Oral cavity:
    - o Oral lesions of TB include chronic non-healing ulcer, non-healing socket, or stomatitis
    - o Oral mucosal sites include tongue (mid-dorsal surface or lateral borders), gingiva, lips, buccal mucosa, and soft and hard palate
    - o Oral tuberculous ulcer:
      - o Usually due to secondary infection of the mucosa from pulmonary TB
      - o Reported prevalence: 0.5–5%
      - o Typically solitary painless angular ulcer with overhanging indurated edges (Figure 13.3 a and b)
      - o Cervical lymph nodes may be enlarged
      - o Primary TB of oral mucosa is extremely rare
      - o Intrabony lesions are lytic and sequestrate with radiographical features of osteomyelitis
      - o Oropharyngeal lymphoid tissue involvement (scrofula) solely due to drinking contaminated milk may occur but is rare
      - o On plain radiography of the chest, primary TB manifests as an area of homogeneous parenchymal consolidation (Figure13.3c)

13.4.5 Microscopic Findings

- Centrally necrotic granulomas with peripheral multinucleated Langhans' giant cells Figure 13.3d–f)
- Positive acid-fast or Ziehl–Neelsen tissue staining of microorganisms from oral lesions and sputum

13.4.6 Differential Diagnosis

- Squamous cell carcinoma ulcer
- Syphilitic ulcer
- Deep mycotic ulcer
- Traumatic ulcer
- Lymphoma (cervical node involvement)

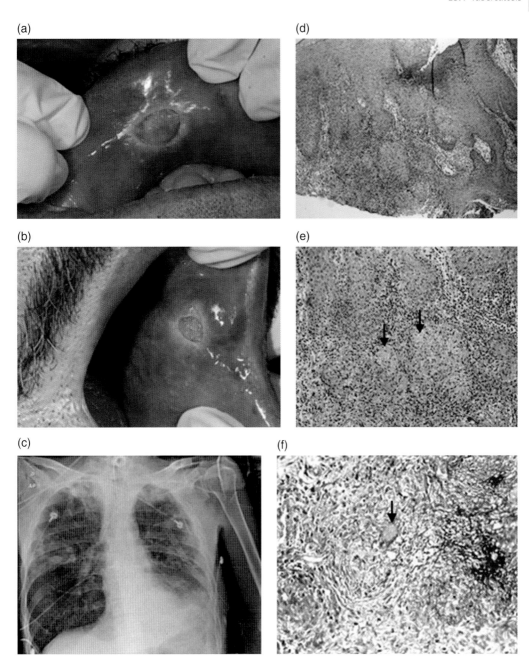

Figure 13.3 (a-f) Oral, radiographic and microscopic features of tuberculosis. (a). Ulcerative lesions with granulomatous center and whitish halo on the upper labial mucosa near the mid line and (b) on the left buccal mucosa near the labial commissure. (c). Chest radiograph showing the presence of active disease manifested as budding tree-like centrilobular nodules in both lungs. (d). Photomicrograph shows granulomas surrounded by intense mixed inflammatory infiltrate, with inflammatory cells inside the epithelium (H&E stain). (e). Well-shaped granulomas surrounded by epithelioid histiocytes and inflammatory cells. Two black arrows indicate incipient necrosis (H&E stain). (f). Ziehl–Neelsen stained section shows giant Langhans cell, with nuclei distributed across the peripheral cytoplasm, in a necklace pattern (black arrow). (*source:* by kind permission of Dr Maria Cristina Munerato, Brazil.)

13.4.7   Diagnosis

- History (medical, dental, social, family and lesional history)
- Clinical findings
- Microbiology: culture, Ziehl–Neelsen stained sputum and histopathology of the lesion
- Tuberculin skin test: two-step Mantoux test

13.4.8   Management

- Systemic chemotherapy: isoniazid, rifampin, streptomycin, and other anti-tuberculous drugs (to be administered by specialists)
- Oral lesions respond to systemic treatment

13.4.9   Prognosis

- Good prognosis for those adequately treated
- Prognosis is fair in immunosuppressed patients
- Multi-drug resistant organisms may be present which present difficulties for the clinicians

Recommended Reading

Bandara, H.M.H.N. and Samaranayake, L.P. (2019). Viral, bacterial, and fungal infections of the oral mucosa: types, incidence, predisposing factors, diagnostic algorithms, and management. *Periodontology 2000* 80 (1): 148–176.

Dahlén, G. (2009). Bacterial infections of the oral mucosa. *Periodontol 2000* 49: 13–38.

Li, X., Kolltveit, K.M., Tronstad, L., and Olsen, I. (2000). Systemic diseases caused by oral infection. *Clinical Microbiology Reviews* 13: 547–558.

Neville, B.W., Damm, D.D., Allen, C.M., and Chi, C.A. (2016). Bacterial infections. In: *Oral and Maxillofacial Pathology*, 4e, 164–186. St Louis, MO: Elsevier.

Odell, E.W. (2017). Diseases of the oral mucosa: mucosal infections. In: *Cawson's Essentials of Oral Pathology and Oral Medicine*, 9e, 235–250. Edinburgh: Elsevier.

Preshaw, P.M., Alba, A.L., Herrera, D. et al. (2012). Periodontitis and diabetes: a two-way relationship. *Diabetologia* 55 (1): 21–31.

14

Fungal Infections of the Oral Mucosa

CHAPTER MENU
14.1 Candidosis (Candidiasis) 14.2 Histoplasmosis 14.3 Blastomycosis: Key Features

14.1 Candidosis (Candidiasis)

14.1.1 Definition/Description

- Oral candidosis (oral candidiasis) is a fungal infection caused by several species of candida that are normally present (as commensal organisms) in the mouths of nearly one third of normal population
- Carrying candidal species in the oral cavity does not cause clinical disease; infection becomes evident in those with local or systemic predisposing factors
- Candidal yeasts are not pathogenic; invasive hyphal forms cause disease
- The most pathogenic candidal species include: *Candida albicans, C. glabrata, C. tropicalis, and C. krusei*
- The majority of oral candidosis infections are caused by *C. albicans*
- Oral candidosis includes a spectrum of presentations, including:
  - Pseudomembranous candidosis (thrush)
  - Erythematous candidosis (Acute atrophic candidosis)
  - Denture-induced stomatitis (chronic atrophic candidosis, denture sore mouth)
  - Chronic hyperplastic candidosis (candidal leukoplakia)
  - Median rhomboid glossitis
  - Angular cheilitis (perleche, cheilosis, or angular stomatitis)
  - Chronic mucocutaneous candidosis

14.1.2 Frequency

- The oral carriage of candida organisms is reported to be 30–45% in the general healthy adult population

Handbook of Oral Pathology and Oral Medicine, First Edition. S. R. Prabhu.
© 2022 John Wiley & Sons Ltd. Published 2022 by John Wiley & Sons Ltd.
Companion website: www.wiley.com/go/prabhu/oral_pathology

- Oral candidosis is common among those with predisposing/risk factors. Some examples are:
  - Approximately 5–7% of infants develop oral candidosis
  - Its prevalence in people with AIDS is estimated to be 9–31%
  - Candidosis is prevalent close to 20% in cancer patients

14.1.3   Aetiology/Risk Factors

- Causative agent: *Candida* species, particularly *C. albicans*
- Risk factors:
  - Patients on broad-spectrum antibiotics
  - Those with impaired immune system
  - HIV infection
  - Infants
  - Elderly individuals
  - Those with endocrinopathy (e.g. diabetes mellitus)
  - Anaemia and patients with leukemia
  - Steroid inhaler users
  - Patients with xerostomia
  - Poor oral hygiene
  - Denture wearers
  - Those with debilitating illness

14.1.4   Clinical features

- Pseudomembranous candidosis:
  - Asymptomatic or mild symptoms: burning sensation and taste disorder
  - White cream-coloured curd-like plaques or flecks loosely adherent to the oral mucosa (Figure 14.1)
  - Buccal mucosa palate and dorsal tongue are frequently involved
  - Plaques can be wiped off with gauge or mirror head exposing the underlying erythematous mucosa

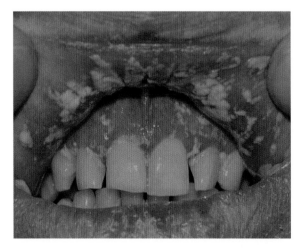

Figure 14.1   Pseudomembranous candidosis of the gingiva and lips (*source:* reproduced with permission from the National HIV Curriculum, David Spach, 5 September 2020. Retrieved from www.hiv.uw.edu).

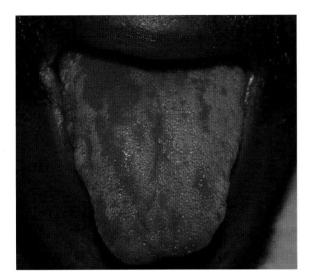

Figure 14.2   Erythematous candidosis of the tongue (*source:* reproduced with permission from the National HIV Curriculum, David Spach, 5 September 2020. Retrieved from www.hiv.uw.edu).

- Erythematous (atrophic) candidosis:
  - History of the use of broad-spectrum antibiotics (acute antibiotic stomatitis)
  - Burning mouth sensation is common
  - Loss of filiform papillae resulting in red or 'bald' areas on the tongue on the dorsum of the tongue (Figure 14.2)
- Angular cheilitis:
  - Infection at the commissures of the lips (Figure 14.3)
  - May be seen in infants with pseudomembranous candidosis, denture wearers, people who are HIV positive, and those with hyperplastic candidosis
  - Painful fissuring and inflammation of one or both commissures are characteristic
  - Fissuring may extend on to the skin in the elderly
  - Occasionally in immunodeficient persons, infection is mixed: *C. albicans* and *Staphylococcus aureus* are involved
- Denture stomatitis:
  - Occurs in 50–60% of denture wearers
  - History of the continuous use of removable denture (maxillary denture in particular)
  - Varying degree of erythema confined to the denture-bearing maxillary mucosal surface (Figure 14.4a)
  - Palatal erythema may be focal and pin-pointed, diffuse, or nodular in appearance due to papillary hyperplasia. (Figure 14.4b)
  - Usually asymptomatic
  - Occasional petechiae seen on the mucosa
- Chronic hyperplastic candidosis:
  - White patch that cannot be removed by scraping is located usually on the anterior buccal mucosa
  - Most patients are smokers
  - May resemble speckled leukoplakia (Figure 14.5)
  - A small percentage of lesions may carry malignant potential

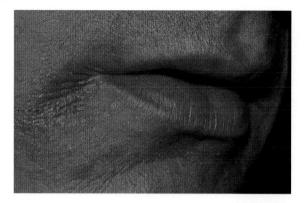

Figure 14.3 Angular cheilitis (*source:* reproduced with permission from the National HIV Curriculum, David Spach, 5 September 2020. Retrieved from www.hiv.uw.edu).

(a)

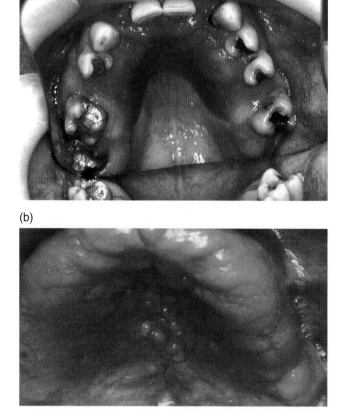

(b)

Figure 14.4 Denture stomatitis. (a) Diffuse erythema of the mucosa in contact with the partial denture. (b) Diffuse palatal erythema with papillary hyperplasia.

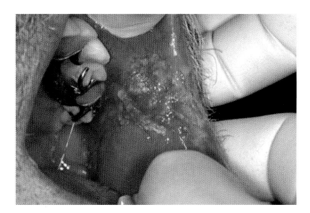

Figure 14.5 Chronic hyperplastic candidosis of the labial commissure. Well-demarcated, raised irregular fixed white patch is seen on a red background.

- Median rhomboid glossitis:
  - Seen as a red patch in the mid-line of the dorsum of the tongue at the junction of the anterior two thirds with the posterior one third (Figure 14.6)
  - Lesion is usually diamond shaped
  - Symptomless lesion
  - Surface may be nodular/lobulated
  - Matching patch on the palatal mucosa is occasionally present

14.1.5 Microscopic features

- Pseudomembranous candidosis: scrapings stained with Gram or periodic acid–Schiff stains show masses of tangled fungal hyphae, exfoliated epithelial cells and neutrophils
- Erythematous/atrophic candidosis and median rhomboid glossitis: scrapings may not show candidal hyphae. Histology shows atrophic epithelium with sparce candidal hyphae in its superficial layers
- Candidal leukoplakia: mildly parakeratotic epithelium, scanty candidal hyphae in the superficial epithelial layers, hyperplastic rete ridges, and rarely mild epithelial dysplasia. Connective tissue shows chronic inflammatory cell infiltrate (see chapter 19)

14.1.6 Differential diagnosis

- Pseudomembranous candidosis
  - White-coated tongue
  - Thermal and chemical burns
  - Lichenoid reactions
  - Leukoplakia
  - Diphtheria
- Erythematous candidosis:
  - Mucositis
  - Denture stomatitis

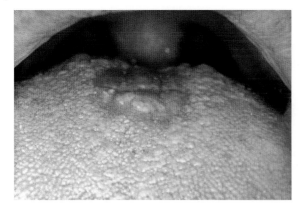

Figure 14.6 Median rhomboid glossitis. Note a lobulated bald lesion located at the junction of the anterior two thirds with the posterior one third on the dorsum of the tongue.

- – Erythema migrans
- – Thermal burns
- – Erythroplakia
- – Anaemia
- Angular cheilitis
  - – Candidal leukoplakia
  - – Chemical injury
  - – Contact mucositis
  - – Actinic, glandular, granulomatous, exfoliative and plasma cell cheilitis
  - – Herpes labialis
- Denture stomatitis:
  - – Smoker's palate
  - – Mucosal allergy
  - – Erythroplakia
  - – Thermal burn
- Chronic hyperplastic candidosis:
  - – Leukoplakia
  - – Lichen planus
  - – Angular cheilitis
  - – Squamous cell carcinoma
- Median rhomboid glossitis:
  - – Erythroplakia
  - – Geographic tongue
  - – Granular cell tumour
  - – Candidal leukoplakia
  - – Chemical injury
  - – Contact mucositis
  - – Secondary syphilis

Diagnosis

- All forms of oral candidosis:
  - – History (medical history including predisposing conditions)

- Clinical findings
- Microbiology: scrapings from the lesions and stained with periodic acid–Schiff stain and for culture
- Biopsy and histopathology for hyperplastic candidosis
- Haematology: full blood count, iron, folate, and fasting blood glucose levels

14.1.7 Management

- Topical therapy:
  - Pseudomembranous and erythematous candidosis:
    - Clotrimazole troches 10 mg, one troche to be dissolved in the mouth and swallowed, five times daily (not to be chewed)
    - Nystatin oral suspension 100 000 units/ml, 5 ml. To be rinsed for three minutes and expectorated, four times daily
  - Erythematous candidosis
    - Nystatin oral suspension 100 000 units/ml, 1–5 ml four times a day after food and swallowed; treatment for 5–14 days depending on the severity of the infection
      or
    - Amphotericin B 10 mg lozenge to be sucked and swallowed four times after food for 7–14 days
  - Angular cheilitis:
    - Nystatin–triamcinolone acetonide ointment to be applied to the affected area after meals and at bedtime until symptoms subside
    - Miconazole 2% cream to be applied sparingly to the corners of the mouth after meals and at bedtime for 14 days and to be continued for 14 days after symptoms resolve
  - Denture-induced stomatitis (denture sore mouth):
    - Ketoconazole cream 2% (15 g tube). A thin coat to be applied to the inner surface of the denture and to the affected mucosal area after meals and at bedtime
  - Chronic hyperplastic candidosis (candidal leukoplakia):
    - Miconazole 2% cream to be applied sparingly to the lesion after meals and at bedtime for 14 days and to be continued for 14 days after symptoms resolve, plus systemic antifungal (fluconazole) therapy
    - Fluconazole 100 mg tablets (15 tablets), two tablets on the first day and one tablet daily for 14 days
  - Median rhomboid glossitis:
    - Treatment is not required for all cases
    - Treatment should be carried out only after identifying candida in the scrapings
    - Biopsy should not be attempted
    - Miconazole 2% cream to be applied sparingly to the lesion after food and at bedtime for 14 days and to be continued for 14 days or until scrapings are negative for candida
- Systemic therapy (for severe forms of candidosis):
  - Fluconazole 100 mg tablets (15 tablets), two tablets on the first day and one tablet daily until gone
  - Ketoconazole 200 mg tablets. (14 tablets), one tablet every day with breakfast for 14 days. To be taken with meal or orange juice
- Special considerations:
  - To prevent immediate recurrence medication should be continued for a few days after disappearance of clinical signs

- o Identifying systemic predisposing factors and their treatment (by specialists) is of paramount importance
- o Salivation should be within normal limits
- o Creams and ointments are ideal for denture wearers
- o Patients should be advised to remove dentures prior to going to bed
- o Dentures may be soaked in a sodium hypochlorite solution for 15 minutes and rinsed before use
- o Periodic denture fit assessment should be carried out (reline, rebase, or a new denture)
- o Patients to be educated about denture hygiene
- o Withdrawal of antibiotic may be necessary (in consultation with the medical practitioner)
- o Systemic antifungal agents to be used with caution in patients with impaired liver function
- o Liver function tests should be carried out periodically for those on ketoconazole for an extended period

14.1.8 Prognosis

- Prognosis is fair to good, depending on patient compliance and elimination of underlying predisposing factors

14.2 Histoplasmosis

14.2.1 Definition/description

- A systemic infection caused by the fungus *Histoplasma capsulatum*

14.2.2 Frequency

- Common in the United States
- Less common in other parts of the world

14.2.3 Aetiology/risk factors

- Natural habitat is soil
- Transmission through spore inhalation

14.2.4 Clinical features

- Three forms of disease occur: acute, chronic, and disseminated
- Acute histoplasmosis: fever, headache, malaise, and non-productive cough
- Chronic histoplasmosis: lungs are mainly affected; cough, fever, weight loss, dyspnoea, and haemoptysis
- Disseminated histoplasmosis: systemic spread to extrapulmonary sites, including oral mucosa
- People who are HIV positive are vulnerable
- Oral manifestations of disseminated histoplasmosis include:
  - Transmission of infection to oral sites is via the haematogenous route
  - Oral lesions: solitary ulceration on the palate, tongue, and buccal mucosa
  - Ulcers are indurated with firm and rolled margins (often mimicking malignant ulcer; Figure 14.7)

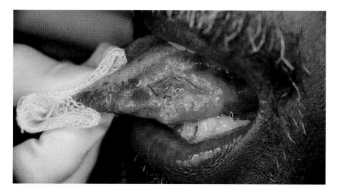

Figure 14.7 Oral histoplasmosis appearing as an ulcerative lesion mimicking squamous cell carcinoma (*source:* by kind permission of Kartikeya Patil, JSS Dental College and Hospital, JSS University, Mysore India).

14.2.5   Microscopic features

- Granulomatous inflammation with multinucleated giant cells (haematoxylin and eosin stain)
- Organisms are detected with periodic acid–Schiff-stained lesions

14.2.6   Differential diagnosis

- Squamous cell carcinoma
- Tuberculous ulcers
- Deep mycotic ulcers
- Chronic traumatic ulcer
- Tertiary syphilitic ulcer

14.2.7   Diagnosis

- Histopathology, culture, and serology (detection of antigen and antibody) are diagnostic

14.2.8   Management

- Acute disease is self-limiting; symptomatic treatment is adequate
- Treatment for chronic histoplasmosis: intravenous administration of amphotericin B
- Disseminated histoplasmosis is treated with amphotericin B, ketoconazole, fluconazole or itraconazole
- Spontaneous recovery in some patients

14.2.9   Prognosis

- Generally, prognosis is good with adequate treatment
- Oral lesions respond to systemic treatment

14.3 Blastomycosis: Key Features

- Caused by *Blastomyces dermatitidis*
- Relatively common in the United States; uncommon in other parts
- Male to female ratio 9 : 1
- Transmission through inhalation of spores from the soil
- Two forms of blastomycosis occur: acute and chronic
- Acute disease resembles pneumonia
- Chronic form resembles pulmonary tuberculosis; also involves the skin
- Oropharyngeal involvement occurs in chronic blastomycosis: granulomatous ulcerative lesions occur caused by local inoculation of the fungus
- Oral ulcers resemble those of squamous cell carcinoma or tuberculous ulcers
- Diagnosis by culture of sputum, cytology and histopathology of lesions
- Potassium hydroxide preparation of the scraped lesional tissue offers rapid diagnosis
- Treatment is with systemic antifungal agents
- Good prognosis for adequately treated patients
- Disease may be fatal if not treated
- Oral lesions respond to systemic treatment

Recommended Reading

Bandara, H.M.H.N. and Samaranayake, L.P. (2019). Viral, bacterial, and fungal infections of the oral mucosa: types, incidence, predisposing factors, diagnostic algorithms, and management. *Periodontology 2000* 80 (1): 148–176.

Farah, C.S., Lynch, N., and McCullough, M.J. (2010). Oral fungal infections: an update for the general practitioner. *Australian Dental Journal* 55 (1 Suppl): 48–54.

Kong, E.F., Kuchaříková, S., Van Dijck, P. et al. (2015). Clinical implications of oral candidiasis: host tissue damage and disseminated bacterial disease. *Infection and Immunity* 83: 604–613.

Neville, B.W., Damm, D.D., Allen, C.M., and Chi, C.A. (2016). Fungal and protozoal diseases. In: *Oral and Maxillofacial Pathology*, 4e, 191–213. St Louis, MO: Elsevier.

Odell, E.W. (2017). Diseases of the oral mucosa: mucosal infections. In: *Cawson's Essentials of Oral Pathology and Oral Medicine*, 9e, 235–250. Edinburgh: Elsevier.

Patil, K., Mahima, V.G., and Prathibha Rani, R.M. (2009). Oral histoplasmosis. *Journal of Indian Society Periodontology* 13 (3): 157–159.

15

Viral Infections of the Oral Mucosa

15.1 Primary Herpetic Gingivostomatitis (Primary Herpes)

15.1.1 Definition/Description

- Primary herpetic gingivostomatitis is caused by an initial infection with the herpes simplex virus (HSV) type I
- Characterized by painful, erythematous, and swollen gingivae

15.1.2 Frequency

- Herpetic gingivostomatitis is the most common clinical manifestation of HSV primary infection, occurring in 15–30% of cases
- Common in children. Rarely, adults are infected

Handbook of Oral Pathology and Oral Medicine, First Edition. S. R. Prabhu.
© 2022 John Wiley & Sons Ltd. Published 2022 by John Wiley & Sons Ltd.
Companion website: www.wiley.com/go/prabhu/oral_pathology

15.1.3 Aetiology/Risk Factors

- HSV type 1 (90–95%) and type 2 (5–10%) are the causative agents
- Physical contact with the contaminated source (oral secretions) is the mode of transmission
- Incubation period: three to six days

15.1.4 Clinical Features

- Up to 90% experience subclinical infection or are asymptomatic
- About 1% of those infected develop symptoms, which are often minimal
- Most infections occur between six months and five years of age (peak between two and three years)
- Onset is abrupt with fever, headache, malaise, and tender cervical lymph node enlargement
- Both keratinized and non-keratinized mucosa are affected
- Gingivitis with swollen and erythematous gingiva followed by appearance of pin-head vesicles on the tongue, lips, and gingiva (Figure 15.1a)
- Vesicles are intraepithelial, rupture leaving erosions/ulcers covered by yellow fibrin
- Occasionally vermillion border involvement and satellite lesions on the perioral skin are seen

(a)

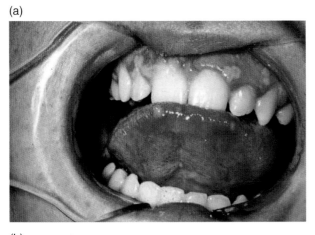

(b)

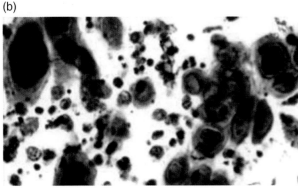

Figure 15.1 Primary herpetic gingivostomatitis. (a) Blisters and erosive lesions on the gingiva and tongue. (b) Tzanck smear shows herpes virus infected cells with enlarged nuclei and marginated chromatin. Also note inflammatory cell infiltrate.

- Acute stage lasts for five to seven days; severe infection lasts longer
- Symptoms usually subside within two weeks
- Viral shedding continues for about three weeks (contagious)

15.1.5 Differential Diagnosis

- Herpangina
- Hand, foot, and mouth disease
- Varicella
- Herpes zoster (shingles)

15.1.6 Microscopic Features

- Vesicles are intraepithelial
- At the floor of the vesicle and in direct smears (Tzanck smear) infected cells with enlarged nuclei and marginated chromatin (ballooning degeneration) are seen (Figure 15.1b)
- Multinucleated giant cells are common
- In addition, inflammatory cell infiltrate is seen in an ulcer

15.1.7 Diagnosis

- History
- Clinical presentation
- Diagnosis is clinical and, in most cases, does not require laboratory confirmation
- Laboratory diagnosis for confirmation include:

  - Smear: cytology preparation demonstrates multinucleated virus infected giant epithelial cells (Tzanck test)
  - Biopsy: histopathology shows intraepithelial vesicles or early virus-induced (cytopathic) epithelial changes
  - Viral culture
  - Serology for antibody titres: rising antibody titre, reaching a peak in two to three weeks
  - Polymerase chain reaction (PCR) test of blister fluid or scraping from base of erosion. PCR testing looks for viral genetic material

15.1.8 Management

- Simple oral analgesia including paracetamol and ibuprofen for pain and fever
- Topical analgesics (e.g. lidocaine [lignocaine] hydrochloride 2%) for pain
- Chlorhexidine (0.12%) mouth rinses
- Systemic antiviral agents to be administered in the first 48 hours:
  - Acyclovir 200 mg 400 mg three times daily for seven days
  - Valacyclovir 500 mg 1000 mg twice daily for five days
  - For severe infection: aciclovir 10 mg/kg (max. 400 mg) intravenously eight-hourly until there are no new lesions; these patients need hospitalization

- Bed rest
- Soft diet and hydration
- Nutritional supplements (available over the counter)

15.1.9 Prognosis

- Good
- Complications include eczema herpeticum, herpetic whitlow (often in children who suck their thumbs), lip adhesions and secondary infection
- Serious complications are rare; may include keratoconjunctivitis, pneumonitis, meningitis, and encephalitis
- Lifelong latency of the virus can occur in the ganglia of the nerves supplying the infected area
- Reactivation can occur with cold, trauma, stress, or immunosuppression
- About 15–45% of patients may develop recurrent infections (herpes labialis)

15.2 Herpes Labialis

15.2.1 Definition/Description

- Also known as cold sore, secondary herpetic stomatitis, and recurrent herpetic stomatitis
- Herpes labialis is the secondary infection with HSV-1 characterized by the vesicular lesions of the vermillion border and adjacent skin
- Herpes labialis is caused by reactivation of the latent virus in the nerve ganglion

15.2.2 Frequency

- Common; 15–45% of the population is affected

15.2.3 Aetiology/Risk Factors

- HSV 1
- Reactivation of latent virus in an immune individual whose neutralizing antibodies from the primary infection are not able to protect
- Virus travels along the nerve to a new site (such as the lip)
- Ultraviolet light, stress, cold, and immunosuppression can trigger recurrence

15.2.4 Clinical Features

- Prodromal sensation of tingling, paraesthesia, burning, or pain at the site of recurrence
- Erythema followed by clusters of multiple fragile vesicles appear, commonly on the mucocutaneous junction of the lips and adjoining skin (Figure 15.2)
- Vesicles rupture within an hour of their appearance causing virus-filled exudate
- Crust/scab forms over the lesions after two to three days
- The process lasts for over 10 days and lesions heal leaving no scar
- Recurrence rate: approximately two recurrence episodes annually
- Intraoral involvement is rare in immunocompetent individuals; hard palate or attached gingiva are preferred intraoral sites for secondary infection
- Lesions are more severe in immunocompromised patients
- Recurrent herpes can trigger erythema multiforme in some patients

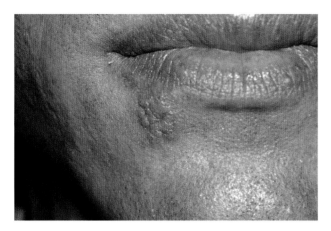

Figure 15.2 Herpes labialis. Note the typical focal cluster of vesicular lesions with a surrounding slightly erythematous base on the facial skin and lower lip (*source:* reproduced with permission from the National HIV Curriculum, University of Washington by David Spach, 5 September 2020. Retrieved from www.hiv. uw.edu).

15.2.5 Differential Diagnosis

- Herpes zoster
- Hand, foot, and mouth disease (in children)
- Erythema multiforme
- Herpangina

15.2.6 Diagnosis

- History
- Clinical presentation
- Diagnosis is clinical and, in most cases, does not require laboratory confirmation
- Viral culture/PCR test on vesicular fluid or scraping of the base of ulcers are confirmatory. Not routinely required
- Cytology of the smear (direct immunofluorescence). Not routinely required

15.2.7 Management

- Topical antiviral treatment:
  - Penciclovir cream 1%; dab on to lesion every two hours during waking hours for four days, beginning when symptoms first occur
- When recurrence is triggered by exposure of lips to sunlight, application of sunscreen to the lip (sun protection factor 15 or higher) is useful as a preventive measure
- Topical penciclovir or aciclovir cream for early prodromal stage is effective in reducing severity
- Acyclovir may be used for prophylaxis for seropositive transplant patients
- Ganciclovir for patients who are HIV positive

15.2.8 Prognosis

- Excellent
- Healing without scarring within two weeks
- Protracted healing in patients who are HIV positive

15.3 Varicella (Chickenpox)

15.3.1 Definition/Description

- Chickenpox is a highly contagious disease caused by primary infection with varicella zoster virus
- Causes acute fever and blistered rash
- Commonly affects children

15.3.2 Frequency

- Common worldwide in children younger than 12 years
- Endemic in some parts of the world

15.3.3 Aetiology/Risk Factors

- Caused by varicella zoster virus
- Transmission by airborne droplets or by direct contact with the infected person
- Incubation is 14–16 days
- Infants, adolescents, adults, pregnant women, and immunocompromised people are at risk for more severe disease

15.3.4 Clinical Features

- Maculopapular skin rash usually appearing first on the chest, back, and face, then spreads over the entire body
- Mild flu-like fever and sore throat are common
- Perioral skin and vermilion of the lips may be involved
- Oral manifestations of chickenpox include small vesicular lesions/eroded ulcers with red margin
- Oral sites include buccal mucosa, tongue, gingiva, and palate, as well as the pharyngeal mucosa
- Symptoms typically last four to seven days

15.3.5 Differential Diagnosis

- Dermatitis herpetiformis
- Bullous pemphigoid
- Erythema multiforme
- Drug eruptions
- Impetigo

15.3.6 Diagnosis

- History
- Clinical examination
- Diagnosis is clinical and, in most cases, does not require laboratory confirmation
- Laboratory tests for confirmation include:

  – PCR detects the varicella virus in skin lesions
  – Serology (immunoglobulins M and G) is most useful in pregnant women

15.3.7 Management

- Chickenpox is a self-limiting infection
- Symptomatic treatment may be required
- Aciclovir is useful in reducing the duration of symptoms

15.3.8 Prognosis

- Once infected, individual gets lifetime immunity
- Chickenpox is a self-limiting disease; prognosis is generally good for affected children
- In adults, chickenpox may occasionally cause serious complications, which include cerebellar ataxia, encephalitis, viral pneumonia, haemorrhagic conditions, septicaemia, toxic shock syndrome, necrotizing fasciitis, osteomyelitis, bacterial pneumonia, and septic arthritis
- Following the initial chickenpox illness, varicella zoster virus establishes latency in the sensory nerve ganglia and may reactivate later in life as shingles (herpes zoster)
- Vaccination is the best protection against chickenpox

15.4 Herpes Zoster (Shingles)

15.4.1 Definition/Description

- Herpes zoster is a secondary/recurrent varicella infection caused by reactivation of the latent virus in neurons of cranial nerve ganglia, dorsal root ganglia, and autonomic ganglia along the entire neuroaxis
- Herpes zoster usually occurs in adults or older individuals who have had a primary varicella (chicken pox) infection in childhood

15.4.2 Frequency

- Approximately one in three people will develop herpes zoster during their lifetime
- Most common in the elderly and immunocompromised individuals worldwide

15.4.3 Aetiology/Risk Factors

- Causative agent: varicella zoster virus (a primary infection causes chickenpox)
- Risk/predisposing factors include old age, immunosuppressive drugs, HIV infection, radiation, malignancy, alcohol abuse, stress, and traumatic manipulation of tissues during dental treatment

15.4.4 Clinical Features

- Prodromal phase:
  - Burning, tingling, itching or prickly sensation in the skin/mucous membrane innervated by the affected sensory nerve (dermatome)
  - Fever, headache, and malaise may accompany

- Acute phase:

  - One to four days later, skin and/or mucosa develops clusters of vesicles on an erythematous base following path of the affected nerve (Figure 15.3)
  - Lesions do not cross the midline
  - Within three to four days vesicles become pustular and rupture leaving ulcers
  - 7–10 days later crusts develop on the affected skin
  - Healing takes place with or without scarring
  - Oral lesions: usually occur in the trigeminal nerve, involvement stopping at midline
  - In prodromal phase, pain mimics odontogenic pain
  - Crops of mucosal vesicles may extend to the skin of the affected quadrant
  - Cervical lymph nodes are enlarged and tender
  - Virus can be transmitted to non-immune individuals (non-vaccinated or those who did not have chickenpox in childhood). These individuals can develop primary infection (chickenpox) but not herpes zoster

15.4.5 Differential Diagnosis

- Primary herpes simplex infection
- Recurrent intraoral herpes simplex infection
- Herpangina
- Pemphigus vulgaris
- Mucous membrane pemphigoid

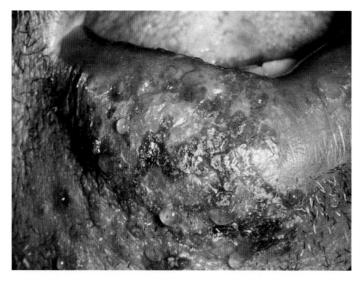

Figure 15.3 Herpes zoster; clusters of vesicular lesions confined to the right lower face and lip. (By kind permission of Professor Newell Johnson, Brisbane, Australia)

15.4.6   Microscopic Features

- Vesicles are intraepithelial
- At the floor of the vesicle and in direct smears, infected cells with enlarged nuclei and margin-ated chromatin (ballooning degeneration) are seen
- Multinucleated giant cells are common
- In addition, inflammatory cell infiltrate is seen in an ulcer

15.4.7   Diagnosis

- History
- Clinical findings (readily recognizable)
- Cytologic smear that shows cytopathic features (Tzanck test)
- Viral culture and PCR test of fluid from the vesicle
- Serology for viral antibody detection
- Biopsy with direct fluorescent examination using fluorescein-labelled varicella zoster virus antibody

15.4.8   Management

- Mild cases: symptomatic treatment with analgesics and soothing creams for skin lesions
- Severely affected cases or in immunocompromised patients or patients with extensive disease, antiviral drugs to be started (in the first 48–72 hours)
  - Acyclovir 800 mg five times daily for seven days
  - Valacyclovir 500 mg, 1 g three times daily for seven days
- Systemic corticosteroids (prednisolone) with antiviral agents help in controlling/preventing post-herpetic neuralgia
- Pain control

15.4.9   Prognosis

- Generally good
- Recurrences are more likely in immunosuppressed patients
- Reactivation of varicella zoster virus in the geniculate ganglion may cause Ramsay Hunt syndrome
- Ramsay Hunt syndrome is characterized by cutaneous lesions of the external auditory canal and involvement of the facial and auditory nerves of the same side causing facial paralysis, hearing deficits and vertigo
- About 15% of patients with herpes zoster develop postherpetic neuralgia, which is characterized by persistent pain after resolution of the rash (for a period of one to three months)
- Elderly and immunocompromised individuals are vulnerable. Pain is of burning, throbbing and stabbing type, usually resolving within two months to a year

15.5   Infectious Mononucleosis (Glandular Fever)

15.5.1   Definition/Description

- Infectious mononucleosis is the primary acute infection in young adults caused by Epstein–Barr virus (human herpes virus 4)
- Also known as glandular fever, 'mono' and 'kissing disease'

15.5.2 Frequency

- Common in young adults
- In military personnel on active duty and college students, annual incidence for infectious mononucleosis ranges from 11 to 48 cases per 1000 persons

15.5.3 Aetiology/Risk Factors

- Epstein–Barr virus transmitted via the infected saliva
- Incubation period is four to eight weeks

15.5.4 Clinical Features

- Sore throat
- Fever
- Myalgia
- Malaise
- Headache
- Generalized lymphadenopathy (posterior cervical nodes in particular)
- Tonsillitis
- Maculopapular skin rash
- Hepatomegaly and splenomegaly
- Petechiae at the junction of hard and soft palate (Figure 15.4)
- Thrombocytopenia

15.5.5 Differential Diagnosis

- Idiopathic thrombocytopenia
- Cytomegalovirus infections
- Bacterial/viral pharyngitis
- Lymphoma
- Symptoms of acute HIV infection
- Other viral infections

15.5.6 Laboratory Tests

- Positive Paul Bunnel test
- In an acute infection, heterophile antibodies that agglutinate sheep erythrocytes are produced. This process forms the basis for the monospot rapid latex agglutination test

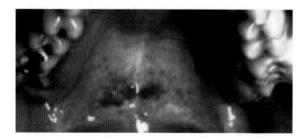

Figure 15.4 Infectious mononucleosis. Note palatal petechiae at the junction of hard and soft palate.

15.5.7 Diagnosis

- History
- Clinical examination
- Blood examination for heterophile antibody test (Paul Bunnel test, monospot test)

15.5.8 Management

- No specific treatment (infection is self-limiting)
- Symptomatic treatment may be necessary for fever, headache, and myalgia

15.6 Oral Hairy Leukoplakia: Key Features

- Oral hairy leukoplakia occurs in up to 20% of individuals whose immune status is severely compromised
- Rarely occurs in patients with immunosuppression after organ transplantation
- Epstein–Barr virus is strongly associated
- The tongue is the common intraoral site
- Clinically presents as a white, corrugated, fixed lesion seen on the lateral surfaces of the tongue (Figure 15.5); often bilateral
- Lesion is asymptomatic and cannot be rubbed off with gauge
- Differential diagnosis includes candidosis, allergic contact stomatitis, frictional keratosis, and lichen planus
- Characteristic histopathologic findings include cellular nuclear changes (acanthosis, Cowdry type A inclusions (round eosinophilic material surrounded by a clear halo), absence of an inflammatory infiltrate, regions of ballooning cells, and epithelial hyperplasia
- Oral hairy leukoplakia is not a potentially malignant disorder
- Treatment is usually not required for asymptomatic cases. Topical therapy with podophyllin resin combined with acyclovir cream is useful for symptomatic patients
- In most people who are HIV positive, antiretroviral therapy will cause the lesions to resolve

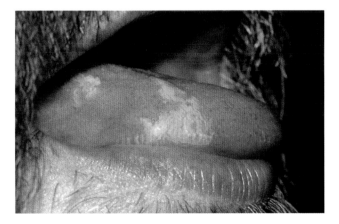

Figure 15.5 Oral hairy leukoplakia of the tongue (*source:* reproduced with permission from the National HIV Curriculum, University of Washington by David Spach, 5 September 2020. Retrieved from www.hiv.uw.edu).

15.7   Cytomegalovirus Infection: Key Features

- Cytomegalovirus (CMV) is a member of the herpes virus family (HSV-5)
- CMV infection causes symptoms similar to those of infectious mononucleosis
- Can cause disease in neonates and immunocompromised individuals
- 90% of CMV infections are asymptomatic
- Oral infection with CMV causes large solitary oral ulcerations particularly in those who are HIV positive
- In neonates, CMV infection can cause developmental tooth defects
- CMV ulcers are treated with aciclovir
- CMV can reside latently in salivary gland cells

15.8   Herpangina: Key Features

- Herpangina is a viral disease caused by the members of the coxsackievirus group A (1–16) or group B (1–5) of the genus *Enterovirus*
- Usually affects young children in summer
- Subclinical and asymptomatic in most patients
- Soft palate and tonsillar area show macular erythematous areas followed by blisters and one to six small ulcers (Figure 15.6)
- Pharyngitis, fever, dysphagia, malaise, cough, and lymphadenitis are common
- Lesions self-limiting in about two weeks
- Diagnosis: history, clinical findings, and culture studies/PCR tests
- Treatment: symptomatic

15.9   Hand, Foot, and Mouth Disease

15.9.1   Definition/Description

- A common coxsackievirus (A10 or A16) infection in childhood characterized by vesicular and erythematous on hands and feet and ulceration in the mouth

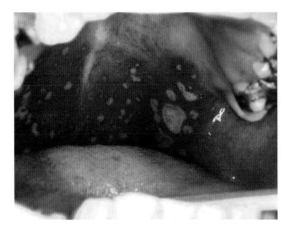

Figure 15.6   Herpangina. Note multiple ulcers on the soft palate.

15.9.2   Frequency

- Common infection (in childhood)

15.9.3   Aetiology

- Enterovirus (coxsackievirus A 10 and A16 and enterovirus 71)

15.9.4   Clinical Features

- Incubation period is less than one week
- Vesicular rash on the extremities (palms, soles, and feet; Figure 15.7a)
- Small ulcers (1–30) in the anterior mouth on the non-keratinizing mucosa (Figure 15.7b)
- Mild systemic effects (pharyngitis, sore throat, and mild fever)
- Resolves within a week

15.9.5   Differential Diagnosis

- Herpangina
- HSV infection
- Acute lymphoreticular pharyngitis (an enterovirus infection)

15.9.6   Diagnosis

- History of concomitant skin and mucosal lesions
- Clinical findings
- Antibody titre (rise during convalescence)

15.9.7   Management

- Symptomatic treatment only
- Use of aspirin in children is contraindicated to avoid Reye's syndrome, rare, serious condition that causes confusion, swelling in the brain and liver damage

(a)   (b)

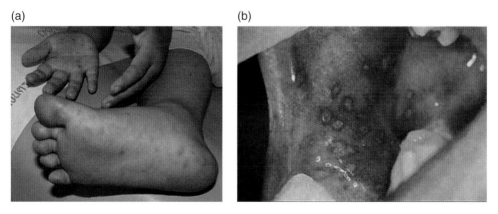

Figure 15.7   Hand, foot, and mouth disease. (a) Note vesicular lesions on hands and the foot. (b) Mucosal vesiculo-ulcerative lesions.

15.9.8   Prognosis

- Good

15.10   Squamous Papilloma

15.10.1   Definition/Description

- A benign proliferation of stratified squamous epithelium characterized by papillary growth

15.10.2   Frequency

- Common; 7–8% of all growths in children
- Occurs at any age; common in children and those of 50–60 years of age

15.10.3   Aetiology/Risk Factors

- Human papillomavirus (HPV types 6 and 11)

15.10.4   Clinical Features

- Sites of predilection: soft and the hard palate, tongue, and lips
- The lesion:
  - Solitary, soft, painless, pedunculated exophytic mass
  - Finger-like projections: wart-like (papillary) or blunted (cauliflower) (Figure 15.8a)
  - Colour: normal, white, or slightly red
  - Traumatized projections result in bleeding

15.10.5   Microscopic Features

- Proliferation of finger-like projections of the keratinized epithelium (Figure 15.8b)
- Fibrovascular connective tissue extends into the projections
- Cytological signs of viral infection are absent

(a)   (b)

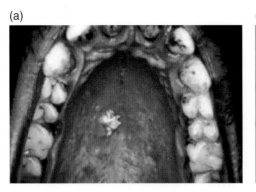
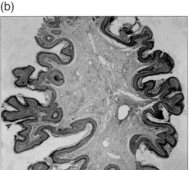

Figure 15.8   (a) Palatal squamous cell papilloma. (b) Photomicrograph of papilloma showing narrow stalks with numerous blunt and pointed finger-like projections.

15.10.6   Differential Diagnosis

- Verruca vulgaris
- Condyloma acuminatum
- Multifocal epithelial hyperplasia

15.10.7   Diagnosis

- History
- Clinical findings
- Microscopic findings

15.10.8   Management

- Surgical excision

15.10.9   Prognosis

- Good
- No recurrence if adequately removed

15.11   Condyloma Acuminatum: Key Features

- Condyloma acuminatum is an HPV (types 6 and 11)-induced proliferation of stratified squamous epithelium of the anogenital and oral mucosa
- Condyloma acuminatum is a common sexually transmitted disease accounting for 1% of sexually active individuals
- May affect any age group but usually diagnosed in teenagers and young adults
- Labial mucosa, lingual frenum, and soft palate are preferred sites
- Condyloma presents as multiple, sessile, pink, and well-demarcated soft lesions with blunt projections (Figure 15.9)

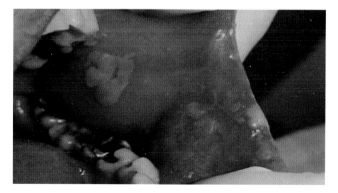

Figure 15.9   Condyloma acuminatum presenting as multiple pink coloured sessile projections on the buccal mucosa.

- Histologically presents acanthotic stratified squamous epithelium with minimal keratinization and thin connective tissue core
- Differential diagnosis includes verruca vulgaris, squamous papilloma, and focal epithelial hyperplasia
- Management includes surgical removal
- Lesions have no malignant potential

15.12   Multifocal Epithelial Hyperplasia: Key Features

- Also known as Heck's disease
- Benign proliferation of the stratified squamous epithelium induced by HPV (types 13 and 32)
- Genetic factors may be involved
- Common in Native Americans and Inuit
- Commonly seen in children and adolescents
- Labial, lingual, and buccal mucosa and gingiva are preferred sites of occurrence
- White to pale pink, papillomatous, painless, soft nodules are characteristic (Figure 15.10)
- Histopathology reveals acanthosis of the surface epithelium with broad and elongated rete ridges and keratinocytes may show altered nuclei resembling mitotic figures (mastoid cells)
- Differential diagnosis includes verruca vulgaris and condyloma acuminatum
- Spontaneous regression may occur after months or years
- Surgical treatment for diagnostic and aesthetic reasons
- Lesions have no malignant potential

15.13   Verruca Vulgaris: Key Features

- Verruca vulgaris (common wart) is a benign HPV (types 2, 4 and 40)-induced skin lesion that may rarely appear in the oral mucosa
- May affect individuals of any age; children are commonly affected
- Oral lesions are usually autoinoculated from skin lesions (fingers in particular)

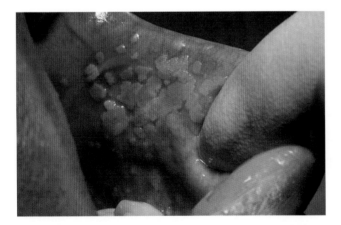

Figure 15.10   Multifocal epithelial hyperplasia (Heck's disease).

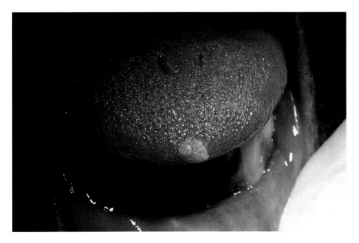

Figure 15.11   Verruca vulgaris seen as white cauli-flower like lesion on the tip of the tongue.

- Vermilion border, lip commissures, and anterior tongue are preferred sites
- Presents as sessile, painless, soft, white, cauliflower-like lesions (Figure 15.11)
- May be single or multiple
- Histologically characterized by hyperkeratosis and prominent granular cell layer arranged in finger like projections with connective tissue core
- HPV-altered epithelial cells with pyknotic nuclei are common
- Differential diagnosis includes condyloma acuminatum, multifocal epithelial hyperplasia, verruciform xanthoma and squamous papilloma
- Treatment is surgical excision

15.14   Measles: Key Features

- Oral lesions in measles are secondary to the systemic viral infection
- Measles is a childhood infection caused by the virus in the family Paramyxoviridiae
- Rare in recent years due to widespread vaccination
- Occasional outbreaks occur in winter or spring months
- Transmission by respiratory droplets
- Lymphoid hyperplasia is common in infected children
- Runny nose (coryza), cough, and conjunctivitis accompanied by fever are common in early stages
- Small blue-white macules surrounded by erythema appear on the buccal and labial mucosa. These are called Koplik spots
- Maculopapular erythematous rash occurs on the face followed by trunk and extremities
- Rash appears in the second stage of the infection, whereas desquamation of involved skin is a feature of the third stage of infection
- If the child with measles is severely malnourished, oral candidosis and necrotizing ulcerative gingivitis may occur
- Measles in the immunocompromised patients can occasionally be fatal
- History and clinical findings are useful in diagnosis; immunoglobulin M antibody assay is confirmatory

- Hydration, bed rest and non-aspirin antipyretic medication is an effective symptomatic treatment
- Prevention of measles is by measles, mumps, and rubella vaccination: (first dose between 12 and 15 months and second dose between 4 and 6 years)
- 99% of individual develop immunity after the second dose

Recommended Reading

Bandara, H.M.H.N. and Samaranayake, L.P. (2019). Viral, bacterial, and fungal infections of the oral mucosa: types, incidence, predisposing factors, diagnostic algorithms, and management. *Periodontology 2000* 80 (1): 148–176.

Clarkson, E., Mashkoor, F., and Abdulateef, S. (2017). Oral viral infections. *Dental Clinics* 61: 351–363.

Neville, B.W., Damm, D.D., Allen, C.M., and Chi, C.A. (2016). Viral infections. In: *Oral and Maxillofacial Pathology*, 4e, 218–239. St Louis, MO: Elsevier.

Odell, E.W. (2017). Diseases of the oral mucosa: mucosal infections. In: *Cawson's Essentials of Oral Pathology and Oral Medicine*, 9e, 235–250. Edinburgh: Elsevier.

Prabhu, S.R. (2019). Benign mucosal blisters, erosions and ulcers. In: *Clinical Diagnosis in Oral Medicine: A case based approach*, 154–201. New Delhi: Jaypee Brothers Medical Publishers.

Slots, J. (2009). Oral viral infections of adults. *Periodontology 2000* 49: 60–86.

16

Non-infective Inflammatory Disorders of the Oral Mucosa

16.1   Recurrent Aphthous Stomatitis

16.1.1   Definition/Description

- A common inflammatory condition characterized by multiple recurrent, painful, round ulcers with circumscribed margins, surrounded by erythematous halo and a central yellow or grey floor
- Also known as recurrent aphthous ulcers (as discussed below) or canker sores

16.1.2   Frequency

- Affects 20–25% of the population
- Three-month recurrence rates are as high as 50%

16.1.3   Aetiology/Risk Factors

- The exact cause is not known

Handbook of Oral Pathology and Oral Medicine, First Edition. S. R. Prabhu.
© 2022 John Wiley & Sons Ltd. Published 2022 by John Wiley & Sons Ltd.
Companion website: www.wiley.com/go/prabhu/oral_pathology

- Many implicated factors include hormonal changes, trauma, drugs, food hypersensitivity, nutritional deficiency, stress, and tobacco
- Genetic predisposition has been noted (family history in about 30% of patients)
- Immunodysfunction may be a factor (antibody-dependent cellular cytotoxicity reaction)
- Predisposing factors include:
  - Stress, anxiety, hormonal changes (during menstruation for example), dietary factors and trauma
  - Iron and folate deficiency (20% of patients)
  - Neutropenia
  - Sodium lauryl sulfate in oral health products
  - Cessation of smoking
  - Crohn's disease and coeliac disease in about 3% of cases
  - Behcet's disease
  - Reactive arthritis
  - Immune deficiency
  - Bone marrow suppression
  - Food allergy
  - Vitamin B12 and zinc deficiency

16.1.4 Clinical Features

Three main clinical types: minor, major, and herpetiform recurrent aphthous ulcers

- Minor recurrent aphthous ulcers:
  - Also known as Mikulicz ulcer
  - The most common type of recurrent aphthous stomatitis
  - Common in people 10–40-years of age
  - Single/multiple (up to five) small round/oval ulcers 2–4 mm in diameter
  - Floor of ulcer is yellow/grey surrounded by an erythematous halo (Figure 16.1a)
  - Commonly found on lips, cheeks, floor of the mouth, labial, or buccal sulci, and ventral surface of the tongue (non-keratinizing mucosa)
  - Rarely found on the dorsum of the tongue and hard palate (keratinizing mucosa)
  - Self-limiting; heal in 7–10 days with no scarring and recur at intervals of one to four months
- Major recurrent aphthous ulcers:
  - Also known as Sutton's disease
  - Usually single, rarely multiple (two to three in number)
  - Larger ulcer 1 cm or greater in diameter often surrounded by erythematous halo (Figure 16.1b)
  - Deep ulcers with ragged edges and elevated margins (mimicking squamous cell carcinoma)
  - More painful than minor recurrent aphthous stomatitis
  - Any mucosal surface (keratinizing and non-keratinizing)
  - Heal slowly often with scarring in 10–40 days
  - Ulcers recur more frequently
- Herpetiform recurrent aphthous ulcers:
  - Occur in slightly older age group
  - Common in females

(a) (b) (c) (d)

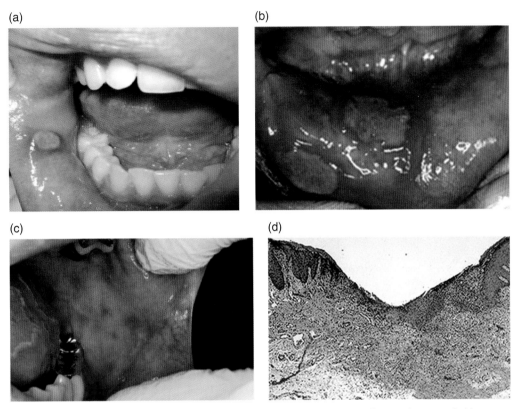

Figure 16.1 (a) Minor recurrent aphthous ulcer. Note round ulcer with grey floor and surrounded by erythematous halo. (b) Major aphthous ulcer. Note large ulcers with ragged edges. Elevated margins and erythematous halo surrounding them. (c) Herpetiform recurrent aphthous ulcers. Note multiple small ulcers on the buccal mucosa with erythematous halo surrounding them. (d) Photomicrograph of an aphthous ulcer. The surface is covered by stratified squamous epithelium with an ulcer in the centre. Intense mixed inflammatory cell infiltrate is seen in the connective tissue. There are no specific diagnostic microscopic findings (*Source:* images a-c, by kind permission of David Clark, Faculty of Dentistry, University of Toronto, Ontario, Canada).

- Vesiculation followed by ulceration
- No association with herpes simplex virus infection; ulcers mimic herpes simplex virus erosions
- Cluster of ulcers 1–2 mm in diameter (Figure 16.1c)
- Multiple painful ulcers: 10–100 in number
- Occur on non-keratinizing/keratinizing mucosa
- Heal within 7–14 days leaving no scar
- Recur very frequently

16.1.5 Differential Diagnosis

- Traumatic ulcer
- Recurrent herpes simplex virus lesions
- Recurrent ulcers in cyclic neutropenia

- Recurrent aphthous ulcers with Behcet's disease
- Ulcers in Crohn's disease
- Smoking related aphthous ulcers
- Recurrent ulcers of erythema multiforme

16.1.6   Microscopic Features

- Ulcers have no specific microscopic features
- Break in the epithelium is present suggesting ulceration
- Prior to ulceration (prodromal stage) lymphocytic infiltration is present
- Acute and chronic mixed inflammatory cell infiltrate is seen in the ulcerated lesion (Figure 16.1d)

16.1.7   Diagnosis

- History
- Clinical findings (usually diagnostic)
- Haematology to rule out underlying systemic disorders

16.1.8   Management

- The aim of treatment of recurrent aphthous stomatitis is to decrease symptoms, reduce ulcer number and size, and increase disease-free periods
- Topical therapy:
  - Prodromal/pre-ulcerative stage:
    - Hydrocortisone 1% cream/ointment topically two to three times daily after meals
    - Fluocinonide 0.05% gel/cream; to be applied to early lesions after meals and at bedtime
    - Benzydamine 1% gel topically two to three times daily after meals (for pain relief)
  - Ulcerative stage:
    - Dexamethasone elixir 0.5 mg/5 ml (100 ml) to be used as a rinse; 5 ml 'swish and spit' for two minutes four times a day; to be discontinued when lesions become asymptomatic
    - Triamcinolone acetonide in Orabase 0.1% (5 g tube); thin layer to be applied to dried ulcers after each meal and at bedtime until healed
    - Tetracycline capsules 250 mg. One capsule to be dissolved in 180 ml of water and used as a rinse four times a day for five days
    - Viscous lidocaine 2% to be applied to the ulcers as needed
- Systemic therapy:
  - Prednisone 5 mg; 5 tablets in the morning for five days, and then 5 tablets in the morning every other day until gone
  - For very severe cases, prednisone 10 mg (26 tablets). 4 tabs in the morning for 5 days and then to be decreased by one tablet on each successive day until gone.
  - Colchicine 0.5 mg to be taken each morning with breakfast for one week
  - Thalidomide 100 mg one to two times daily for three to eight weeks, depending on the severity of symptoms. Contraindicated in pregnancy
- For severe, persistent, and chronic aphthous ulcers other medications in use are azathioprine, pentoxifylline, levamisole, and dapsone
- If underlying systemic disorders are present, they should be treated by specialists
- Close collaboration with patient's physician is recommended when systemic medications are used

16.1.9 Prognosis

- Fair to good control with corticosteroids in most cases

16.2 Oral Lichen Planus

16.2.1 Definition/Description

- Lichen planus is an inflammatory chronic cell-mediated immune response that affects both skin and oral mucosa

16.2.2 Frequency

- Skin: affects 1–2% of general population. Of these, up to one third of patients have only skin involvement
- Oral: affects 0.1–2.2% of population. Of these, up to one third have only oral lesions
- Both skin and mucosa: one third of patients have skin as well as mucosal involvement
- Other areas of involvement: genital mucosa and nails

16.2.3 Aetiology

- Exact cause not known
- Probably immunologically mediated T-cell disorder targeting basal keratinocytes; antigen unknown
- Link between hepatitis C and lichen planus has been reported; exact mechanism unknown; could be an immunological cross reaction or T cell immune response against hepatitis C virus

16.2.4 Clinical Features

- Most patients with lichen planus are middle-aged adults
- Female predominance is seen
- Skin lichen planus:
  - Purple, pruritic (itchy), papules usually on flexor surfaces of extremities with fine lace-like network of white lines (Wickham striae)
- Oral lichen planus:
  - Presents in five different clinical forms:
    - Reticular: a network of raised white lines or striae (most common form) (Figure 16.2a)
    - Papular: white papular lesions (Figure 16.2b)
    - Plaque-like: white patch similar to leukoplakia (Figure 16.2c)
    - Atrophic/erosive/ulcerative: red patch similar to erythroplakia (Figure 16.2d)
    - Bullous: blisters and small tags of epithelium resembling mucous membrane pemphigoid (rare)
  - Oral lesions are bilateral and often symmetric in distribution
  - Tends to develop in sites of trauma (Koebner phenomenon)
  - Posterior buccal mucosa is commonly involved, followed by the tongue, gingiva (desquamative gingivitis) and lips
  - White lesions (papular, reticular and plaque types) are often asymptomatic
  - Atrophic and erosive lesions are sore; intolerant to acidic and spicy drinks/foods

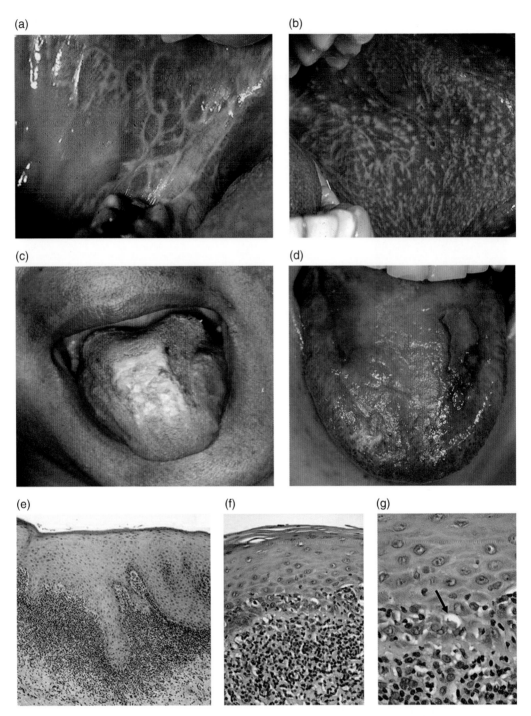

Figure 16.2 Oral lichen planus. Clinical types: (a). Reticular type showing network of raised white lines (striae) giving a lacy pattern. (b) papular type with multiple white papular lesions, (c) plaque type showing a white patch (associated with pigmentation) and (d) erosive (atrophic/ulcerative) type on the dorsum of the tongue. Photomicrographs of oral lichen planus show: (e) epithelial proliferation and a dense band-like infiltrate of lymphocytes underneath the epithelium, (f) vacuolar degeneration of the basal cell layer and (g) civatte bodies (black arrow). *source:* images a, b, d–g by kind permission of Associate Professor Mark Schifter, University of Sydney, Sydney, NSW, Australia; image c reproduced with permission from Ramdas, K., Lucas, E., Thomas, G. et al. 2008. *A Digital Manual for the Early Diagnosis of Oral Neoplasia*. Lyon: IARC. Available from http://screening.iarc.fr/atlasoral.php?lang=1.)

16.2.5   Microscopic Features

- Hyperkeratosis/parakeratosis (reticular, papular and plaque types)
- Band-like lymphocytic infiltration at the epithelium–connective tissue interface (Figure 16.2e)
- Basal cell degeneration and apoptosis (Figure 16.2f) and 'sawtooth' appearance of rete ridges
- Civatte bodies (eosinophilic hyaline spherical bodies seen in or just beneath the epidermis, formed by necrosis of individual basal cells) (Figure 16.2g)
- Separation of epithelium from lamina propria due to basal cell destruction
- Atrophic epithelium (atrophic type)

16.2.6   Differential Diagnosis

- Lichenoid lesions
- Leukoplakia
- Erythroplakia
- Lupus erythematosus
- Mucous membrane pemphigoid

16.2.7   Diagnosis

- History
- Clinical findings
- Biopsy and histopathological findings
- Direct immunostaining (detection of tissue fibrinogen and cytoid bodies at interface)

16.2.8   Management

- Asymptomatic patients need no treatment
- Reassurance and improvement of oral hygiene are essential
- Patients with mild to moderate symptoms are treated with topical corticosteroids or tacrolimus (immunosuppressant)
- Patients with severe or ulcerative symptoms are treated with systemic corticosteroids
- Topical steroids:
  - Fluocinonide gel 0.05%; lesion to be coated with a thin film after each meal and at bedtime
  - Betamethasone cream (0.1%); apply after each meal and at bedtime
- Topical tacrolimus:
  - Tacrolimus 0.1% ointment; to be applied to the affected sit(s) twice daily as directed
- Intralesional therapy:
  - Triamcinolone acetonide 5–10 mg/ml; 1–3 ml. intralesional injection per session with sessions at three to four week intervals
- Systemic steroids:
  - Prednisone 10 mg; 40 mg in the morning for five days and then to be decreased by 10 mg each successive day
- Other drugs:
  - Other drugs in use include azathioprine, mycophenolate–mofetil and cyclosporin. Not to be used routinely because of their potential adverse effects. A physician should be consulted

16.2.9   Prognosis

- Fair to good
- Disorder tends to be chronic and cyclic; may last for years
- Rare malignant transformation seen predominantly in erosive/ulcerative form

16.3   Oral Lichenoid Lesions

16.3.1   Definition/Description

- Oral lichenoid lesion (OLL) is a chronic inflammatory lesion of the oral mucosa that occurs as an allergic response to dental materials, certain medications, and in patients with graft-versus-host disease, chronic hepatitis C and those individuals vaccinated against hepatitis B
- Also known as oral lichenoid drug reactions

16.3.2   Frequency

- Prevalence is approximately 2.4% in general population
- Mostly occur in women, with an average age of 53 years

16.3.3   Aetiology/Risk Factors

- Oral lichenoid lesions are caused by known triggers such as restorative materials and drugs:
  - Restorative materials include amalgam, gold, and composites
  - Drugs causing hypersensitivity reaction include sulfasalazine, angiotensin-converting enzyme inhibitors, non-steroidal anti-inflammatory drugs (NSAIDs), beta-blockers, gold, antimalarial sulfonylurea compounds and other drugs

16.3.4   Clinical Features

- Unilateral lesions with mild pain/tenderness
- Lesions appear with central atrophy and peripheral erythema and white striae similar to those of erosive lichen planus (Figure 16.3)
- Lesions may be seen in contact with the restorative material. In such circumstances, buccal mucosa, lateral surfaces of tongue and gingiva are commonly involved
- Any mucosal site may be involved for drug hypersensitivity reactions

16.3.5   Microscopic Features

- Epithelial changes include focal parakeratosis, focal interruption of the granular layer, and the presence of cytoid bodies in the granular and keratinized layers
- Liquefaction degeneration of the basal cell layer
- Band-like layer of lymphocytic infiltrate in the connective tissue

16.3.6   Differential Diagnosis

- Oral lichen planus
- Lichenoid lesions of graft-versus-host disease

Figure 16.3   Oral lichenoid lesion on the right buccal mucosa (*source:* by kind permission of Anura Ariyawardana JCU Cairns, Australia).

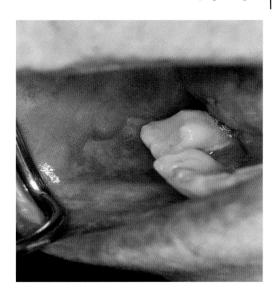

- Lichenoid drug reactions
- Lichenoid contact lesions
- Oral lesions of lupus erythematosus

16.3.7   Diagnosis

- History
- Clinical examination
- Biopsy/microscopic examination
- Patch testing to confirm contact allergen

16.3.8   Management

- Identification and elimination of causative agent/change of drug
- Topical corticosteroid or tacrolimus applications (as for oral lichen planus; see section 16.2.8)

16.3.9   Prognosis

- Good if treated adequately
- A small percentage of lichenoid lesions carry malignant potential

16.4   Pemphigus Vulgaris

16.4.1   Definition/Description

- Pemphigus is a blistering autoimmune disorder that affects the skin and mucous membranes. There are several types of pemphigus which vary in severity. These include:
    - Pemphigus vulgaris (common)
    - Pemphigus foliaceus (least severe)
    - Paraneoplastic pemphigus (complication of lymphoma)

16.4.2 Pemphigus Vulgaris

- Pemphigus vulgaris is the most common types of blistering autoimmune diseases
- Commonly is characterized by the formation of vesicles or bullae on the skin and mucous membranes

16.4.3 Frequency

- An incidence of 1–10 cases per 1 million people worldwide

16.4.4 Aetiology/Risk Factors

- An autoimmune disease
- IgG class of antibodies are directed against desmoglein 1 or 3 proteins of the desmosomes in the epithelium
- Circulating antibodies bind to epithelial desmosomes and cause detachment of the cells, which results in the formation of intraepithelial vesicles

16.4.5 Clinical Features

- Women aged 40–60 years are predominantly affected
- People of Jewish and Indian origin are predisposed
- Oral blisters occur on the non-keratinizing mucosa (buccal mucosa, ventral tongue, floor of the mouth) in over 60% of cases
- Skin lesions usually follow oral lesions
- Blisters are filled with clear fluid
- Blisters rupture within a short time leaving painful erosions/shallow ulcers (Figure 16.4a)
- Lateral sliding force or gentle stroking on the uninvolved skin or mucosa can produce a surface slough or induce vesicle formation (Nikolsky's sign)

16.4.6 Microscopic Features

- Loss of intercellular adherence of suprabasal prickle cells
- Clefts immediately superficial to the intact basal cell layer (Figure 16.4b)
- Nonadherent prickle cells float in blister fluid (Tzanck cells; Figure 16.4c)
- Direct immunofluorescence is positive in all cases; test reveals:
  - Immunoglobulins G (IgG), C3, or A localization to intercellular spaces of the epithelium (Figure 16.4d)
- Indirect immunofluorescence test is positive in 80% of cases

16.4.7 Differential Diagnosis

- Mucous membrane pemphigoid
- Erythema multiforme
- Erosive lichen planus
- Lichenoid drug reaction
- Paraneoplastic pemphigus
- Chronic ulcerative stomatitis
- Recurrent herpes lesions in immunocompromised patients

(a)

(b)

(c)

(d)

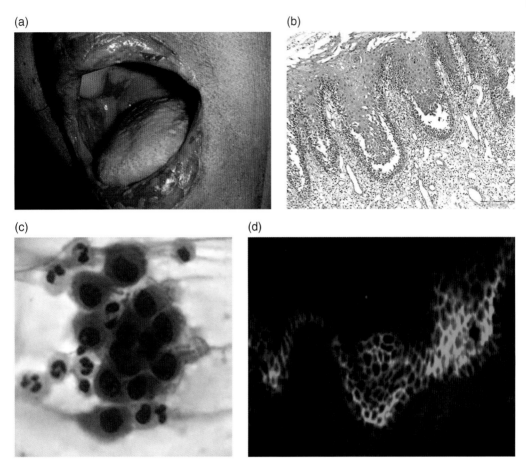

Figure 16.4 Pemphigus vulgaris. (a) Clinical photograph showing blisters and ulcers on the lips and, on the right buccal mucosa and palate (b) Histology shows acantholysis in the lower spinous cell layers and suprabasal cleft at the tips of the epithelial rete ridges. (c) Cytological smear shows grouping of acantholytic keratinocytes observed by the Tzanck method. (d) Direct immunofluorescence examination showing moderate intensity for the IgG and C3 markers. (*Sources:* images a,c,d By kind permission of Dr Adriana Maria Porro, Department of Dermatology, Federal University of Sao Paulo, Sao Paulo, Brazil; image b, by kind permission of Nada Suliman, Anne Astrøm, Raouf Ali et al. 2013. Clinical and histological characterization of oral pemphigus lesions in patients with skin diseases: a cross-sectional study from Sudan. *BMC Oral Health* 13: 66. doi: 10.1186/1472-6831-13-66.)

16.4.8 Diagnosis

- History
- Clinical findings, including positive Nikolsky's sign
- Biopsy of the perilesional tissue for microscopic and direct and indirect immunofluorescence tests (confirmatory)

16.4.9 Management

- Management is aimed at controlling the symptoms of the disorder
- Management to be coordinated with patient's physician
- The cornerstone of treatment remains systemic corticosteroids

- Corticosteroid-sparing therapies (azathioprine and mycophenolate mofetil, high-dose intravenous immunoglobulins, immunoadsorption, and rituximab) are useful.
- First line of treatment:
  - Initial treatment with prednisone 10 mg at a dose of 0.5–1.5 mg/kg/day with breakfast
  - Stepped tapering of prednisone by a 25% reduction bi-weekly is recommended
  - Manage the adverse effects of prednisone
- Steroid-sparing drug therapy:
  - Azathioprine 1–3 mg/kg per day
  - Mycophenolate mofetil 500 mg. 1.5 g twice daily
- Topical or intralesional corticosteroid therapy following an initial favourable response to systemic therapy is useful
- Plasmapheresis plus immunosuppression for severe cases
- Symptomatic and supportive treatment

16.4.10 Prognosis

- No permanent cure
- Symptoms can be controlled
- About 5% mortality rate
- Oral lesions respond more slowly than skin lesions

16.5 Mucous Membrane Pemphigoid

16.5.1 Definition/Description

- An autoimmune subepithelial blistering disease predominantly affecting the mucous membranes associated with antibodies that target the basement membrane zone
- In this disorder IgG class antibodies are directed against the basement membrane zone antigens

16.5.2 Frequency

- The reported incidence is approximately 1.16–2.00 per million population
- Prevalence is 1 in 40 000

16.5.3 Aetiology

- Antibodies directed against basement membrane zone antigens (namely, bullous pemphigoid 180 antigen, integrins, laminin and type VII collagen)

16.5.4 Clinical Features

- Blisters and ulcers of the mucous membranes:
  - Oral mucosa 92%
  - Ocular up to 80%
  - Other mucosal sites: genital, nasopharyngeal, anogenital, and laryngeal mucosa

- Skin involvement up to 20%; predominantly head and neck, and upper trunk
- Middle-aged to elderly patients (50–70 years) are most affected, with women affected more often than men
- Short-lived vesicles/bullae leaving painful ulcers on gingiva, buccal mucosa, palate, and the tongue
- Blisters may be filled with blood
- Ulcers may show flaps or tags of epithelium at their edges (Figures 16.5a and b)
- Gingival involvement is seen as desquamative gingivitis (sometimes the only sign)
- A positive Nikolsky's sign on clinically normal mucosa
- Healing is slow (over a few weeks)
- Ocular (inside the eye lids and over the sclera) heal with scarring, often causing adhesion between the lids and the sclera (cicatricial pemphigoid)

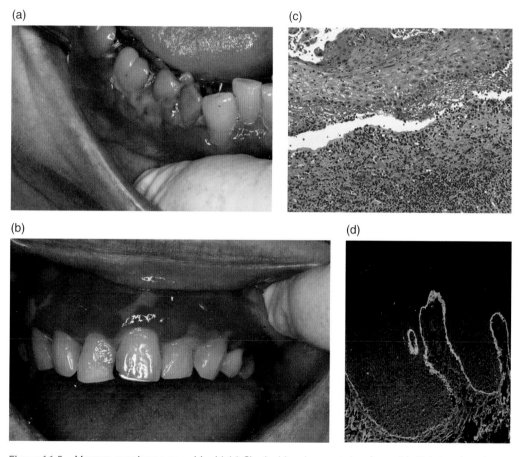

Figure 16.5 Mucous membrane pemphigoid. (a) Gingival involvement showing epithelial slough and erythema. (b) Mucous membrane pemphigoid of the gingiva presenting as desquamative gingivitis. (c) Photomicrograph showing aggregates of erythrocytes in the subepithelial space. The underlying connective tissue contains neutrophils, lymphocytes, and plasma cells. (d) Immunofluorescence findings show linear, shaggy deposits of IgG antibody along the basement membrane zone. (*Image sources:* a and b By kind permission of Associate Professor Nagamani Narayana, UNMC. Nebraska USA); d: by kind permission of Dr Molly Housley Smith, Assistant Professor and division chief of oral and maxillofacial pathology, University of Kentucky College of Dentistry, Kentucky, USA.)

- Scarring may eventually lead to blindness
- Oral mucosal lesions usually do not cause scarring

16.5.5 Microscopic Features

- Loss of attachment and separation of full thickness of epithelium form the connective tissue at the basement membrane zone (Figure 16.5c)
- The blister is subepithelial
- Connective tissue is infiltrated by inflammatory cells

16.5.5.1 Immunofluorescence Findings

- Direct immunofluorescence is positive in 80% of cases
- Linear band of IgG and complement 3 are present at the basement membrane zone in almost all cases (Figure 16.5d)
- Indirect immunofluorescence test is negative or circulating antibodies are at very low levels

16.5.6 Differential Diagnosis

- Pemphigus vulgaris
- Erythema multiforme
- Erosive lichen planus
- Lupus erythematosus
- Epidermolysis bullosa acquisita

16.5.7 Diagnosis

- History
- Clinical findings
- Microscopy and immunofluorescence tests

16.5.8 Management

- Topical therapy:
  - Fluocinonide gel 0.05% (30 g tube). Lesion to be coated with thin film after each meal and at bedtime
  - Dexamethasone elixir 0.5 mg (100 ml); to be rinsed with 5 ml for two minutes four times a day and spit out. Discontinue when lesions become asymptomatic
  - Tacrolimus 0.1% ointment (30 g tube). to be applied to the affected sites twice daily
- Systemic therapy:
  - Prednisone 10 mg (260 mg); 40 mg in the morning for five days and decrease by 10 mg on each successive day
- Other immunosuppressive drugs (azathioprine)
- Cytotoxic agents (cyclophosphamide)
- Intravenous immunoglobulin administration
- Multidisciplinary management is required

16.5.9 Prognosis

- Guarded/variable

16.6 Erythema Multiforme

16.6.1 Definition/Description

- An acute, self-limited, and sometimes recurring skin condition considered to be a type-IV hypersensitivity reaction associated with certain infections, medications, or other various triggers

16.6.2 Frequency

- Globally, approximately 1.2–6 cases per million individuals

16.6.3 Aetiology

- A cell-mediated hypersensitivity reaction
- May be triggered by herpes simplex virus infection (cold sore), genital recurrent herpes, mycoplasma pneumonia, varicella zoster infection, drugs such as sulphonamides, antibiotics, analgesics, phenolphthalein containing laxatives, barbiturates, radiation and chemotherapy

16.6.4 Clinical Features

- Most patients in the 20–40 years age group
- Male predisposition
- Two forms: minor and major
- Minor:
  - Only skin involvement
  - Less severe
- Major:
  - Skin, oral, nasal, and genital involvement
  - Symptoms are severe
  - Acute onset, preceded by vague joint pains and fever
  - In severe cases, bullous lesions may occur
  - Conjunctival involvement may cause lacrimation, photophobia, burning eyes, or visual impairment
  - Oral lesions: inflamed patches, multiple irregular blisters and shallow ulcers occur anteriorly on the labial, buccal, and lingual mucosa
  - Lips may show bleeding tendencies, labial ulcers ooze fibrin and form haemorrhagic crusts (Figure 16.6a)
  - 'Target lesions' or 'iris lesions' (well-defined red macules with a bluish cyanotic centre); appear on the extremities and spread centrally (Figure 16.6b)
  - Lesions may be self-healing within two to four weeks but may recur at an interval of several months

16.6.5 Microscopic Features

- Histological features are characteristic but not diagnostic
- Skin biopsy shows epidermal necrosis and subepidermal bulla formation
- Oral lesions show basal cell degeneration and apoptosis of the epithelium
- Presence of intraepithelial vesicle
- Lymphocytic and acute inflammatory cell infiltrate below the epithelium

(a)　　　　　　　　　　　　　　　　　(b)

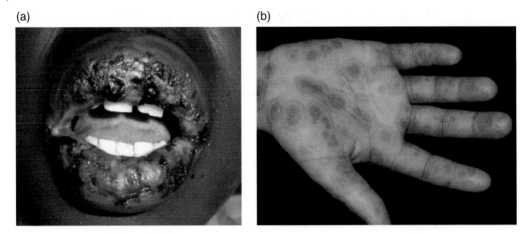

Figure 16.6 Erythema multiforme. (a) Erythematous lesions with haemorrhagic crusts are seen on the vermillion. (b) Typical 'iris'/'target' lesions seen on the palm.

16.6.6 Differential Diagnosis

- Viral infection primary herpetic stomatitis
- Pemphigus vulgaris
- Major aphthous ulcers (when only mucosa is involved)
- Erosive lichen planus
- Mucous membrane pemphigoid

16.6.7 Diagnosis

- History of previous episodes of trigger
- Clinical findings (characteristic target lesions and multiple site involvement)
- Biopsy (when only mouth is affected) and histopathology

16.6.8 Management

- Minor: symptomatic and supportive treatment with adequate hydration, liquid diet, analgesics, and topical corticosteroid agents adequate
- Major: systemic corticosteroids, parenteral fluid, replacement, antipyretics required
- If evidence of an antecedent viral infection or trigger exists, systemic antiviral drugs during the disease or as a prophylactic measure are helpful
- Steroid therapy:
  - Prednisone 10 mg; 60 mg in the morning until lesions recede, then decrease by 10 mg on each successive day. Do not exceed 14 days of therapy
- Suppressive antiviral therapy (if triggered by herpes simplex virus infection):
  - Acyclovir 200 mg (42 tablets); 200 mg every four hours for seven days, or as prophylaxis, 200 mg twice daily

16.6.9 Prognosis

- Generally good
- Recurrences are common

16.7   Lupus Erythematosus: Key Features

- Lupus erythematosus is a chronic autoimmune connective tissue disorder with two main clinical types: systemic lupus erythematosus (SLE) and chronic cutaneous lupus erythematosus (CCLE; also known as discoid lupus erythematosus)
- Oral lesions occur in both forms of the disorder
- In SLE, in addition to systemic findings such as fever, weight loss and arthritis, a characteristic facial rash having a pattern of butterfly occurs over the malar area and the nose
- In CCLE, systemic features are minimal or absent; scaly erythematous patches are common on the exposed skin in the head and neck region
- 20% of patients with SLE may show palatal or buccal mucosal lesions similar to those of oral lichenoid lesions
- Oral lesions of the CCLE are similar to erosive lichen planus-like lesions characterized by an ulcerated or atrophic, erythematous central zone surrounded by radiating white striae (Figure 16.7)
- Clinical, histopathological and direct immunofluorescence studies of the lesional tissue are useful diagnostic tools
- Oral lesions of chronic cutaneous lupus erythematosus may respond to topical corticosteroid applications but those of SLE may be resistant
- SLE requires a systemic approach to treatment. Medications available include antimalarial drugs, NSAIDs, corticosteroids, immunosuppressive agents, and cytotoxic drugs
- For further information see Chapter 19 (section 19.8)

16.8   Traumatic Ulcer: Key Features

- Common
- Usually single
- Can occur as acute or chronic ulcer
- Causes include physical, thermal, or chemical injuries
- Trauma prone areas: lip, buccal mucosa, or mucosa adjacent to denture flange
- Rarely self-inflicted
- Occasionally iatrogenic
- Occasionally large due to biting after dental local anaesthetic injections

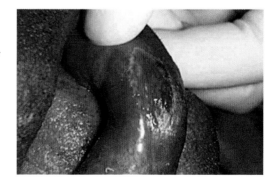

Figure 16.7   Lupus erythematosus. Oral lesion in chronic cutaneous lupus erythematosus (*source:* Reproduced with permission from Ramdas, K., Lucas, E., Thomas, G. et al. 2008. *A Digital Manual for the Early Diagnosis of Oral Neoplasia.* Lyon: IARC. Available from http://screening.iarc.fr/atlasoral.php?lang=1;).

- Silver nitrate or hypochlorite mucosal contact during dental procedures can cause chemical ulceration
- Prolonged contact with aspirin held for toothache against the alveolus can cause aspirin burn and ulceration (an example of chemical burn)
- Traumatic ulcer is tender, with yellowish-grey floor covered with fibrin and with red margin (Figure 16.8a)
- Variable amount of inflammation is present without induration
- Histopathology reveals connective tissue composed of a mixed inflammatory cell infiltrate. (Figure 16.8b)
- Elimination of the cause is effective
- Traumatic ulcer heals within 7–10 days
- After elimination of the cause, if ulcer does not heal in 10 days, biopsy is required to rule out other causes (such as malignancy, tuberculosis, or syphilitic ulcer)

16.9   Oral Lesions in Behcet's Disease/Syndrome

16.9.1   Definition/Description

- A systemic disorder characterized by oral recurrent aphthous stomatitis, genital ulceration, uveitis, arthritis, and other systemic manifestations

16.9.2   Frequency

- Common in Asia and the Middle East; uncommon in western populations

16.9.3   Aetiology

- Exact cause is not known
- Non-infectious inflammation of blood vessels (vasculitis)

(a)

(b)

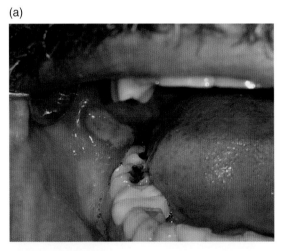 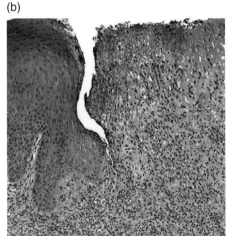

Figure 16.8   Traumatic ulcer. (a) Clinical photograph shows a traumatic ulcer coated with pseudomembrane and surrounded by inflammatory halo. (b) Photomicrograph shows the thickened fibrinopurulent covering and connective tissue composed of a mixed inflammatory cell infiltrate.

- A multisystem disease secondary to an immune dysfunction
- Genetic predisposition noted

16.9.4   Clinical Features

- A chronic disorder; occasionally life threatening
- Affects mostly adult men aged 20–40 years
- Oral recurrent aphthous ulcers and genital recurrent ulcers are common
- Ocular lesions include uveitis and retinal vascular changes
- Arthritis of weight-bearing bones
- Skin lesions include erythema nodosum
- Sensory and motor disturbances (due to vasculitis in the central nervous system) occur

16.9.5   Differential Diagnosis

- Erythema multiforme
- Crohn's disease
- Reiter's syndrome
- Mucous membrane pemphigoid
- Erosive lichen planus

16.9.6   Diagnosis

- History
- Clinical findings (such as oral recurrent aphthous stomatitis, genital ulcers, and ocular changes)
- Pathergy test: appearance of an erythematous papule greater than 2 mm in diameter. 24–48 hours or more after sterile needle-prick test is positive

16.9.7   Management

- Multidisciplinary approach
- Cyclosporin, tacrolimus, and systemic corticosteroids
- Immunosuppressive agents
- Thalidomide and topical tacrolimus for oral lesions

16.9.8   Prognosis

- Guarded
- In treated patients, disease may eventually burn out
- Complications may include blindness, rupture of blood vessels, thrombosis, and embolism

16.10   Oral Lesions in Crohn's Disease

16.10.1   Definition/Description

- Also known as regional enteritis, Crohn's disease is an idiopathic, chronic, relapsing, inflammatory immunologically mediated condition
- Crohn's disease is a form of inflammatory bowel disease

16.10.2   Frequency

- Global inflammatory bowel disease estimation:400–500 people per 100 000
- Prevalence increasing

16.10.3   Aetiology/Risk factors

- Unknown
- Immunologically mediated
- Genetic factors associated

16.10.4   Clinical Features

- First becomes evident in teenage years
- Second peak after 60 years of age
- Abdominal cramping, pain, nausea, diarrhoea and occasional fever, weight loss, and anaemia
- Oral lesions are usually non-specific, such as:
  - Diffuse mucosal nodules
  - Cobble stone appearance of the mucosa
  - Deep mucosal linear ulcers in the buccal vestibule
  - Aphthous-like ulcers
  - Gingival erythematous macules and patches
  - Occasional association of pyostomatitis vegetans

16.10.5   Differential Diagnosis

- Major recurrent aphthous ulcers
- Blastomycosis
- Tuberculous ulcers
- Syphilitic ulceration (tertiary syphilis)

16.10.6   Diagnosis

- History of intestinal and oral symptoms
- Clinical findings
- Biopsy of oral lesion: microscopic findings such as non-caseating granulomatous inflammation

16.10.7   Management

- Multidisciplinary approach
- Systemic corticosteroids
- Oral lesions: intralesional corticosteroid injections
- NSAIDs
- Occasional metronidazole

16.10.8   Prognosis

- Guarded
- Linked to intestinal response to treatment

16.11 Oral Lesions in Reactive Arthritis: Key Features

- Also known as Reiter's disease, reactive arthritis is an immunologically mediated disease characterized by arthritis, urethritis, conjunctivitis, and occasional stomatitis
- Immunological reaction is triggered by micro-organisms such as enterococci and sexually transmitted chlamydia
- Prevalence is approximately 10%
- Young adults with equal frequency in both sexes
- Non-gonococcal urethritis, conjunctivitis, and arthritis are consistent features
- 40% of patients develop oral lesions such as erosion, red patches, or ulcerations on the buccal, palatal, or labial mucosa
- History, clinical examination, and serology are important diagnostic tools
- Antibiotics, NSAIDs and immunosuppressive agents are effective
- Topical corticosteroids are useful for oral lesions

16.12 Uremic Stomatitis: Key Features

- Oral complication of renal failure
- Caused by long-standing uraemia in patients with renal failure
- Four forms of uremic stomatitis are recognized:
  - Ulcerative
  - Haemorrhagic
  - Nonulcerative pseudomembranous
  - Hyperkeratotic
- Non-ulcerative pseudomembranous form and hyperkeratotic form are of oral significance
- The nonulcerative, pseudomembranous form presents as painful diffuse erythema covered by a thick whitish-grey pseudomembrane
- The hyperkeratotic form presents as multiple, painful, white hyperkeratotic lesions with thin projections
- The tongue and the floor of the mouth are more frequently affected
- Xerostomia, uriniferous breath door, unpleasant taste, and a burning sensation are common symptoms
- Candidiasis and viral and bacterial infections are common oral complications
- The diagnosis is based on the history, the clinical features, urinalysis, and blood urea level determination
- May subside after renal dialysis
- Symptoms may respond to hydrogen peroxide rinse
- Palliative treatment: ice chips and topical application of lidocaine
- Prognosis of oral lesions: good

16.13 Chronic Ulcerative Stomatitis: Key Features

- Oral manifestations: lesions resembling lichen planus
- A rare autoimmune mucosal disorder characterized by lichen planus-like lesions
- Affects predominantly females

- Clinically and histologically similar to lichen plans
- Shallow ulcers, erosions, and erythema seen on tongue, buccal mucosa, and gingiva
- Symptomatic with pain and burning sensation
- Direct immunofluorescence shows autoantibodies to squamous epithelial nuclear proteins (chronic ulcerative stomatitis protein)
- Corticosteroids are less effective
- Hydroxychloroquine is effective

16.14   Radiation-Induced Mucositis: Key Features

- Inflammation of the mucosa due to damage caused by ionizing radiation for cancer therapy
- Nearly 80% of patients undergoing radiotherapy for cancer present with radiation mucositis
- Severity of mucositis is dependent on the type of radiation, volume of the irradiated tissue, dose of radiation per day, and the cumulative dose
- Mucosal erythema, atrophy, necrosis, ulceration, and pseudomembrane formation (Figure 16.9)
- Mucosal pain is the main complaint
- Dysphagia is also common
- Mucositis starts usually within two weeks of the start of radiation therapy
- Non-keratinizing mucosa is affected more frequently
- Herpetic and candidal infections may occur during the course of mucositis
- Transient or permanent xerostomia or hyposalivation is a common finding
- Diagnosis: history of radiation and clinical findings
- Differential diagnosis includes erythema multiforme, erythematous candidosis, chemotherapy-induced stomatitis, aphthous ulceration, herpetic infection, and neutropenic ulcers to be considered
- Management: pain control, nutritional support, oral decontamination, palliation of dry mouth are important therapeutic interventions for oral mucositis
- Oral lesions usually heal within two to three weeks
- Maintaining good oral hygiene is the main preventive approach

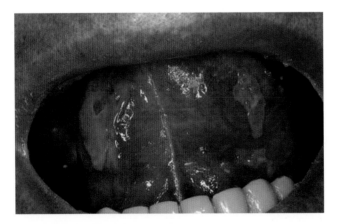

Figure 16.9   Radiation-induced mucositis. Note pseudomembrane and ulcerative lesions on the ventral surface of the tongue (*source:* by kind permission of Vlaho Brailo, Department of Oral Medicine, School of Dental Medicine, University of Zagreb, Croatia).

16.15   Medication-Induced Oral Ulceration: Key Features

- Many kinds of drugs cause oral ulcerations
- Groups of ulcerogenic drugs include cytotoxic drugs used for cancer therapy, beta-blockers, immunosuppressants, anticholinergic bronchodilators, platelet aggregation inhibitors, vasodilators, protease inhibitors, antibiotics, NSAIDs, anti-retroviral agents, and anti-hypertensive drugs (e.g. potassium channel activator nicorandil).
- Widespread mucositis followed by ulcerations (Figure 16.10)
- Ulcers may be single or multiple
- Any mucosal site can be involved
- Ulcers are usually large, flat, and white in appearance and usually not indurated
- Symptomatic treatment and consultation with physician
- Corticosteroids may not be effective
- Ulcers heal when drugs are changed or withdrawn

16.16   Stevens–Johnson Syndrome and Toxic Epidermal Necrolysis

16.16.1   Definition/Description

- Stevens–Johnson syndrome (SJS) and toxic epidermal necrolysis (TEN) are severe mucocutaneous reactions, most triggered by medication
- Mucous membranes are affected in over 90% of patients, usually at two or more distinct sites (ocular, oral, and genital)
- SJS is the less severe condition, in which skin detachment is less than 10% of the body surface
- TEN involves detachment of greater than 30% of the body surface area

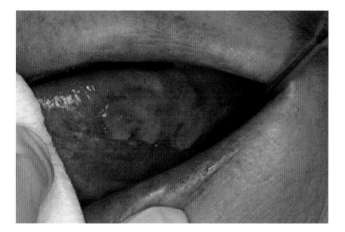

Figure 16.10   Medication induced oral ulceration. Widespread mucositis of the non-keratinized mucosa of the lateral ventral side of the tongue induced by chemotherapy (*source:* by kind permission of Dr Emmanuelle Vigarios, University Cancer Institute Toulouse Oncopole, Toulouse, France).

16.16.2 Frequency

- Uncommon
- Estimated incidence: one to two per million per year

16.16.3 Aetiology/Risk Factors

- Type IV hypersensitivity, mediated by immunological effect caused by medication
- Some aetiological drugs include: carbamazepine, allopurinol, NSAIDs, phenytoin, phenobarbital, penicillins, and other antibiotics
- People with the following conditions are at greater risk of SJS/TEN:
  - Bone marrow transplant
  - Systemic lupus erythematosus
  - HIV
  - Other chronic diseases of joints and connective tissue

16.16.4 Clinical Features

- 4–28 days from the beginning of drug use to the onset of signs and symptoms
- The highest risk in the first two months of treatment with risk drugs on a continuous basis
- Both diseases can start with prodromal symptoms lasting up to one week, such as fever, sore throat, coughing, eye burning, myalgia and arthralgia. After this period there may be a discrete maculopapular rash
- There may be atypical target lesions on the back of the hands, palms, sole of the foot, extensor surface of the limbs, neck, face, ears and perineum, with prominent involvement of trunk and face
- The rash usually spares the palmoplantar areas
- Extensive sloughing of necrotic skin (Nikolsky's sign is positive in perilesional skin)
- Painful oral ulcers

16.16.5 Differential Diagnosis

- Chickenpox
- Staphylococcal epidermolysis
- Staphylococcal scalded skin syndrome
- Autoimmune bullous disease

16.16.6 Diagnosis

- History, including medical
- Clinical examination:
  - percentage of involvement of skin and other areas less the 10% of skin is SJS
  - more than 30% of skin involvement is TENS
  - 10–30% skin involvement is SJS/TEN combined

16.16.7   Management

- Hospitalization is essential
- Identification of causative drug and stopping its use
- Pain medication
- Antihistamines
- Appropriate antibiotics
- Corticosteroids
- Immunoglobulins

16.16.8   Prognosis

- Mortality is around 7.5%

Recommended Reading

Cocca, S. and Viviano, M. (2017). Stevens–Johnson syndrome and abuse of anabolic steroids. *Journal of the Korean Association of Oral and Maxillofacial Surgeons* 43: 57–60.

Joseph, T.I., Vargheese, G., George, D., and Sathyan, P. (2012). Drug induced oral erythema multiforme: a rare and less recognized variant of erythema multiforme. *Journal of Oral and Maxillofacial Pathology* 16 (1): 145–148.

Lodi, G., Scully, C., Carrozzo, M. et al. (2005). Current controversies in oral lichen planus: report of an international consensus meeting. Part 2. Clinical management and malignant transformation. *Oral Surgery, Oral Medicine, Oral Pathology, Oral Radiology, and Endodontics* 100: 164–178.

Mays, J.W., Sarmadi, M., and Moutsopoulos, N.M. (2012). Oral manifestations of systemic autoimmune and inflammatory diseases: diagnosis and clinical management. *Journal of Evidence-Based Dental Practice* 3: 265–282.

Neville, B.W., Damm, D.D., Allen, C.M., and Chi, C.A. (2016). Dermatologic diseases. In: *Oral and Maxillofacial Pathology*, 4e, 690–748. St Louis, MO: Elsevier.

Odell, E.W. (2017). Diseases of the oral mucosa: non-infective stomatitis. In: *Cawson's Essentials of Oral Pathology and Oral Medicine*, 9e, 255–279. Edinburgh: Elsevier.

Porro, A.M., Seque, C.A., Ferreira, M.C.C., and Enokihara, M.M.S.S. (2019). Pemphigus vulgaris. *Anais Brasileiros de Dermatologia* 94 (3): 264–278.

Prabhu, S.R. (2019). Benign mucosal blisters, erosions and ulcers. In: *Clinical Diagnosis in Oral Medicine: A case based approach*, 154–201. New Delhi: Jaypee Brothers Medical Publishers.

Schifter, M., Fernando, S.L., and Li, J. (2013). Oral lichen planus. In: *Skin Biopsy – Diagnosis and Treatment* (ed. S.L. Fernando). London: IntechOpen. Available from: https://doi.org/10.5772/56482., https://www.intechopen.com/books/skin-biopsy-diagnosis-and-treatment/oral-lichen-planus.

Schifter, M., Yeoh, S.C., Coleman, H., and Georgio, A. (2010). Oral mucosal diseases: the inflammatory dermatoses. *Australian Dental Journal* 55: 23–38.

Suliman, N., Astrøm, A., Ali, R. et al. (2013). Clinical and histological characterization of oral pemphigus lesions in patients with skin diseases: a cross sectional study from Sudan. *BMC Oral Health* 13: 66.

Vigarios, E., Epstein, J.B., and Sibaud, V. (2017). Oral mucosal changes induced by anticancer targeted therapies and immune checkpoint inhibitors. *Support Care Cancer* 25: 1713–1739.

17

Non-neoplastic Mucosal Swellings

17.1   Irritation Fibroma (Traumatic Fibroma)

17.1.1   Definition/Description

- Irritation/traumatic fibroma is a hyperplastic connective tissue reactive lesion in response to chronic irritation or trauma

17.1.2   Frequency

- Common

17.1.3   Aetiology

- Low-grade irritation from cheek or lip biting
- Occasionally, long-standing mature pyogenic granuloma

17.1.4   Clinical Features

- Smooth-surfaced, firm, pink, slow-growing, nodular mass (Figure 17.1a)
- Mostly sessile, rarely pedunculated, usually round or oval

Handbook of Oral Pathology and Oral Medicine, First Edition. S. R. Prabhu.
© 2022 John Wiley & Sons Ltd. Published 2022 by John Wiley & Sons Ltd.
Companion website: www.wiley.com/go/prabhu/oral_pathology

(a)

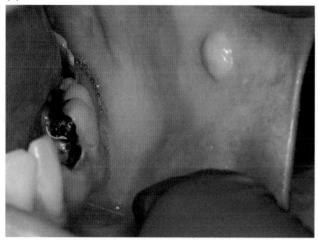

(b)

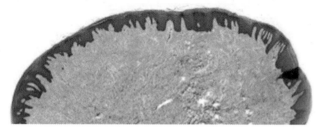

Figure 17.1 (a) Clinical photograph of irritation (traumatic) fibroma of the buccal mucosa (*source:* by kind permission of Dr Nagamani Narayana UNMC, Nebraska, USA.) (b) Photomicrograph showing fibroma with parakeratosis and dense collagenous tissue.

- Few millimetres to a couple of centimetres in size
- Painless mass, non-tender
- Rarely ulcerated or keratotic surface due to secondary trauma
- Buccal mucosa, lateral borders of the tongue, and lower labial mucosa are preferred sites

17.1.5 Microscopic Features

- A mass of fibrous densely collagenous connective tissue covered by stratified squamous epithelium (Figure 17.1b)
- Non capsulated at the periphery
- Overlying epithelium may show atrophy of rete ridges with or without keratotic surface
- Scattered chronic inflammatory cells in the fibrous connective tissue

17.1.6 Differential Diagnosis

- Pyogenic granuloma
- Neurofibroma

- Granular cell tumour
- Benign salivary gland tumour
- Lipoma

17.1.7   Diagnosis

- History
- Clinical findings
- Microscopic findings

17.1.8   Management

- Surgical excision
- Attention to the known source of irritation

17.1.9   Prognosis

- Excellent

17.2   Denture-Induced Granuloma (Epulis Fissuratum)

17.2.1   Definition/Description

- Denture-induced granuloma is characterized by folds of tumour-like hyperplastic fibrous connective tissue caused by overextended flange of ill-fitting partial or complete denture

17.2.2   Frequency

- Common among denture wearers

17.2.3   Aetiology/Risk Factors

- Trauma derived from overextended denture flange/ill-fitting denture

17.2.4   Clinical Features

- Exuberant folds of tissue usually located on vestibular mucosa associated with the facial aspect of denture flange; usually painless unless inflamed (Figure 17.2)
- Female predilection seen
- Common in the anterior region
- Occasionally ulcerated deep into the folds in contact with the inferior border of the flange
- Less commonly seen as a leaf-like pink pedunculated flattened fibrous growth beneath upper denture on the hard palate (leaf fibroma)

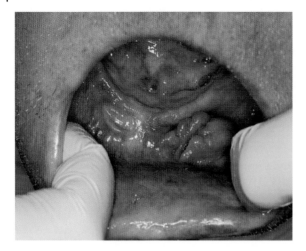

Figure 17.2 Denture induced granuloma of the mandibular vestibule. Note exuberant folds of tissue located on the vestibular mucosa (*source:* by kind permission of Dr Anura Ariyawardana, JCU, Cairns, Australia).

17.2.5   Microscopic Features

- Hyperparakeratotic and hyperplastic surface epithelium
- Occasionally, pseudoepitheliomatous epithelial hyperplasia mimicking carcinoma may be seen
- Folds of underlying fibrovascular hyperplastic fibrous connective tissue
- Variable amount of chronic inflammatory cell infiltrate in the connective tissue

17.2.6   Differential Diagnosis

- Irritation fibroma
- Squamous cell carcinoma
- Benign soft tissue tumours

17.2.7   Diagnosis

- History
- Clinical findings
- Microscopic findings

17.2.8   Management

- Surgical excision
- New dentures after excision of tissue

17.3   Fibrous Epulis (Peripheral Fibroma): Key Features

- A common tumour-like lesion of the gingiva, located in the interdental papilla as a hyperplastic response to local irritation
- Also known as peripheral fibroma

- 'Epulis' is the term used for gingival masses only
- For further information see Chapter 5 (section 5.9)

17.4 Pyogenic Granuloma: Key Features

- Also called gingival angiogranuloma or pregnancy epulis
- A highly vascular, localized inflammatory tumour-like lesion with abundant granulation tissue
- When this occurs in pregnant women, the condition is called pregnancy epulis or pregnancy tumour
- For further information see Chapter 5 (section 5.12)

17.5 Peripheral Giant Cell Granuloma: Key Features

- Also called giant cell epulis
- A tumour-like reactive hyperplastic lesion of the gingival margin located anterior to the permanent molars
- For further information see Chapter 5 (section 5.11)

17.6 Peripheral Ossifying Fibroma: Key Features

- A tumour-like non-neoplastic ossifying fibrous lesion on the gingiva derived from periodontal ligament as a result of local irritation or trauma
- For further information see Chapter 5 (section 5.10)

17.7 Traumatic Neuroma

17.7.1 Definition/Description

- A reactive proliferation of neural tissue as a result of damage of the nerve bundle

17.7.2 Frequency

- Less than 1% in general population

17.7.3 Aetiology/Risk Factors

- Damage to the nerve
- Traumatic surgery
- Reactive hyperplasia of the nerve tissue

17.7.4 Clinical Features

- Can occur at any intraoral site
- Common in the mental foramen area, tongue, and lip

- Diagnosed frequently in the middle-aged adults
- Slight female preponderance
- Smooth surfaced nodular lesion
- Pain or anaesthesia of the involved area

17.7.5   Microscopic Features

- Proliferation of mature myelinated and unmyelinated nerve bundles within fibrous connective tissue
- Dense collagenous or myxoid connective tissue
- Mild inflammatory cell infiltrate

17.7.6   Differential Diagnosis

- Neuroma
- Fibrous polyp
- Benign salivary gland tumours
- Atypical facial pain

17.7.7   Diagnosis

- History
- Clinical findings
- Microscopy

17.7.8   Management

- Surgical excision

17.7.9   Prognosis

- Excellent
- Recurrence very rare

17.8   Squamous Papilloma: Key Features

- A benign human papilloma virus (types 6 and 11)-induced proliferation of stratified squamous epithelial cells
- Can affect any age
- Accounts for 7–8% of all oral mucosal masses in children
- Palate, tongue, and lips are preferred sites
- Presents as soft, pedunculated, painless exophytic growth with numerous pointed or blunt finger-like projections (Figure 17.3)
- Usually solitary, lesion may be white or pink in colour

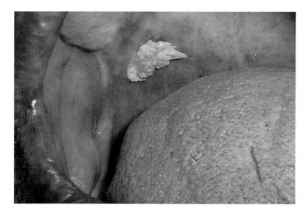

Figure 17.3   Squamous papilloma of the soft palate presenting as a papillary white lesion.

- Differential diagnosis includes verruca vulgaris, condyloma acuminatum, and verruciform xanthoma
- Histopathological features include proliferations of keratinized stratified squamous cell epithelium seen as finger-like projections with fibrovascular connective tissue core
- Inflammation is in the connective tissue is minimal
- Squamous papilloma has no malignant potential
- Surgical excision is adequate
- Recurrence is unlikely

17.9   Congenital Epulis: Key Features

- Rare
- Also known as congenital granular cell tumour or granular cell epulis
- A non-neoplastic lesion
- Arises from primitive gingival perivascular mesenchymal cells
- Cause unknown
- Seen only in the newborn at the time of birth
- Usually does not increase in size postnatally
- Female predilection (90%)
- Commonly involves maxillary alveolar ridge
- Usually single pedunculated lesion, occasionally lobulated
- Pink smooth-surfaced mass
- Interferes with feeding or respiration
- Differential diagnosis: haemangioma, lymphangioma, fibroma, granuloma, and neuroectodermal tumour of infancy
- Microscopy: histological similarity of granular cells to granular cell tumours
- Small lesions may regress after birth
- Treated by surgical removal
- No recurrence

Recommended Reading

Odell, E.W. (2017). Benign mucosal swellings. In: *Cawson's Essentials of Oral Pathology and Oral Medicine*, 9e, 369–376. Edinburgh: Elsevier.

Savage, N.W. and Daly, C.G. (2010). Gingival enlargements and localized gingival overgrowths. *Aust Dent J* 55 (91 Suppl): 55–60.

Scully, C. (2013). Lumps and swellings. In: *Oral and Maxillofacial Medicine: The basis of diagnosis and treatment*, 3e, 103–106. Edinburgh: Churchill Livingstone.

18

Benign Neoplasms of the Oral Mucosa

CHAPTER MENU

18.1   Lipoma
18.2   Schwannoma (Neurilemmoma)
18.3   Granular Cell Tumour
18.4   Haemangioma
18.5   Lymphangioma
18.6   Leiomyoma (Vascular Leiomyomas): Key Features
18.7   Rhabdomyoma: Key Features

18.1   Lipoma

18.1.1   Definition/Description

- A benign neoplasm of the adipose tissue

18.1.2   Frequency

- Common in the trunk and proximal areas of the extremities
- Less than 4.4% of all benign oral mesenchymal neoplasms
- Uncommon in the mouth

18.1.3   Aetiology

- Possible causes
  - Heredity
  - Fatty degeneration
  - Hormonal abnormalities
  - Injuries

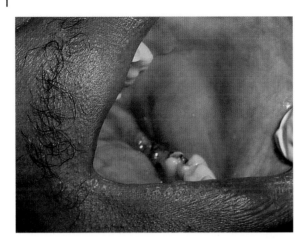

Figure 18.1 Lipoma of the left buccal mucosa presenting as a soft fluctuant mass. *Source:* Reproduced with permission from Ramdas, K., Lucas, E., Thomas, G. et al. 2008. *A Digital Manual for the Early Diagnosis of Oral Neoplasia.* Lyon: IARC. Available from http://screening.iarc.fr/atlasoral.php?lang=1

18.1.4 Clinical Features

- Age group: mostly 60 years and over
- Common intraoral sites: buccal mucosa/buccal vestibule (50% of all intraoral lipomas)
- Other: lip, tongue, palate, and floor of the mouth
- Asymptomatic until they reach a large size
- Usually soft, smooth-surfaced nodular, occasionally fluctuant, and yellowish slow growing mass (Figure 18.1)
- Pedunculated or sessile

18.1.5 Microscopic Features

- Collection of mature fat cells
- Thin fibrous wall
- Occasional significant fibrous component (fibrolipoma)
- Significant small blood vessels (angiolipoma)
- Spindle cell lipoma presents mucoid background (myxoid lipoma)

18.1.6 Differential Diagnosis

- Fibroma
- Neuroma
- Traumatic neuroma
- Pleomorphic adenoma

18.1.7 Diagnosis

- History
- Clinical findings
- Microscopic findings

18.1.8 Management

- Conservative local excision

18.1.9   Prognosis

- Excellent
- No recurrences

18.2   Schwannoma (Neurilemmoma)

18.2.1   Definition/Description

- A benign neoplasm of Schwann cells in the neural sheath

18.2.2   Frequency

- 25–48% occur in the head and neck region
- Spinal nerve roots and the cervical, sympathetic, vagus, and ulnar nerves commonly involved
- Rare in the mouth

18.2.3   Aetiology/Origin

- Proliferation of Schwann cells in the perineurium
- Arises in association with a nerve trunk and as it grows it pushes the nerve aside

18.2.4   Clinical Features

- Age group: young and middle aged people affected
- Location: tongue, followed by palate, floor of mouth, buccal mucosa, gingiva, lips, and vestibular mucosa (Figure 18.2a)
- Solitary, smooth, submucosal swelling
- Asymptomatic and slow growing
- Occasionally mild pain

18.2.5   Microscopic Features

- Encapsulated with a thin fibrous wall
- Tumour consists of two types of cells:
  - Antoni type A: fascicles of spindle-shaped Schwann cells, palisading around central acellular eosinophilic area (Verocay bodies) (Figure 18.2b)
  - Antoni type B type: cells are less organized, fusiform widely separated and dispersed loosely with a network of delicate reticulated fibres (Figure 18.2b)
- Positive immunohistochemical staining for S-100

18.2.6   Differential Diagnosis

- Fibro-epithelial polyp
- Irritation fibroma
- Granular cell tumour
- Lipoma

(a)　　　　　　　　　　　　　　　　　　(b)

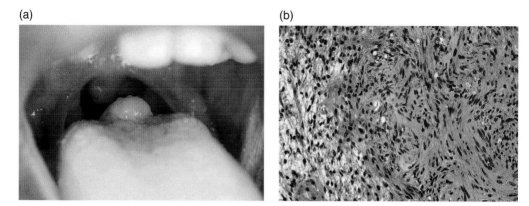

Figure 18.2   Schwannoma. (a) Schwannoma of the base of the tongue (*source:* by kind permission of Dr Rana Sukvinder, Department of Dentistry, Dr Rajendra Prasad Government Medical College, Kangra, Himachal Pradesh, India). (b) Photomicrograph (haematoxylin and esosin ×10) showing cellular Antoni A area on the right and paucicellular Antoni B area on the left (*Source:* Nephron, https://commons.wikimedia.org/w/index.php?curid=17748282. Licensed under CC BY-SA 3.0).

- Mucocele
- Benign salivary gland tumours

18.2.7   Diagnosis

- History
- Clinical findings
- Microscopic findings

18.2.8   Management

- Conservative surgical excision

18.2.9   Prognosis

- Good
- No recurrences

18.3   Granular Cell Tumour

18.3.1   Definition/Description

- A common benign tumour of the oral cavity, possibly derived from Schwann cells
- Characterized by tumour mass composed of eosinophilic cytoplasm and granular cells

18.3.2   Frequency

- Frequently found in the head and neck region (45–65% of all sites affected by the tumour)
- Of these, 70% are in the oral cavity

18.3.3 Aetiology/Origin

- Peripheral nerve sheath origin

18.3.4 Clinical Features

- Age group: second and sixth decade of life
- Tongue, cheek mucosa, and hard palate frequent sites
- Asymptomatic solitary pink or yellow solitary nodule (Figure 18.3)
- Occasionally painful

18.3.5 Microscopic Features

- Proliferation of large, polygonal neoplastic cells with cytoplasmic granules
- Eosinophilic cytoplasm
- Small and eccentrically located nucleus
- Pseudoepitheliomatous hyperplasia
- Lacks a capsule

18.3.6 Differential Diagnosis

- Fibro epithelial polyp
- Irritation fibroma
- Schwannoma
- Traumatic neuroma
- Lipoma
- Benign salivary gland tumours

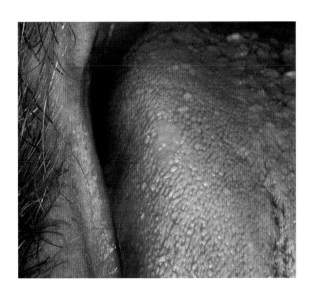

Figure 18.3 Granular cell tumour; nodular lesion located on the dorsum of the tongue. *Source:* Steven Brett Sloan 2018. Oral Granular Cell Tumors - Medscape Reference. https://emedicine.medscape.com › 1079023-overview.

18.3.7 Diagnosis

- History
- Clinical findings
- Microscopic findings

18.3.8 Management

- Surgical excision

18.3.9 Prognosis

- Good
- May have a malignant potential

18.4 Haemangioma

18.4.1 Definition/Description

- A benign tumour of endothelial origin
- History of rapid growth followed by involution
- Some believe that this is a hamartomatous/developmental lesion

18.4.2 Frequency

- Common in infancy: 4–5% of one-year-old children

18.4.3 Aetiology/Origin

- Endothelial proliferation of blood vessels

18.4.4 Clinical Features

- Tumours of infancy/childhood in most cases
- Common in white populations and in females
- 60% of all cases in the head and neck region
- Usually solitary lesions (80%)
- Two types:
  - Capillary (many capillaries)
  - Cavernous haemangioma (large, blood-filled vessels or sinusoids)
- Intraoral sites: tongue, lips, buccal mucosa, gingiva, and palatal mucosa
- Soft, solitary, flat or nodular (sessile) mass
- Smooth or lobulated surface, purple or deep red in colour (Figure 18.4a)
- Blanch on application of pressure (diascopy positive)

18.4.5   Microscopic Features

- Capillary haemangioma: mass of fine capillaries lined by endothelium supported by connective tissue and covered by surface epithelium
- Cavernous haemangioma: dilated thin-walled blood-filled vessels or sinusoids covered by surface epithelium (Figure 18.4b)

18.4.6   Differential Diagnosis

- Haemangioma
- Pyogenic granuloma
- Lymphangioma (filled with traces of blood)
- Kaposi's sarcoma
- Haemangiopericytoma

18.4.7   Diagnosis

- History
- Clinical findings

18.4.8   Management

- Most require no intervention
- Regression seen
- Up to 20% require surgical intervention, intralesional injection of sclerosing agent, laser ablation, or cryosurgery
- Note: incisional biopsy of haemangioma for diagnostic purposes is not recommended since it may lead to a fatal outcome from excessive bleeding

(a)   (b)

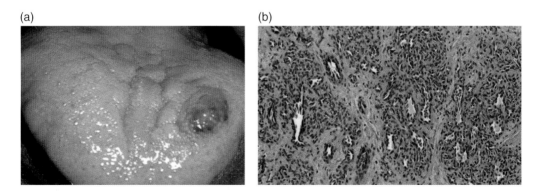

Figure 18.4   Cavernous haemangioma (a) Cavernous haemangioma of the tongue (*source:* by kind permission of Dr Krishna Kripal, Raja Rajeswari Dental College and Hospital, Bangalore, Karnataka, India). (b) Photomicrograph shows dilated thin-walled blood-filled vessels or sinusoids covered by surface epithelium. *Source:* By kind permission of Professor Vijay Shankar, Adichunchanagiri Institute of Medical Sciences,Mandya District, Karnataka, India.

18.4.9 Prognosis

- Oral haemangiomas have an overall favourable prognosis, as these lesions are benign, and only a minority will require treatment

18.5 Lymphangioma

18.5.1 Definition/Description

- A benign tumour that occurs due to proliferation of lymphatic vessels
- Some believe that this is a hamartomatous/developmental lesion

18.5.2 Frequency

- Common in the head and neck region
- Majority occur in the first two years of life

18.5.3 Aetiology/Origin

- Proliferation of lymphatic vessels

18.5.4 Clinical Features

- Usually seen in infancy
- Head and neck are common locations
- Common intraoral site: anterior two thirds of the tongue (causing macroglossia)
- Presentation: translucent, smooth, or nodular (with pebbly surface) lesion (Figure 18.5a)
- Asymptomatic
- May resolve spontaneously

18.5.5 Microscopic Features

- Dilated lymphatic vessels covered by surface epithelium (Figure 18.5b)

(a)　　　　　　　　　　　　　　　　　(b)

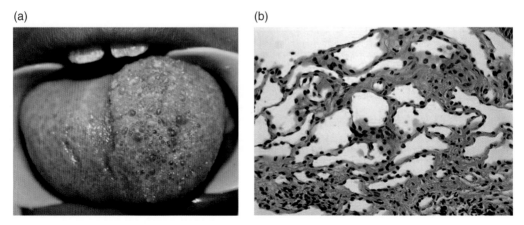

Figure 18.5   Lymphangioma of the tongue. (a) Lymphangioma of the tongue. (b) Photomicrograph showing numerous lymphatic vessels. (*Source:* image (a) Healthjade.net)

18.5.6 Differential Diagnosis

- Haemangioma
- Neurofibroma

18.5.7 Diagnosis

- History
- Clinical findings

18.5.8 Management

- Some lesions do not require treatment
- When treatment is required, surgery or sclerotherapy recommended

18.5.9 Prognosis

- The prognosis is good for most patients, although large tumours of neck/tongue may result in airway obstruction, leading to complications
- Recurrence after surgery is common

18.6 Leiomyoma (Vascular Leiomyomas): Key Features

- Benign tumour of smooth muscle of the skin, gastrointestinal tract or uterus
- In the mouth, they are usually derived from the smooth muscle of the vessel walls (vascular leiomyomas)
- Oral leiomyomas are rare
- Slow-growing firm nodular lesion
- Asymptomatic
- Normal in colour or bluish hue
- Sites: lips, tongue, palate, and buccal mucosa
- Interlacing bundles of spindle shaped cells with blunt ended nuclei
- Positive for vimentin and smooth muscle actin
- Management: local surgical excision

18.7 Rhabdomyoma: Key Features

- Benign neoplasm of striated muscle
- Rare neoplasm
- Middle aged/older adults
- Oral sites: floor of the mouth, soft palate and base of the tongue
- Nodular mass, can grow to a large size
- Differential diagnosis: irritation fibroma, neurilemmoma, granular cell tumour
- Histopathology: large polygonal granular cells with eosinophilic cytoplasm, focal cells with cross striations seen, positive for myoglobin and desmin
- Management: surgical excision
- Recurrence in 10–42% of cases

Recommended Reading

Bhayya, H., Pavani, D., Tejaswi, A., M.L., and Geeta, P. (2015). Oral lymphangioma: a rare case report. *Contemporary Clinical Dentistry* 6 (4): 584–587.

Kripal, K., Rajan, S., Ropak, B., Jayanti, I. (2013).Cavernous haemangioma of the tongue. 2013: 898692.

Neville, B.W., Damm, D.D., Allen, C.M., and Chi, C.A. (2016). Soft tissue tumours. In: *Oral and Maxillofacial Pathology*, 4e, 473–515. St Louis: Elsevier.

Odell, E.W. (2017). Diseases of the oral mucosa: soft tissue tumours. In: *Cawson's Essentials of Oral Pathology and Oral Medicine*, 9e, 377–380. Edinburgh: Elsevier.

Prabhu, S.R. (2019). Benign mucosal swellings. In: *Clinical Diagnosis in Oral Medicine: A case based approach*, 205–239. New Delhi: Jaypee Brothers Medical Publishers.

Torres-Domingo, S., Bagan, J.V., Jiménez, Y. et al. (2008). Benign tumors of the oral mucosa: a study of 300 patients. *Medicina Oral, Patología Oral y Cirugía Bucal* 13 (3): E161–E166.

19

Oral Potentially Malignant Disorders

19.1 Erythroplakia

19.1.1 Definition/Description

- A red patch or a plaque that cannot be clinically or pathologically diagnosed as any other definable lesion

19.1.2 Frequency

- Uncommon to rare

19.1.3 Aetiology/Risk Factors

- Tobacco use, alcohol consumption
- Betel quid chewing among non-drinkers and non-smokers
- Often no known cause (idiopathic)

Handbook of Oral Pathology and Oral Medicine, First Edition. S. R. Prabhu.
© 2022 John Wiley & Sons Ltd. Published 2022 by John Wiley & Sons Ltd.
Companion website: www.wiley.com/go/prabhu/oral_pathology

19.1.4 Clinical Signs and Symptoms

- Middle-aged/older people
- Male preponderance
- Asymptomatic
- Occasional burning sensation
- Floor of the mouth, lateral and ventral surfaces of the tongue, soft palate, and buccal mucosa
- Well-demarcated, erythematous patch with a soft velvety texture (Figure 19.1a)
- Occasionally combined with a white lesion (erythroleukoplakia)

19.1.5 Microscopic Features

- Atrophic and non-keratinized epithelium
- In 75–90% of lesions severe epithelial dysplasia (carcinoma in situ; Figure 19.1b)
- Frank malignancy (squamous cell carcinoma) in 50% of cases on first biopsy
- Signs of chronic inflammation in the connective tissue
- Some of the most important microscopic characteristics of dysplasia are:
  - Loss of polarity of basal cells
  - Increased nuclear cytoplasmic ratio
  - Irregular epithelial stratification
  - Increased number of abnormal mitotic figures and their presence in the superficial epithelium
  - Cellular and nuclear pleomorphism
  - Keratinization of single cell groups
  - These features are suggestive of malignant potential

19.1.6 Differential Diagnosis

- Non-specific mucositis
- Lichen planus
- Erythematous candidosis

(a)

(b)

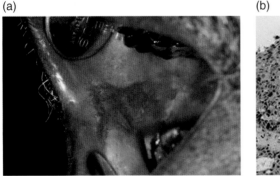 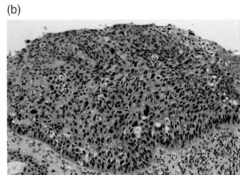

Figure 19.1 (a) Erythroplakia of the buccal mucosa (*source:* reproduced with permission from Ramdas, K., Lucas, E., Thomas, G. et al. 2008. *A Digital Manual for the Early Diagnosis of Oral Neoplasia.* Lyon: IARC. Available from http://screening.iarc.fr/atlasoral.php?lang=1). (b) Histopathological features show severe dysplasia (carcinoma in situ) with abnormal cytological features occupying the entire thickness of the epithelium; 70–90% of erythroplakia lesions show these features.

- Lupus erythematosus
- Vascular lesions
- Geographic tongue/erythema migrans
- Median rhomboid glossitis
- Lichenoid lesion
- Drug reactions
- Contact stomatitis

19.1.7 Diagnosis

- History of tobacco and alcohol habits
- Clinical findings
- Biopsy to assess degree of dysplasia

19.1.8 Management

- Guided by the histopathological diagnosis:
  - Surgical excision or laser ablation for dysplastic lesions
  - Aggressive treatment for squamous cell carcinoma
  - Long-term follow-up
  - Cessation of tobacco, betel quid, and alcohol use

19.1.9 Prognosis

- Fair to good, depending on the degree of dysplasia

19.1.10 Special Considerations

- A potentially malignant lesion
- 50% of erythroplakia lesions turn out to be malignant in the first biopsy
- The remaining 50% show dysplasia of varying degree

19.2 Leukoplakia

19.2.1 Definition/Description

- A white patch or plaque that cannot be characterized clinically or pathologically as any other disease
- Predominantly a white patch of questionable risk, having excluded other known diseases or disorders that carry no increased risk for cancer

19.2.2 Frequency

- Global prevalence 1–5%
- Higher prevalence in the Indian subcontinent

19.2.3 Aetiology/Risk Factors

- 75% associated with tobacco use (smoking, chewing, and snuff dipping)
- Betel quid use
- Areca nut chewing
- Alcohol consumption in excess
- Human papilloma virus types 16 and 18 (in those who do not use tobacco in any form or drink alcohol)
- *Candida albicans* (candidal leukoplakia): aetiological association is debated
- Herbal sanguinaria used in tooth paste or mouth rinse
- Chronic sun exposure (for lower-lip leukoplakia)
- Idiopathic

19.2.4 Clinical Features

- Asymptomatic
- Usually in persons above 40 years of age
- Male predilection (70%)
- Six times more common among smokers than non-smokers
- Common on the lateral margins of the tongue and floor of the mouth in western populations
- Common on the buccal mucosa and lower buccal sulcus in Asian populations
- White patch cannot be scraped off with gauge or mouth mirror
- White patch does not blanch or disappear on stretching
- Two main clinical types of leukoplakia occur: Homogeneous and non-homogeneous.
  - Homogeneous leukoplakia arises as a white patch slightly elevated, thin, white to grey, uniform, and can present well-defined borders or may gradually mix with normal adjacent mucosa (Figure 19.2a)
  - Non-homogeneous:
    - Mixed with red patch with predominantly white surface (erythroleukoplakia/speckled leukoplakia) (Figure 19.2b)
    - Nodular (granular) leukoplakia (Figure 19.2c).
    - Verrucous (exophytic) leukoplakia (Figure 19.2d)
    - Proliferative verrucous leukoplakia (Figure 19.2e)

19.2.5 Microscopic Features

- Epithelial features in oral leukoplakia are highly variable
- Basic microscopic features include hyperkeratosis (of ortho or parakeratotic type), epithelial acanthosis, and chronic inflammatory infiltrates in lamina propria (Figure 19.2f)
- Histological evidence of epithelial dysplasia seen in leukoplakia is suggestive of malignant potential
- Some of the most important microscopic architectural disturbances of dysplasia include the following:
  - Loss of polarity of basal cells
  - Increased nuclear cytoplasmic ratio
  - Irregular epithelial stratification

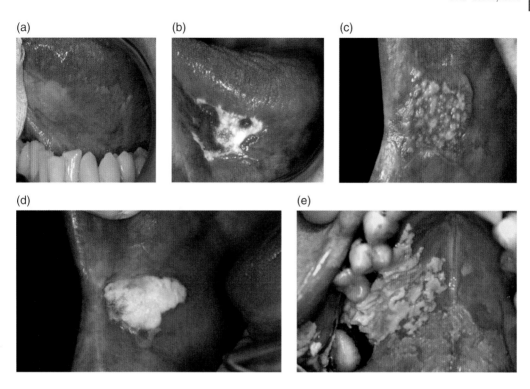

Figure 19.2 (a-e)   Clinical types of leukoplakia. (a) Homogeneous leukoplakia. (b) Non-homogeneous leukoplakia (Erythroleukoplakia). (c) Non-homogeneous leukoplakia (nodular/granular type). (d) Non-homogeneous leukoplakia (Verrucous type). (e) proliferative verrucous leukoplakia. (*Source:* Images a-d By kind permission of Professor Isaac vander Waal, Netherlands and image e, reproduced with permission from Ramdas, K., Lucas, E., Thomas, G. et al. 2008. *A Digital Manual for the Early Diagnosis of Oral Neoplasia.* Lyon: IARC. Available from http://screening.iarc.fr/atlasoral.php?lang=1.

- Increased number of abnormal mitotic figures and their presence in the superficial epithelium
- Cellular and nuclear pleomorphism
- Keratinization of single cell groups

- Dysplastic changes can be graded as mild, moderate, or severe
  - Architectural disturbances affecting the lower third of the epithelium with cytological atypia suggest mild dysplasia (Figures 19.2g)
  - Architectural disturbances affecting greater than two thirds of the epithelium with pronounced cytological atypia suggest severe dysplasia (Figure 19.2h)
  - Architectural disturbances affecting the full thickness of epithelium with pronounced cytological atypia is suggestive of carcinoma in situ (Figure 19.2i)

19.2.6   Differential Diagnosis

- List includes all chronic white lesions that cannot be rubbed off with gauge
- The following lesions must be clinically ruled out before a diagnosis of leukoplakia is made:
  - Frictional keratosis (lesions due to cheek and tongue biting)

(f)   (g)

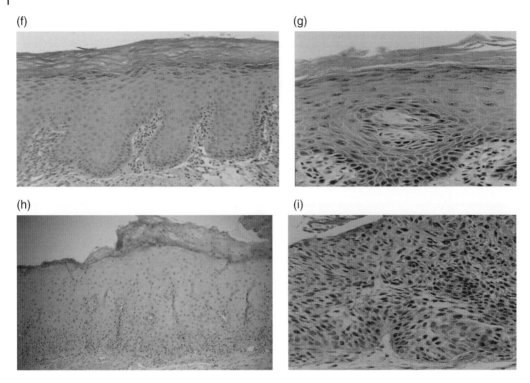

(h)   (i)

Figure 19.2 (f-i) Photomicrographs of oral leukoplakia. (f) shows epithelial hyperplasia with increased number of basal/parabasal cells and a hyperkeratotic surface. Regular stratification is observed. There is no cytological atypia. (g) Note mild dysplasia. Architectural disturbances affecting the lower third of the epithelium and cytological atypia are seen. (h) photomicrograph shows moderate to severe dysplasia. Note architectural disturbances affecting more than two thirds of the epithelium and pronounced atypia is present. (i) Photomicrograph showing microscopic features of carcinoma in situ: architectural disturbances are observed in the full thickness of epithelium with pronounced cellular atypia. No superficial keratinization is evident. (*Source:* images f–i, Maria Auxiliadora Vieira do Carmo and Patrícia Carlos Caldeira. 2013. Binary system of grading epithelial dysplasia in oral leukoplakias. In: *Carcinogenesis*, ed. Kathryn Tonissen, IntechOpen, doi: 10.5772/54466).

- Lichen planus (plaque or papular types)
- lichenoid lesions
- Smoker's keratosis
- Smokeless tobacco keratosis (tobacco pouch keratosis)
- Submucous fibrosis
- Sublingual keratosis
- Actinic keratosis (lower lip)
- Candidal leukoplakia (chronic hyperplastic candidosis)
- Syphilitic leukoplakia (rare)
- Hairy leukoplakia
- Hereditary intraepithelial dysplasia
- White sponge nevus
- Leukoedema

19.2.7 Diagnosis

- History
- Clinical examination
- Biopsy (mandatory to rule out dysplastic changes)

19.2.8 Management/Prevention

- Surgical excision, laser ablation, cryosurgery, electrosurgery
- Topical application of cytotoxic drugs such as bleomycin
- Systemic retinoid (vitamin A alone or in combination with beta-carotene) to prevent recurrence
- Cessation of tobacco habits
- Avoidance of excessive alcohol consumption
- Follow-up with repeat biopsies

19.2.9 Prognosis

- Good; if the lesion is completely removed and causative habits are eliminated

19.2.10 Special Considerations

- Leukoplakia is essentially a clinical term with no histological connotation
- Leukoplakia is a potentially malignant lesion
- It is not possible to determine clinically which area of leukoplakia carries malignant potential
- The risk of malignant transformation in leukoplakia ranges from 0.9% to 17.5%.
- Early detection is essential

19.3 Chronic Hyperplastic Candidosis (Candidal Leukoplakia)

19.3.1 Definition/Description

- A white and red, keratotic, fixed, mucosal lesion usually at the labial commissural region associated with chronic *C. albicans* infection

19.3.2 Frequency

- Uncommon
- Prevalence varies from 0.2–11%

19.3.3 Aetiology/Risk Factors

- Causative agent: chronic *C. albicans* infection (hyphal forms)
- Predisposing factors:
  - Reduced vertical dimension
  - Poor denture hygiene

  – Dry mouth
  – Tobacco habits
  – Diabetes
  – Vitamin and iron deficiencies, etc.

19.3.4   Clinical Features

- Well-demarcated, palpable, raised irregular white or red-white lesions (Figure 19.3a)
- Lesions cannot be rubbed off
- Common on the labial commissures, followed by the dorsum of the tongue
- May be associated with median rhomboid glossitis, denture stomatitis or angular cheilitis
- Usually painless; occasionally sore
- More common in adult males, middle aged or older and smokers

19.3.5   Microscopic Features

- Parakeratotic surface epithelium
- Candidal hyphae in the surface epithelium (periodic acid–Schiff stain; Figure 19.3b)
- Epithelial dysplasia in rare instances (in which case diagnosis usually is leukoplakia superimposed with candida)
- Mild connective tissue chronic inflammation

19.3.6   Differential Diagnosis

- All white keratotic lesions that cannot be rubbed off:
  – Leukoplakia (speckled leukoplakia)
  – Frictional keratosis (morsicatio buccarum)
  – Lichen planus
  – Lichenoid lesions

(a) (b)

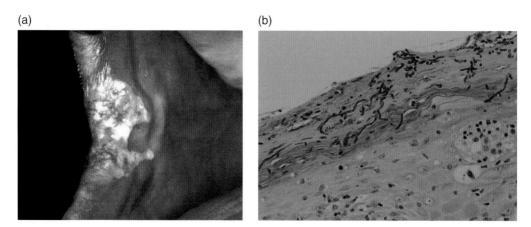

Figure 19.3   (a) Chronic hyperplastic candidosis (candidal leukoplakia) of the labial commissure.
(b). Photomicrograph showing filamentous candidal hyphae in the superficial layers of the epithelium
and the presence of inflammatory cells (periodic acid–Schiff stain).

19.3.7 Diagnosis

- History of symptoms, habits and predisposing factors
- Clinical findings
- Cytology of scrapings for candidal hyphae
- Biopsy (to confirm candidal association and to assess dysplastic changes if any)

19.3.8 Management/Prevention

- Antifungal treatment after confirmation of candidal involvement
- Miconazole topical gel
- Systemic antifungal agent: fluconazole
- Treatment of accompanying fungal infections (e.g. angular cheilitis)
- Management of local and systemic predisposing factors
- Cessation of smoking
- Surgical excision of the lesion (little value)
- Follow-up

19.3.9 Prognosis

- Fair to good

19.3.10 Special Considerations

- Long-term intermittent antifungal therapy may be required
- The risk of malignant transformation of candidal leukoplakia exists but is low

19.4 Palatal Lesions in Reverse Smokers

19.4.1 Definition/Description

- A kind of smoking where the burnt end of a hand-rolled smoking device is put in the mouth. The smoking device is a homemade cigar made by crudely rolling few semi-dried tobacco twigs. Palatal changes in reverse smokers are considered potentially malignant

19.4.2 Frequency

- Reverse smoking is prevalent in some communities in the Philippines, South America, the Caribbean, the Netherlands, Columbia, Sardinia, Venezuela, Panama, and India
- There is a great degree of variation in the prevalence rates from country to country
- Majority of people practising reverse smoking are household workers and a sizable proportion of them are females

19.4.3 Aetiology/Risk Factors

- Tobacco and heat are the main etiologic factors
- The highest intra-oral air temperatures of those using reverse smoking device (known as chutta in India) can reach up 120 degrees C

19.4.4 Clinical Features

- Palate and the dorsum of the tongue are mainly affected
- The palatal changes consist of the following features:
  - Elevated white patches, red patches, hyperpigmented or non-pigmented areas (Figure 19.4) and ulcerations
  - Palatal cancers can arise in this region with pre-existing palatal changes; hence mucosal changes seen in reverse smokers are considered potentially malignant
  - Malignant transformation in lesions associated with reverse smoking ranges from 5.6% to 6.25%

19.4.5 Microscopic Features

- Any of the following changes can be seen:
  - Hyperorthokeratinized epithelium
  - Hyperparakeratinized epithelium
  - Hyperorthokeratinized or parakeratized epithelium with melanin pigmentation in the basal cell layer
  - Inflammatory cells in the connective tissue
  - Mild, moderate, or severe epithelial dysplasia
  - Squamous cell carcinoma

19.4.6 Differential Diagnosis

- All keratotic lesions including leukoplakia
- Smoker's melanosis
- Melanoma
- Kaposi's sarcoma
- Erythroplakia
- Squamous cell carcinoma

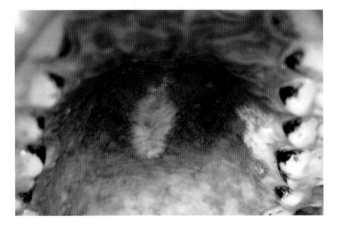

Figure 19.4 Palatal lesions in reverse smokers. Note palatal white keratotic lesions (leukoplakia) and areas of hyperpigmented and depigmented areas in an Indian reverse smoker (*source:* by kind permission of Dr T. Sreenivasa Bharath, Vishnu Dental College, Bhimavaram, Andhra Pradesh, India).

19.4.7 Diagnosis

- History
- Clinical examination
- Microscopic findings

19.4.8 Management

- Cessation of the reverse or customary smoking habit
- No tobacco chewing
- Management (surgical or non-surgical) of the lesions is based on the microscopic assessment
- Periodic follow-up is essential

19.4.9 Prognosis

- Early detection and treatment of the lesions have a good prognosis

19.5 Oral Lichen Planus: Key Features

- Oral lichen planus is a chronic mucocutaneous disorder:
  - A chronic T-cell mediated disorder that affects up to 3–5% of population
  - Of uncertain aetiology
- Clinically, commonly manifests as bilateral white, lacy plaques, located mainly on the buccal mucosa and tongue
- Other clinical subtypes include:
  - Reticular (asymptomatic and most common)
  - Papular (resembling Fordyce spots)
  - Plaque-like (resemble leukoplakia)
  - Atrophic/erosive/ulcerative (sore and erythematous and resemble lichenoid lesion and discoid lupus erythematosus)
  - Bullous (rare, resembles pemphigus and mucous membrane pemphigoid)
  - Atrophic, presenting on the gingiva present as desquamative gingivitis
- Usually, lesions are multiple and have a symmetric/bilateral distribution
- Some patients may present skin lesions of lichen planus
- Biopsy and histopathologic examination are confirmatory
- Histopathologically, oral lichen planus is characterized by the presence of a band-like lymphocytic infiltrate at the interface between the epithelium and connective tissue and by the basal cell degeneration
- Histopathology also aids in identifying the presence of epithelial dysplasia and rarely malignancy
- Oral lichen planus is a potentially malignant disorder:
  - Malignant potential:
    - Around 1.1% of lesions progress into oral squamous cell carcinoma (OSCC), with a higher incidence in smokers, alcohol users, and in those infected with hepatitis C virus
    - Among all subtypes, erosive oral lichen planus is the type that has the highest frequency to progresses to OSCC (Figure 19.5)

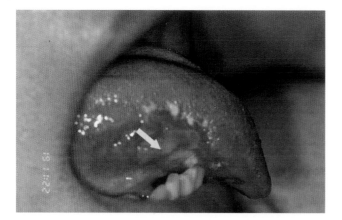

Figure 19.5   Erosive lichen planus with malignant transformation (arrow) on the right lateral margin of the tongue surrounded by white striae (*source:* reproduced with permission from Ramdas, K., Lucas, E., Thomas, G. et al. 2008. *A Digital Manual for the Early Diagnosis of Oral Neoplasia.* Lyon: IARC. Available from http://screening.iarc.fr/atlasoral.php?lang=1).

  o The tongue is the most common oral site that shows malignant transformation
  o On average, it takes 5.5 years for lesions to transform into an established OSCC
  o Numerous biomarkers have been shown to be associated with malignant transformation. These include:
    o Modulators of apoptosis (p53, myeloid cell leukemia 1)
    o Cell-cycle regulators (Bmi1, p16)
    o Tissue remodelling factors (matrix metalloproteinases)
    o Inflammation-related factors (tumour necrosis factor alpha, interleukin 6, and cyclooxygenase-2)
 – There is no increased risk of skin malignancy in patients with cutaneous lichen planus
• For further information see Chapter 16 (section 16.2)

19.6   Oral Submucous Fibrosis

19.6.1   Definition/Description

• Oral submucous fibrosis is characterized by immobility and progressive limitation of the mouth opening resulting from fibrosis of the submucosa

19.6.2   Frequency

• Prevalence in India: 6.4% of the population
• Prevalent in countries where migration from the subcontinent is significant
• Genetic predisposition is linked (for those of Indian origin)

19.6.3   Aetiology/Risk Factors

• Habitual chewing of 'paan' or gutkha
• Paan (betel quid) contains grated areca nut and slaked lime wrapped in a betel leaf (*Piper betel*)
• Gutkha: mixture of powdered areca nut and tobacco

- Areca nut contains alkaloid arecoline that stimulates fibroblasts to produce collagen
- Other risk factors:
  - Excessive chilly consumption
  - Areca nut chewing
  - Vitamin B complex and iron deficiency
  - Autoimmunity
  - Genetic and environmental factors

19.6.4 Clinical Features

- Common in men 20–40 years of age
- Common sites: buccal mucosa, labial mucosa, retromolar pads, soft palate, and floor of the mouth. Rarely, fibrotic changes occur in the pharynx and oesophagus
- Symptoms (from early to late stages):
  - Mucosal burning sensation
  - Hypersalivation ending with xerostomia
  - Mucosal blanching with marble like appearance (Figure 19.6a)
  - Leathery and inelastic mucosa with palpable fibrous bands resulting in restricted mouth opening
  - Difficulty in swallowing
  - Speech and hearing defects
  - Leukoplakia or erythroplakia also may occur

19.6.5 Microscopic Features

- Thin (atrophic) epithelium
- Thickened and hyalinization of the subepithelial connective tissue (Figure 19.6b)

(a)   (b)

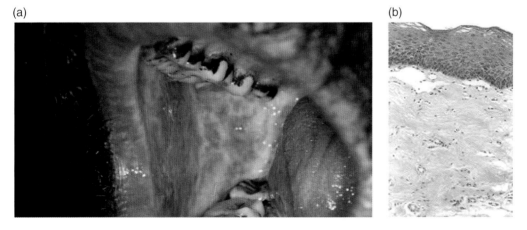

Figure 19.6 Oral submucous fibrosis. (a) Note the characteristic blanching and marble like appearance of the buccal mucosa. (b) Photomicrograph shows atrophic squamous epithelium with collagenization of the sub epithelial tissue with scanty inflammatory cells. (*Source:* images reproduced with permission from Ramdas, K., Lucas, E., Thomas, G. et al. 2008. *A Digital Manual for the Early Diagnosis of Oral Neoplasia.* Lyon: IARC. Available from http://screening.iarc.fr/atlasoral.php?lang=1.)

- Avascular connective tissue
- Neutrophils and eosinophils in the connective tissue (early stages)
- Moderate chronic inflammatory cell infiltrate in the connective tissue (later stages)
- Atrophy of the underlying muscle fibres and replacement with fibrous tissue
- Occasional presence of dysplastic epithelial cells

19.6.6 Differential Diagnosis

- Scleroderma
- Morphea (localized scleroderma)
- Scar tissue
- Reticular lichen planus
- Leukoplakia
- Frictional keratosis
- Temporomandibular joint dysfunction

19.6.7 Diagnosis

- History of betel quid or gutkha chewing habits and symptoms
- Clinical findings
- Biopsy to rule out dysplastic changes

19.6.8 Management

- Cessation of paan/gutkha chewing habit
- Intralesional injections of corticosteroids
- Muscle-stretching exercises
- Surgical excision of the fibrous bands

19.6.9 Prognosis

- Variable
- Relapse is common
- Betel quid with areca nut is a carcinogen
- Oral submucous fibrosis is a potentially malignant disorder; risk of malignant change is 5–8%
- Regular follow-up biopsy of red or white lesions in patients with oral submucous fibrosis is mandatory

19.7 Oral Lichenoid Lesion

19.7.1 Definition/Description

- Oral lichenoid lesion, also known as oral lichenoid reaction, is a lichen planus-like chronic inflammatory lesion of the oral mucosa that occurs as an allergic response to dental materials or to the use of certain medications

19.7.2 Frequency

- 2.4% in general population
- Female predilection
- Majority in adults

19.7.3 Aetiology/Risk Factors

- Topographical association with dental materials (mercury and amalgam, epoxy resins, composite restorations)
- Medications implicated:
  - Nonsteroidal anti-inflammatory drugs
  - Angiotensin-converting-enzyme inhibitors
  - Beta-blockers
  - Oral antidiabetic drugs
  - Antimalarials
  - Antibiotics (metronidazole, penicillins, tetracycline, and sulphonamides)
  - Some tricyclic antidepressants
  - Allopurinol
  - Carbimazole
- Can also be found in association with chronic graft-versus-host disease (GVHD).

19.7.4 Clinical Features

- White or mixed white and red lesions similar to lichen planus (reticular, linear, annular striae or erosive; Figure 19.7)
- White lesions usually asymptomatic

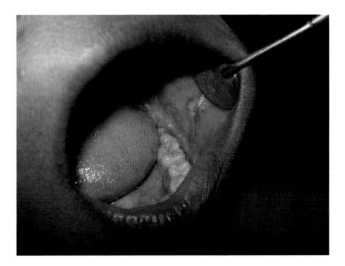

Figure 19.7 Oral lichenoid lesion. Note the lichenoid reaction on the left buccal mucosa due to type IV hypersensitivity reaction to amalgam restoration in the buccal aspect of first and second molars on the left lower jaw (*source:* reproduced with permission from Ramdas, K., Lucas, E., Thomas, G. et al. 2008. *A Digital Manual for the Early Diagnosis of Oral Neoplasia.* Lyon: IARC. Available from http://screening.iarc.fr/atlasoral. php?lang=1).

- Erosive lesions symptomatic
- Buccal mucosa, lateral border of the tongue, and labial mucosa
- Unilateral lesions
- Limited in size

19.7.5 Microscopic Features

- Dense subepithelial lymphohistiocytic infiltrate
- Increased numbers of intraepithelial lymphocytes
- Degeneration of basal keratinocytes
- Degenerating basal keratinocytes form colloid (civatte, hyaline, and cytoid) bodies, which appear as homogenous eosinophilic globules

19.7.6 Differential Diagnosis

- Lichen planus
- Leukoplakia
- Erythema multiforme
- Mucous membrane pemphigoid
- Pemphigus vulgaris

19.7.7 Diagnosis

- History (recent restorations, medications or GVHD)
- Clinical examination
- Skin patch test (if dental materials are suspected as the cause)
- Biopsy to rule out dysplastic changes
- Immunofluorescence tests

19.7.8 Management

- Corticosteroids (as for lichen planus)
- For restoration-related lesions, removal and replacement of restorations with alternatives
- For drug associations, withdrawal, and replacement in consultation with medical practitioner
- If GVHD-related, seek medical consultation
- Maintenance of good oral hygiene

19.7.9 Prognosis

- Good
- Oral lichenoid lesion is a potentially malignant lesion
- The reported malignant transformation varies between 0.5% and 2%

19.8 Lupus Erythematosus

19.8.1 Definition/Description

- Lupus erythematosus is an autoimmune connective tissue disorder characterized by skin lesions and rarely lichen planus-like oral lesions

- Three types:
  - Systemic lupus erythematosus (SLE)
  - Chronic cutaneous lupus erythematosus (CCLE), also known as discoid lupus erythematosus
  - Subacute cutaneous lupus erythematosus (SCLE)

19.8.2 Frequency

- Estimated incidence rates 1–25 per 100 000 in North America, South America, Europe, and Asia
- More common in those of African descent
- Sex predilection: affects females more than males
- Age at onset 15–55 years

19.8.3 Aetiology/Risk Factors

- Unknown
- Multifactorial: immunological, genetic, hormonal, environmental factors

19.8.4 Clinical Signs and Symptoms

- Fatigue, skin rashes (malar rash), fevers, and pain or swelling in the joints, sun sensitivity and oral ulcers
- Oral lesions in approximately 20% of patients; common in CCLE.
- Oral lesions are:
  - Unilateral
  - Symptomatic if ulcerated
  - Lichen planus-like with mucosal erosion/ulceration and surrounding white striae (Figure 19.8)
- Palate is the preferred site (lichen planus spares this site)

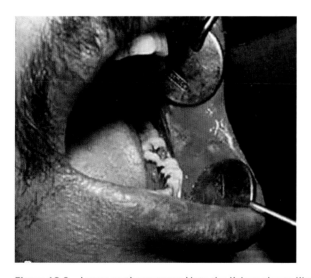

Figure 19.8 Lupus erythematosus. Note the lichen planus like lesion on the left buccal mucosa in a patient with discoid erythematosus (*source:* reproduced with permission from Ramdas, K., Lucas, E., Thomas, G. et al. 2008. *A Digital Manual for the Early Diagnosis of Oral Neoplasia.* Lyon: IARC. Available from http://screening.iarc.fr/atlasoral.php?lang=1).

19.8.5   Microscopic Features

- Epithelium hyperplastic
- Keratin extends in to rete ridges
- Thickening of the basement membrane zone
- Mild fibrosis around blood vessels
- Chronic inflammatory infiltrate extends deep into connective tissue and is perivascular
- Immunofluorescence test: granular deposits of immunoglobulins and complement (C3) along the basement membrane zone

19.8.6   Differential Diagnosis

- Oral lesions of lupus erythematosus with:
  - Lichen planus
  - Oral lichenoid lesions
  - Leukoplakia
  - Erythema multiforme
  - Mucous membrane pemphigoid
  - Pemphigus

19.8.7   Diagnosis

- History of disease (systemic or cutaneous)
- Clinical examination of the oral lesions
- Biopsy of erosive lesions to rule out dysplastic changes
- Immunofluorescence studies (lupus band test)
- Detection of autoantibodies (in SLE)
- Raised erythrocyte sedimentation rate, anaemia, leukopenia in SLE

19.8.8   Management

- Systemic corticosteroids and immunosuppressant drugs for SLE
- Topical applications of corticosteroid agents for oral lesions
- Low doses of antimalarial drug (hydroxychloroquine)
- Intralesional corticosteroid injections
- Avoid excessive sun (ultraviolet) exposure

19.8.9   Prognosis

- Good response in CCLE
- Variable outcome in SLE
- Oral lesions of lupus erythematosus carry a very low malignant potential

19.9   Actinic Keratosis of the Lip (Actinic Cheilitis)

19.9.1   Definition/Description

- Actinic keratosis of the lip is a keratotic scaly white potentially malignant lesion commonly occurring as a result of intense and chronic sun damage to the skin and lips in susceptible patients
- Synonyms used include actinic cheilitis, solar cheilosis, sailor's lip, farmer's lip

19.9.2 Frequency

Common among fair-complexioned outdoor people with a male: female ratio of 10:1.

19.9.3 Aetiology/Risk Factors

- Chronic sun damage: ultraviolet radiation (range: 290–320 nm) to the lower lip of people who are fair complexioned

19.9.4 Clinical Signs and Symptoms

- Asymptomatic in most cases
- Vermilion of the lower lip
- Irregular scaly plaques; often crusted and fissured (Figure 19.9a)
- Areas of atrophic areas
- Indistinct mucocutaneous junction

19.9.5 Microscopic Features

- Hyperkeratosis
- Atrophy of epithelium
- Irregular budding and basilar atypia (Figure 19.9b)
- Epithelial dysplasia (mild to moderate or severe) in some cases
- Signs of elastosis in the submucosa

(a) (b)

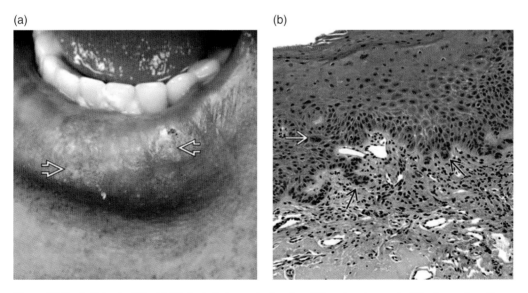

Figure 19.9 Actinic cheilitis. (a) Clinical photograph showing diffuse involvement of the lower lip with associated crusting (arrows). (b) Photomicrograph shows mucosal acanthosis with overlying parakeratosis. There is irregular budding and basilar atypia, with many of the cells showing enlarged, hyperchromatic-staining nuclei (arrows). (*Source:* images by kind permission of Dr Cao Xuan Cu.)

19.9.6   Differential Diagnosis

- Thermal/chemical burns
- Exfoliative cheilitis
- Squamous cell carcinoma

19.9.7   Diagnosis

- History of outdoor/sun exposure
- Clinical signs
- Biopsy to rule out dysplastic changes

19.9.8   Management

- Avoidance of sun exposure
- Use of sunscreens
- Surgical removal of the lesions
- Laser ablation
- Topical 5-fluorouracil application
- If already malignant, resection and reconstructive surgery

19.9.9   Prognosis

- Good prognosis
- Long term follow-up
- Avoid exposure to the sun
- A potentially malignant lesion; malignant transformation around 3.7%

19.10   Graft-Versus-Host Disease

19.10.1   Definition/Description

- GVHD is one of the most frequent and serious complications of hematopoietic stem cell transplantation which usually affects multiple organs and tissues including the oral tissues
- Two forms exist: acute and chronic

19.10.2   Frequency

- The acute form is observed in 50–70% and chronic form is seen in 30–50% of all allogenic transplant patients
- In the chronic form of GVHD, the oral cavity is one of the most commonly affected regions
- The prevalence of oral GVHD lesions ranges between 45% and 83%

19.10.3   Aetiology/Risk Factors

19.10.3.1   Risk Factors
- Human leukocyte antigen incompatibility or the absence of blood ties between the donor and recipient
- Advanced age of the donor and recipient

- A female donor and male recipient
- Childbirth (parity) in female donors (allosensitization)
- The transplantation of mobilized peripheral blood cells
- The infusion of donor lymphocytes

19.10.4   Clinical Features

- In the chronic form of GVHD, the oral cavity is one of the most affected regions
- Skin: lichen planus-like lesions
- Mouth: lichen planus-like lesions, hyperkeratotic plaques, restricted mouth opening
- Genitalia: lichen-type lesions
- Gastrointestinal tract: oesophageal web and strictures
- Joints: stiffness

19.10.5   Microscopic Features

- Oral lesions:
  - Dyskeratotic epithelial cells
  - Apoptosis and an inflammatory infiltrate of lichenoid appearance beneath the epithelial basal lamina
  - Fibrosis secondary to collagen deposits

19.10.6   Differential Diagnosis

- Oral lesions:
  - Oral lichen planus
  - Lichenoid lesions
  - Morphea
  - Submucous fibrosis
  - Leukoplakia

19.10.7   Diagnosis

- History of haematopoietic stem cell transplant and symptoms and signs
- Clinical examination
- Biopsy to rule out dysplastic changes

19.10.8   Management

- Intensive topical corticosteroid therapy (dexamethasone/triamcinolone gel or rinse)
- Tacrolimus ointment
- Intralesional injection (triamcinolone) for recalcitrant lip lesions
- Follow-up

19.10.9   Prognosis

- Serious and potentially life-threatening condition
- Oral lesions in chronic GVHD are potentially malignant disorders

19.11 Dyskeratosis Congenita

19.11.1 Definition/Description

- A rare, genetic, progressive bone marrow failure syndrome characterized by the triad of reticulated skin hyperpigmentation, nail dystrophy, and oral leukoplakia

19.11.2 Frequency

- Rare; estimated to occur in one in one million people
- Male to female ratio is approximately three to one

19.11.3 Risk Factors/Aetiology

- Loss of chromosomal telomeres
- *TERC*, *TERT*, and *TINF2* gene mutations in autosomal dominant dyskeratosis congenita
- *NOP10*, *TERT*, *NHP2*, and *RTEL1* mutations in autosomal recessive dyskeratosis congenita

19.11.4 Clinical Features

- Mucocutaneous features appear between the ages of 5 years and 15 years
- Skin: reticulated tan to grey hyperpigmentation or hypopigmented macules
- Nails: nail dystrophy, with ridging and longitudinal splitting in 90% of patients
- Oral: mucosal leukoplakia involving buccal mucosa, tongue, and oropharynx in 80% of patients (part of the triad)
- Oral dysplastic red lesions
- Haematological abnormalities
- Symptoms and signs of bone marrow failure
- OSCC in up to one third of cases

19.11.5 Microscopic Features

- Oral leukoplakia:
  - Hyperkeratosis
  - Epithelial hyperplasia
  - Dysplastic epithelium (mild/moderate/severe)
  - Occasionally squamous cell carcinoma arising from leukoplakia

19.11.6 Differential Diagnosis

- Oral lesions: all keratotic white lesions (leukoplakia):
  - Frictional keratosis
  - White sponge nevus
  - Lichen planus (plaque and papular types)
  - Lupus erythematosus

19.11.7 Diagnosis

- Family history, and systemic and oral symptoms
- Clinical examination of skin, nail, and oral mucosa
- Skin: dermatoscope
- Oral lesions: biopsy to identify degree of dysplasia

19.11.8 Management

- Oral lesions: biopsy mandatory to determine dysplastic changes
- Management based on microscopic findings (as for leukoplakia)

19.11.9 Prognosis

- Bone marrow failure is a major cause of death, with approximately 70% mortality rate
- Patients have an increased prevalence of malignant mucosal neoplasms (usually in the third decade of life)

19.12 Sublingual Keratosis: Key Features

- Sublingual keratosis is leukoplakia located in the sublingual region
- Cannot be rubbed off with gauze
- Cause is unknown
- A white lesion with wrinkled surface which extends from the anterior floor of the mouth on to the ventral surface of the tongue
- The lesion is irregular in its outline often showing 'ebbing tide' appearance on its surface (Figure 19.10)
- Sublingual keratosis is considered to be potentially malignant

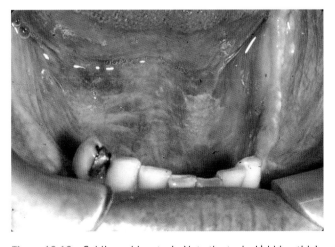

Figure 19.10 Sublingual keratosis. Note the typical 'ebbing tide' appearance of the lesion (*source:* by kind permission of David Wilson, Adelaide, Australia).

- Malignant transformation of these lesions may be as high as 24%
- Specialist referral is indicated for surgical removal of the lesion and follow-up

19.13   Syphilitic Leukoplakia: Key Features

- Syphilitic leukoplakia is a rare mucosal white patch in patients with tertiary syphilis
- Known to carry malignant potential
- For further details see Chapter 23 (section 23.4)

19.14   Darier's Disease: Key Features

- Also known as Darier–White disease, keratosis follicularis
- Darier's disease is a genetic disorder
- Skin and nails may be involved
- Affected skin areas may be itchy and sore and the skin may have an unpleasant odour
- Oral lesions are found in nearly 50% of patients with the disorder
- Palate is the most common site for oral lesions followed by the gingiva, tongue and the floor of the mouth
- Oral lesions vary from mild pink or white papules to large plaques with cobblestone surface mimicking those of pyostomatitis vegetans
- Oral lesions are generally asymptomatic
- Histologically, the lesions present suprabasal splits in the epithelium with acantholytic and dyskeratotic cells observed as corps ronds and corps grains
- Diagnosis of Darier's disease is often made by the appearance of the skin, family history, or genetic testing for the mutation in the *ATP2A2* gene
- Management of oral lesions is as for leukoplakia

Recommended Reading

Cawson, R.A. and Odell, E.W. (2017). Potentially malignant disorders. In: *Cawson's Essentials of Oral Pathology and Oral Medicine*, 9e (ed. E.W. Odell), 299–312. Edinburgh: Churchill Livingstone.

do Carmo, M.A.V., Caldeira, P.C. (2013). Binary system of grading epithelial dysplasia in oral leukoplakias. In: *Carcinogenesis*, ed. Kathryn Tonissen, doi: 10.5772/54466. IntechOpen. Available from: https://www.intechopen.com/books/carcinogenesis/binary-system-of-grading-epithelial-dysplasia-in-oral-leukoplakias

Neville, B.W., Damm, D.D., Allen, C.M., and Chi, C.A. (2016). Epithelial pathology. In: *Oral and Maxillofacial Pathology*, 4e, 331–401. St Louis, MO: Elsevier.

Prabhu, S.R. (2019). Mucosal white and red lesions and disorders with malignant potential. In: *Clinical Diagnosis in Oral Medicine: A case based approach*, 68–124. New Delhi: Jaypee Brothers Medical Publishers.

Prabhu, S.R. and Felix, D.H. (2016). Mucosal white lesions. In: *Handbook of Oral Diseases for Medical Practice* (ed. S.R. Prabhu), 129–514. New Delhi: Oxford University Press.

Saman Warnakulasuriya, Omar Kujan, José M. Aguirre-Urizar, José V. Bagan, Miguel Ángel González-Moles, Alexander R. Kerr, Giovanni Lodi, Fernanda Weber Mello, Luis Monteiro, Graham R. Ogden,

Philip Sloan, Newell W. Johnson.(2020). Oral potentially malignant disorders: A consensus report from an international seminar on nomenclature and classification, convened by the WHO Collaborating Centre for Oral Cancer. https://doi.org/10.1111/odi.13704

Thongprasom, K., Suter, V.G.,.A., and Warnakulasuriya, S. (2016). Oral potentially malignant disorders II: oral lichen planus, oral lichenoid lesions, oral graft-versus-host disease and oral submucous fibrosis. In: *Handbook of Oral Diseases for Medical Practice* (ed. S.R. Prabhu), 331–344. New Delhi: Oxford University Press.

van der Waal, I. (2015). Oral leukoplakia, the ongoing discussion on definition and terminology. *Medicina Oral, Patología Oral y Cirugía Bucal* 20 (6): e685–e692.

Warnakulasuriya, S. (2016). Oral potentially malignant disorders 1. Leukoplakia and erythroplakia. In: *Handbook of Oral Diseases for Medical Practice* (ed. S.R. Prabhu), 319–330. New Delhi: Oxford University Press.

Warnakulasuriya, S. and Tilakaratne, W.M. (eds.) (2014)). *Oral Medicine and Pathology: A Guide to Diagnosis and Management*. New Delhi: Jaypee Brothers Medical Publishers.

Warnakulasuriya, S., Johnson, N.W., and Van Der Waal, I. (2007). Nomenclature and classification of potentially malignant disorders of the oral mucosa. *Journal of Oral Pathology and Medicine* 36 (10): 575–580.

20

Malignant Neoplasms of the Oral Mucosa

CHAPTER MENU

20.1 Squamous Cell Carcinoma and Verrucous Carcinoma
20.2 Melanoma (Malignant Melanoma)
20.3 Kaposi's Sarcoma
20.4 Fibrosarcoma: Key Features
20.5 Rhabdomyosarcoma: Key Features
20.6 Leiomyosarcoma: Key Features

20.1 Squamous Cell Carcinoma and Verrucous Carcinoma

20.1.1 Definition/Description

- Malignant neoplasms of the stratified squamous epithelium of the lip and oral mucosa are known as squamous cell carcinomas
- Oral squamous cell carcinoma is synonymous with the term 'oral cancer'
- Verrucous carcinoma is a variant of squamous cell carcinoma with low-grade malignancy

20.1.2 Frequency

- 95% of all oral cancers are squamous cell carcinomas (OSCC)
- Globally, OSCCs account for 2–4% of all cancers
- Geographical variation exists: around 45% of all cancers in India are OSCCs
- 95% of people with OSCC are older than 40 years
- Lip cancer is prevalent in Australia. Papua New Guinea, Serbia and Ukraine and is low in prevalence in Asia
- Oral verrucous carcinoma accounts for 2–12% of all oral carcinomas

20.1.3 Aetiology/Risk Factors

- Lip squamous cell carcinoma:
  - Sunlight (ultraviolet radiation)
  - Smoking unfiltered cigarettes and 'roll your own cigarettes' are also implicated

Handbook of Oral Pathology and Oral Medicine, First Edition. S. R. Prabhu.
© 2022 John Wiley & Sons Ltd. Published 2022 by John Wiley & Sons Ltd.
Companion website: www.wiley.com/go/prabhu/oral_pathology

- Fair-skinned older outdoor workers and immunocompromised individuals are at increased risk
- Immunosuppression
- OSCC:
  - Multifactorial aetiology
  - 75% of OSCCs are associated with smoking and smokeless tobacco use
  - Excess alcohol consumption: tobacco and alcohol have a synergistic effect
  - Betel quid chewing
  - Areca nut chewing
  - Iron deficiency anaemia (a predisposing factor)
  - Potentially malignant oral disorders (see Chapter 19)
  - Oncogenic human papillomaviruses (HPV) for those who have no tobacco or alcohol habits
  - Chronic candidal infections
  - Radiation
  - Genetic (rare)
- Verrucous carcinoma:
  - Prolonged use of smokeless tobacco (chewing tobacco/snuff dipping) and areca nut chewing in the Indian subcontinent
  - Strong association also exists with alcohol consumption, smoking, and oral microbiota
  - May arise from potentially malignant oral disorders such as oral verrucous leukoplakia, oral lichen planus, oral submucous fibrosis

20.1.4 Clinical Features

- Lip squamous cell carcinoma:
  - 90% occur in the lower lip
  - Male predominance
  - Early presentation: epithelial thickening, induration, crusting, and shallow ulceration (Figures 20.1a and b)
  - Regional lymph node metastasis is a late feature (10% of cases)
- OSCC:
  - Asymptomatic in early stages
  - Common sites: lateral borders and ventral surface of the tongue, floor of the mouth, lingual aspect of the alveolus, retromolar region buccal mucosa
  - In India, buccal mucosa is the most common intraoral site
  - OSCC may manifest in any of the following forms:
    - Exophytic growth such as fungating, cauliflower-like, papillary or verruciform, non-healing ulcers with indurated and everted edges, fissures, white, red, or white and red mixed patches (Figures 20.1b-f)
    - Non-healing tooth sockets
    - Unexplained tooth mobility
    - Trismus
    - Dysphagia
    - Pain in later stages (due to secondary infection or neural infiltration)
    - Cervical lymph node enlargement (due to regional metastasis)
    - May invade bone in advanced stages
    - Weight loss and distant metastasis in advanced stages

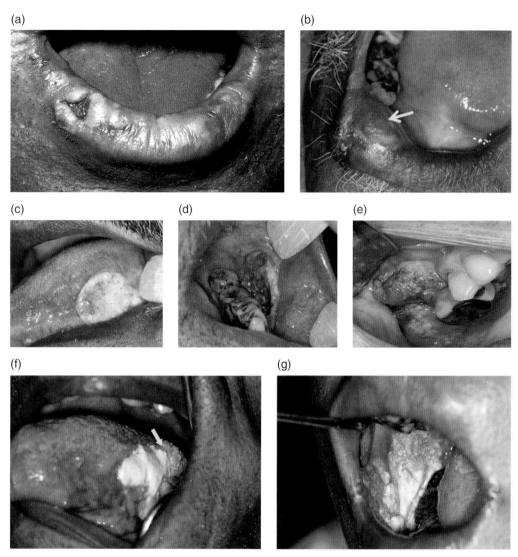

Figure 20.1 Presentation of clinical forms of lip and oral cancer(a-g). (a) Squamous cell carcinoma of the lower lip presenting as an indurated ulcerative white lesion. Note the signs of extensively sun damaged lip. (b) Squamous cell carcinoma of the lower lip presenting as a red lesion (yellow arrow) and ulceration (red arrow). (c) Squamous cell carcinoma of the tongue presenting as a raised white lesion. (d) Squamous cell cancer presenting as a non-healing ulcer with indurated and everted margins. (e) Squamous cell carcinoma presenting as a fungating growth of the gingiva. (f) Squamous cell carcinoma (yellow arrow) arising from oral leukoplakia. (g) Verrucous carcinoma of the buccal mucosa. Note blunt projections of the exophytic mass. *Source:* Image a. Coronation Dental Specialty Group, CC BY-SA 4.0 <https://creativecommons.org/licenses/by-sa/4.0>, via Wikimedia Commons. images b–d, f, g reproduced with permission from Ramdas, K., Lucas, E., Thomas, G. et al. 2008. *A Digital Manual for the Early Diagnosis of Oral Neoplasia.* Lyon: IARC. Available from http://screening.iarc.fr/atlasoral.php?lang=1;

- Verrucous carcinoma:
  - Sites of occurrence: buccal mucosa, tongue, lip gingiva alveolar ridge, and floor of the mouth (Figure 20.1g)
  - Predilection for elderly males
  - Papillary exophytic mass

(h) (i)

(j) (k)

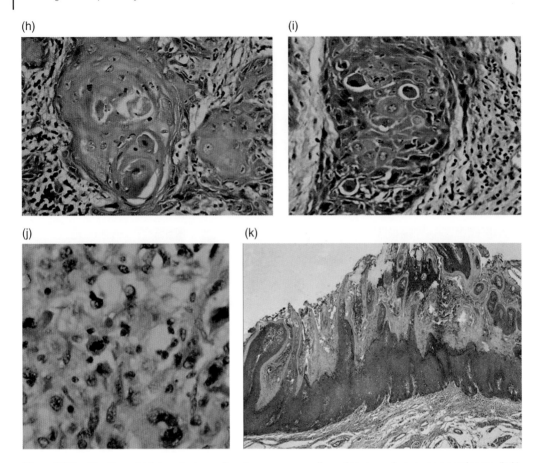

Figure 20.1 (Continued) Histopathology of oral squampous cell carcinoma and verrucous carcinoma (h-k). (h) Photomicrograph showing features of well-differentiated squamous cell carcinoma. Note neoplastic cells with pale eosinophilic cytoplasm forming concentric layers of keratin (keratin pearls). (i) Photomicrograph showing features of moderately differentiated squamous cell carcinoma with evidence of squamous pattern somewhere between the well differentiated (h) and the poorly differentiated (j) examples. (j) Photomicrograph showing poorly differentiated squamous cell carcinoma. The tumour cells have little cytoplasm and are irregular and darkly stained with poor evidence of squamous pattern. (k) Photomicrograph showing features of verrucous carcinoma. Note the enlarged bulb like acanthotic invaginations giving it a 'pushing margin' appearance. image k by kind permission of Dr P. Swetha, Vishnu Dental College, Bhimavaram Andhra Pradesh, India.)

- Slow growing
- Rare regional/distant metastasis

20.1.5 Microscopic Features

- Lip and OSCCs:
  - Proliferating cells with nuclear pleomorphism, increased nuclear to cytoplasmic ratio, increased and abnormal mitosis, and abnormal keratinization
  - Pointed rete ridges infiltrating deep into the connective tissues
  - Three histological grades: well differentiated, moderately differentiated, and poorly differentiated
  - Well differentiated (Figure 20.1h):

- ○ Histological and cytological features closely resemble those of the squamous epithelial lining of the oral mucosa
    - ○ Keratinisation is a prominent feature
    - ○ Few mitotic figures are seen
    - ○ Rare, atypical mitoses or multinucleated epithelial cells
    - ○ Nuclear and cellular pleomorphism is minimal
    - ○ Histologically, most lip cancers are well-differentiated squamous cell carcinomas
  - – Moderately differentiated (Figure 20.1i):
    - ○ Features are intermediate between well-differentiated and poorly differentiated
    - ○ Less keratinisation and more nuclear and cellular pleomorphism
    - ○ More mitotic figures and some are abnormal in form
    - ○ Intercellular bridges are less conspicuous
  - – Poorly differentiated (Figure 20.1j):
    - ○ Slight/poor resemblance to the normal stratified squamous epithelium of the oral mucosa
    - ○ Keratinization is rarely present and intercellular bridges are extremely scarce
    - ○ Mitotic activity is frequent and atypical mitoses can readily be found
    - ○ Cellular and nuclear pleomorphism are obvious and multinucleated cells are frequent
- Verrucous carcinoma:
  - – Histologically, verrucous carcinoma is a well-differentiated squamous cell carcinoma
  - – Shows proliferative epithelial pegs with hyperplastic and blunt drop-shaped ends (Figure 20.1k)
  - – All epithelial pegs in verrucous carcinoma invade the connective tissue with the same depth, forming pushing borders
  - – Low-grade malignant changes seen with minimal epithelial atypia
  - – Lymphocytes and plasma cells are present in the connective tissue

20.1.6 Differential Diagnosis

- Lip and OSCCs:
  - – Hyperplastic/reactive benign lesions (granulomas, fibromas, etc.)
  - – Non-neoplastic chronic ulcerative lesions (e.g. traumatic ulcer, tuberculous ulcer, syphilitic ulcer, necrotizing sialometaplasia)
  - – Oral potentially malignant disorders (leukoplakia, erythroplakia, and other oral potentially malignant disorders)
  - – Verrucous carcinoma
  - – Chronic white or red benign lesions (e.g. frictional keratosis, papilloma, erythematous candidosis)
- Verrucous carcinoma:
  - – Verrucous hyperplasia, including verrucous proliferative leukoplakia
  - – Squamous papilloma
  - – Well-differentiated OSCC

20.1.7 Diagnosis

- History (of risk factors, symptoms, etc.)
- Clinical findings including clinical TNM staging (stages I–IV)
- Biopsy/microscopic findings, including histological grading
- Other: computed tomography, ultrasound and magnetic resonance imaging

20.1.8 Management

- Surgical
- Radiotherapy
- Combined surgery and radiotherapy
- Chemotherapy

20.1.9 Prognosis

- Lip cancers: good prognosis: 90% survive five years
- Oral cancers: Generally good prognosis for TNM stages I and II (over 90% survive the first year and 75% for five years)
- Poor prognosis for TNM stages III and IV (50% die in two years and 60% in five years)
- Recurrences can occur
- Verrucous carcinomas: five-year survival rate of only approximately 50%
- Cessation of tobacco smoking/chewing habits, areca nut chewing, and moderate alcohol consumption, and protected (sunscreen) exposure to solar radiation are essential preventive measures
- Detection and treatment of oral potentially malignant disorders and early diagnosis are of paramount importance

20.2 Melanoma (Malignant Melanoma)

20.2.1 Definition/Description

- Melanoma is a malignant neoplasm of melanocytic origin

20.2.2 Frequency

- Third most common skin cancer
- 5% of total skin cancers and 75% of skin cancer deaths
- Mucosal melanoma rare; less than 1% in Europe and the United States but up to 12% in Japan
- Australia has one of the highest rates of melanoma in the world

20.2.3 Aetiology/Risk Factors

- Cause: ultraviolet radiation from sun exposure
- Risk factors:
  - Fair skin
  - Tendency to sun burn and freckle easily
  - Family history of melanoma
  - Excessive numbers of nevi
  - Immunosuppression

20.2.4 Clinical Features

- Age group: 45–85 years
- Female predilection
- Hard palate and upper alveolar ridge favoured sites
- 30% of melanomas preceded by pre-existing long standing hyperpigmented lesions

- Asymptomatic, dark brown or black patches in early stages; grow laterally
- Nodular growth, ulceration, loosening of teeth and bleeding in later stages (Figure 20.2a)
- In later stages, growth is deeper into the connective tissue and about 50% metastasize to the cervical lymph nodes and 29% to the distant sites
- Most cases diagnosed in the later stages

20.2.5 Microscopic Feature

- In the radial phase, malignant melanocytes cluster along the basement membrane (Figure 20.2b)
- In the vertical phase, malignant melanocytes invade connective tissue
- Spindle-shaped or pleomorphic and hyperchromatic malignant cells with granules of melanin are seen
- Mitotic activity is variable
- Malignant cells invade blood vessels and lymphatics
- Around 10% are amelanotic, with lack of melanin

20.2.6 Differential Diagnosis

- Vascular malformations
- Kaposi's sarcoma
- Haematoma

20.2.7 Diagnosis

- History
- Clinical findings
- Microscopic findings
- Immunohistochemistry

(a) (b)

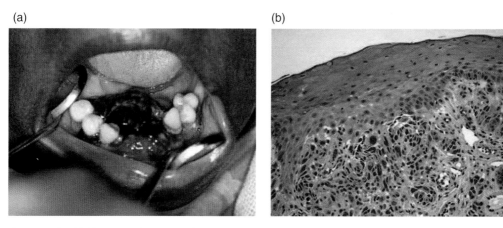

Figure 20.2   Malignant melanoma of the floor of mouth. (a) Note the extensive black mass with a nodular surface involving the lower labial sulcus extending to the floor of mouth (*source:* reproduced with permission from Ramdas, K., Lucas, E., Thomas, G. et al. 2008. *A Digital Manual for the Early Diagnosis of Oral Neoplasia.* Lyon: IARC. Available from http://screening.iarc.fr/atlasoral.php?lang=1). (b) Photomicrograph reveals tumour cells showing affinity for the surface epithelium (merging of tumour and epithelium). Cellular pleomorphism and smudged nuclei with pseudo inclusions are also noted.

20.2.8 Management

- Wide surgical excision with simultaneous neck dissection followed by radical radiotherapy and/ or chemotherapy

20.2.9 Prognosis

- Five-year survival rate for node negative melanomas is 30%; for metastatic lesion 10%
- Early diagnosis is of paramount importance

20.3 Kaposi's Sarcoma

20.3.1 Definition/Description

- A malignant neoplasm of the blood vessels or lymphatics caused by the human herpes virus type 8 (HHV-8; also called Kaposi's sarcoma-associated herpesvirus)
- Four forms of Kaposi's sarcoma have been recognised: classic, African (endemic), immunosuppression-associated and, AIDS-related (epidemic) forms

20.3.2 Frequency

- HIV/AIDS-associated form is common on the skin and oral cavity
- 70% of individuals with AIDS-related Kaposi's sarcoma develop oral lesions

20.3.3 Aetiology

- Aetiological agent is HHV-8

20.3.4 Clinical Features

- Usually asymptomatic; may precede or follow skin lesions
- Predominantly adult males (men who have sex with men) affected (peak incidence 25–59 years of age)
- The hard palate, gingiva, and tongue are frequently affected sites
- Starts as a flat purplish area, enlarges into a nodular mass, ulcerates and bleeds (Figure 20.3a)

20.3.5 Microscopic Features

- Proliferation of endothelial cells with cytological atypia and frequent mitoses (Figure 20.3b)
- Vascular slits and extravascular blood cells

20.3.6 Differential Diagnosis

- Purpura, ecchymosis, haematoma
- Haemangioma
- Melanoma

(a) (b)

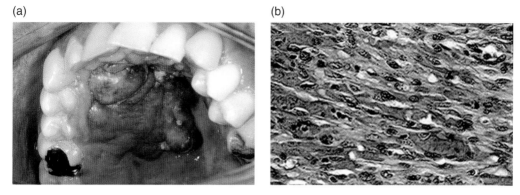

Figure 20.3   Kaposi's sarcoma. (a) Note a purple-coloured nodular mass on the hard palate (*source: reproduced with permission from Ramdas, K., Lucas, E., Thomas, G. et al. 2008. A Digital Manual for the Early Diagnosis of Oral Neoplasia. Lyon: IARC. Available from http://screening.iarc.fr/atlasoral.php?lang=1*).
(b) Photomicrograph shows proliferation of endothelial cells with cytological atypia and slit-like vascular spaces filled with erythrocytes.

- Bacillary angiomatosis
- Pyogenic granuloma

20.3.7   Diagnosis

- History (sexual orientation, HIV infection, symptoms, etc.)
- Clinical findings
- Microscopic findings
- Immunostaining for podoplanin (a marker for lymphatic endothelial cells)
- Immunohistochemical staining for HHV-8 virus

20.3.8   Management

- Small and localized lesions: surgical excision
- Intralesional injection of chemotherapeutic agent (e.g. interferon alpha with didanosine, bleomycin) for widespread lesions
- For advanced cases, systemic chemotherapy with chimeric antigen receptor T-cell therapy for AIDS is useful
- Opportunistic infections, if any, should be treated
- Radiotherapy not recommended (to avoid mucositis)

20.3.9   Prognosis

- Variable

20.4   Fibrosarcoma: Key Features

- A malignant mesenchymal neoplasm derived from fibroblasts that can occur as a soft-tissue mass or as a primary or secondary bone tumour

- Constitutes only 0.05% of fibrosarcomas of all body sites
- Presents as a soft red tumour with or without surface ulceration
- Tongue, gingiva, buccal mucosa, and lip are usual sites
- May affect jaw bones
- Histology is confirmatory
- Microscopic features of a well-differentiated fibrosarcoma include fascicles of spindle-shaped cells ('herringbone pattern'), collagen and variable numbers of mitotic figures
- Poorly differentiated neoplasm shows a large number of mitotic figures, giant cells, and less collagen
- Differential diagnosis includes Kaposi's sarcoma, malignant fibrohistiocytoma, and other connective tissue malignant neoplasms
- Surgical excision is the treatment of choice
- Recurrence occurs in about 50% of cases
- Over all five-year survival rate 20–35%

20.5   Rhabdomyosarcoma: Key Features

- Malignant neoplasm of the skeletal muscle origin
- Two major types: embryonal and alveolar rhabdomyosarcoma
- Common in children and adolescents
- Common in the head and neck region
- Rarely occurs in oral cavity and accounts for 0.04% of all head and neck malignancies
- Male preponderance
- Common intraoral sites: tongue followed by the soft palate, hard palate, and buccal mucosa
- Extraoral: face and orbit commonly affected
- Most cases are painless, sometimes with pain or paraesthesia
- A space-occupying lesion with rapid growth
- Loss of teeth and possible trismus
- Microscopic features include small round tumour cells with hyperchromatic nuclei, skeletal muscle-like cross-striations and giant cells
- Tumour is vimentin and myosin positive
- Local surgical excision followed by chemotherapy
- Five year survival rate is around 66% for embryonal type

20.6   Leiomyosarcoma: Key Features

- Malignant neoplasm of the smooth muscle origin
- Uncommon in the oral soft tissues
- Origin from the smooth muscle cells of the blood vessels and circumvallate papillae
- Presents as a painless or painful rubbery slow growing mass
- Individuals 50–70 years of age are affected
- Microscopic features include fascicles of spindle-shaped cells with abundant cytoplasm with cigar-shaped, blunt-ended nuclei
- Masson trichrome stain shows bright red cytoplasm

- Differential diagnosis includes pyogenic granuloma, leiomyoma, peripheral ossifying fibroma, angiosarcoma and Kaposi's sarcoma
- Radical surgical excision is the treatment of choice
- Reported five-year survival rate is around 55%

Recommended Readings

Johnson, N.W. (2016). Oral carcinoma and other malignant lesions of the mouth and jaws. In: *Handbook of Oral Diseases for Medical Practice* (ed. S.R. Prabhu), 332–345. New Delhi: Oxford University Press.

Johnson, N.W. (2004). Oral cancer. In: *Textbook of Oral Medicine* (ed. S.R. Prabhu), 166–175. New Delhi: Oxford University Press.

Johnson, N.W., Jayasekara, P., Hemalatha, A.A., and Amarasinghe, K. (2011). Squamous cell carcinoma and precursor lesions of the oral cavity: epidemiology and aetiology. *Periodontology* 57: 19–37.

Neville, B.W., Damm, D.D., Allen, C.M., and Chi, C.A. (2016). Epithelial pathology. In: *Oral and Maxillofacial Pathology*, 4e, 331–401. St Louis, MO: Elsevier.

Odell, E.W. (2017). Oral cancer. In: *Cawson's Essentials of Oral Pathology and Oral Medicine*, 9e, 317–339. Edinburgh: Elsevier.

Prabhu, S.R. (2019). Oral cancer (squamous cell carcinoma) and other malignancies. In: *Clinical Diagnosis in Oral Medicine: A case based approach*, 243–265. New Delhi: Jaypee Brothers Medical Publishers.

Shah, J. and Johnson, N.W. (2016). *Textbook of Oral Cancer*, 2e. London: CRC Press.

Swetha, P., Supriya, N.A., and Kumar, G.N. (2013). Characterization of different verrucous mucosal lesions. *Indian Journal of Dental Research* 24: 642–644.

Warnakulasuriya, S. (2011). Squamous cell carcinoma and precursor lesions: prevention. *Periodontology* 57: 38–50.

Part IV

Pathology of the Salivary Glands

21

Non-neoplastic Salivary Gland Diseases

CHAPTER MENU
21.1   Salivary Calculi: Key Features
21.2   Mucoceles (Mucous Extravasation Cysts, Mucous Retention Cysts and Ranula)
21.3   Sjögren's Syndrome
21.4   Sialadenitis: Key Features
21.5   Necrotizing Sialometaplasia: Key Features

21.1   Salivary Calculi: Key Features

- Salivary stone in the salivary gland or duct
- 80% in the submandibular gland
- 8% in the parotid gland
- 2% in the sublingual and minor salivary glands
- Male preponderance
- Common in adults
- Saliva is supersaturated with calcium and magnesium phosphate, which deposits around a nidus, usually cell debris
- Usually unilateral
- Pain and swelling of the gland at mealtime
- Does not cause dry mouth
- Smell and taste of the food is the stimulating factor
- Large stone can be seen on radiography (Figure 21.1)
- Ultrasound is effective in locating the stone
- Small stones can be manipulated out of the duct orifice
- Lithotripsy for larger stones
- Occasionally surgical incision of the duct is required

Handbook of Oral Pathology and Oral Medicine, First Edition. S. R. Prabhu.
© 2022 John Wiley & Sons Ltd. Published 2022 by John Wiley & Sons Ltd.
Companion website: www.wiley.com/go/prabhu/oral_pathology

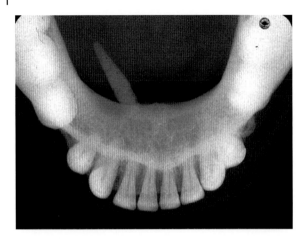

Figure 21.1   Occlusal radiographical image of a sialolith.

21.2   Mucoceles (Mucous Extravasation Cysts, Mucous Retention Cysts and Ranula)

21.2.1   Definition/Description

- A cavity filled with mucous
- Two types: mucous extravasation and mucous retention cysts
- Ranula is a distinctive type of extravasation cyst of the sublingual gland located in the floor of the mouth

21.2.2   Frequency

- Common in the minor salivary glands, less common in the major salivary glands
- Almost never occurs in the upper lip

21.2.3   Aetiology

- Extravasation cyst: trauma causing duct rupture and escape of saliva into the connective tissue
- Retention cyst: obstruction and dilatation of the ducts
- Ranula: damage to or obstruction of one of the ducts of Rivinus, which drain into the sublingual duct or floor of the mouth

21.2.4   Clinical Features

- Mucous extravasation cyst:
  - Minor salivary glands of the lower lip usually involved
  - Common in children
  - Appear as round, fleshy, fluctuant, shiny, bluish swelling mimicking a vesicle (Figure 21.2a)

(a)   (b)

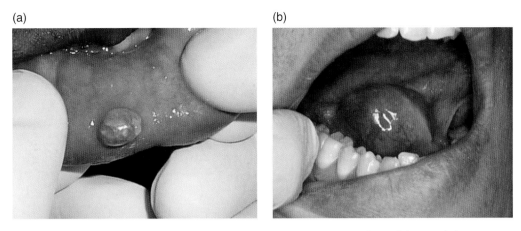

Figure 21.2   Salivary cysts. (a) Mucocele of the lower lip. (b) Ranula of the floor of the mouth (*source:* images by kind permission of Associate Professor Nagamani Narayana, UNMC, Nebraska, USA).

- Mucous retention cysts:
  - Less common
  - Arise in both major (parotid) and minor glands
- Ranula:

  - Extravasation cyst of the sublingual gland
  - Usually unilateral, located in the floor of the mouth (Figure 21.2b)
  - Dome-shaped, soft, fluctuant, bluish cyst of 2–3 cm in diameter
  - Painless in most cases
  - Tongue is elevated and may interfere with speech
  - When the ranula extends through the facial plans, it is usually posterior to the mylohyoid muscle into the neck, and presents as a cervical mass, it is called plunging ranula

21.2.5   Microscopic Features

- Two patterns are seen:
  - Mucous retention cyst: An intact epithelium-lined duct, which is dilated to form a cyst, filled with mucin and inflammatory debris
  - Mucous extravasation cyst: An extravasated mucin within the stroma, often associated with granulation tissue, a brisk inflammatory response, and foamy histiocytes, without epithelium. The macrophages contain phagocytosed mucin

21.2.6   Differential Diagnosis

- Differential diagnosis of ranula:
  - Thyroglossal duct cyst
  - Branchial cleft cyst
  - Cystic hygroma

- Submandibular sialadenitis
- Intramuscular haemangioma
- Cystic or neoplastic thyroid disease

21.2.7 Diagnosis

- History
- Clinical examination
- Microscopy

21.2.8 Management

- Excision for extravasation and retention cysts
- Drainage of the cavity and marsupialisation for ranula

21.2.9 Prognosis

- Mucous extravasation cyst:
  - Recurrence is common
  - If untreated, duct heals with a scar
- Extravasation and retention cysts; recurrence is likely

21.3 Sjögren's Syndrome

21.3.1 Definition/Description

- An autoimmune disorder of salivary glands characterized by dry eyes, dry mouth, and other systemic manifestations
- Two forms occur: primary and secondary

21.3.2 Frequency

- Between 0.2% and 1.2% of the population are affected, with half having the primary form and the other half the secondary form

21.3.3 Aetiology/Risk Factors

- The exact cause is unclear
- Combination of genetic and environmental (possibly viral) factors may play a role
- An autoimmune disorder attack on all exocrine glands, including those of the skin, vagina, lung and pancreas
- Increased prevalence of human leukocyte antigen DR/DQ alleles
- Autoantibody production against nuclear antigens SS-A and SS-B

21.3.4 Clinical Features

- Female predominance; female to male ratio 10 : 1
- Common in middle age

- Diminished production of saliva (dry mouth) and tear production (dry eyes)
- Tongue: dry, red, atrophy of papillae, lobulated dorsum with a cobblestone appearance (Figure 21.3a)
- Oral mucosa: dry, shiny and sore with generalized erythema, often associated with candidal infection and angular stomatitis
- Dental plaque accumulates, leading to dental caries
- Intermittent parotid gland enlargement in some patients, which may lead to suppurative parotitis
- Ocular manifestations:
  – Xerophthalmia
  – Gritty sensation in the eyes
  – In severe cases, conjunctival and corneal ulcerations, and visual impairment
- In the primary Sjögren's syndrome, exocrine gland dysfunction leading to above findings dominates
- In the secondary Sjögren's syndrome, all the above findings plus associated autoimmune conditions such as rheumatoid arthritis or lupus erythematosus
- Bilateral parotid swellings strongly suggest lymphoma

21.3.5 Microscopic Features

Biopsy of labial mucosa consisting of six to eight minor salivary glands:
– Lymphocytic (CD4+) infiltration clustering around small ducts (Figure 21.3b)
– Replacement of the acinar cells
– Sheets and islands of cells around the ducts causing an appearance of myoepithelial sialadenitis

21.3.6 Differential Diagnosis

- Conditions leading to dry mouth including drug adverse effects
- Benign lymphoepithelial sialadenitis
- Lymphoma

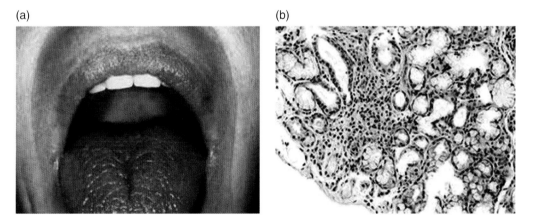

(a)   (b)

Figure 21.3   Sjögren's syndrome. (a) Xerostomia causing lobulated dorsum of the tongue. (b) Photomicrograph of a labial biopsy showing focal lymphoid infiltration in the minor salivary gland associated with Sjögren syndrome (*source:* KGH, https://commons.wikimedia.org/wiki/File:Sjogren%27s_syndrome_(2).jpg#/media/File:Sjogren's_syndrome_(2).jpg. Licensed under CC BY-SA 3.0).

- Sarcoidosis
- Hepatitis C
- HIV infection
- Graft-versus-host disease
- Systemic vasculitis

21.3.7 Diagnosis

- History
- Clinical findings
- Salivary flow rate
- Tear secretion (Schirmer test)
- Sialogram or ultrasound findings ('snowstorm' appearance on sialogram) to exclude obstructions or strictures; useful test but not specific
- Microscopic findings of labial salivary gland biopsy
- Blood tests: erythrocyte sedimentation rate and circulating CD4+ and CD8+ lymphocyte ratio
- Serological demonstration of associated SS-A or SS-B antibodies

21.3.8 Management

- Frequent small sips of water
- Use of oral moisturizing agents
- Pilocarpine for severe dry mouth
- Systemic corticosteroids for severe symptoms
- Control of dental plaque and caries (topical fluoride applications oral hygiene maintenance)
- Treatment of candida infection if present
- Periodic follow-up: check for lymphomas and candidal infections
- Referral to specialists (ophthalmologist, rheumatologist)

21.3.9 Prognosis

- Variable
- The risk of development of lymphoma exists in those with primary Sjögren's syndrome

21.4 Sialadenitis: Key Features

- Common cause of acute parotid swelling
- Children commonly infected
- Caused by paramyxovirus (mumps virus)
- Highly infectious; spreads by saliva
- Incubation period of 21 days
- Headache, fever, malaise, and tense, painful, swollen, parotid glands
- Infection in adults may cause complications such as orchitis and oophoritis, pancreatitis, arthritis, and nephritis
- Rise in immunoglobulin M antibodies in unvaccinated individuals is diagnostic of mumps
- Measles-mumps-rubella vaccination given at one and four years of age is a preventive measure

Figure 21.4 Sialometaplasia of the hard palate (*source:* Mohammad 2018, https://commons.wikimedia.org/wiki/File:Sialometaplasia.jpg. Licensed under CC BY-SA 4.0).

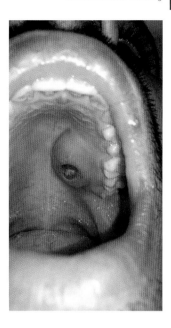

21.5   Necrotizing Sialometaplasia: Key Features

- A tumour-like lesion that affects the palatal minor salivary glands due to ischaemia secondary to trauma
- Clinically appears as a non-healing ulcerated necrotic lesion 1–3 cm in diameter on the hard palate, usually at the site of trauma (e.g. local anaesthetic injection site; Figure 21.4)
- Some predisposing factors include smoking, use of alcohol, denture wearing, recent surgery, traumatic injuries, respiratory infections, systemic diseases (HIV), bulimia, and anorexia
- Painless lesion often mimics salivary gland carcinoma or squamous cell carcinoma
- Histology reveals pseudoepitheliomatous hyperplasia of the overlying epithelium and varying amount of inflammation in the connective tissue
- The treatment is symptomatic
- Lesions will undergo spontaneous healing within two to three months

Recommended Reading

Eveson, J.W. and Speight, P. (2006). Non-neoplastic lesions of the salivary glands: new entities and diagnostic problems. *Diagnostic Histopathology* 12: 22–30.

Neville, B.W. (2016). Salivary gland pathology. In: *Oral and Maxillofacial Pathology*, 4e (eds. D.D. Damm, C.M. Allen and C.A. Chi), 422–464. St Louis, MO: Elsevier.

Odell, E.W. (2017). Diseases of the oral mucosa: non-neoplastic diseases of salivary glands. In: *Cawson's Essentials of Oral Pathology and Oral Medicine*, 9e, 341–352. Edinburgh: Elsevier.

Wilson, K.F., Meier, J.D., and Ward, P.D. (2014). Salivary gland disorders. *American Family Physician* 89 (11): 882–888.

22

Salivary Gland Neoplasms

22.1   World Health Organization Histological Classification of Salivary Gland Tumours (2017)

- Malignant epithelial tumours:
  - Acinar cell carcinoma
  - Mucoepidermoid carcinoma
  - Adenoid cystic carcinoma
  - Polymorphous low-grade adenocarcinoma
  - Epithelial–myoepithelial carcinoma
  - Clear cell adenocarcinoma,
  - Basal cell adenocarcinoma
  - Sebaceous carcinoma
  - Sebaceous lymphadenocarcinoma, cystadenocarcinoma
  - Low-grade cribriform cystadenocarcinoma, mucinous adenocarcinoma
  - Oncocytic carcinoma
  - Salivary duct carcinoma
  - Adenocarcinoma
  - Myoepithelial carcinoma
  - Carcinoma ex pleomorphic adenoma
  - Carcinosarcoma
  - Metastasizing pleomorphic adenoma
  - Squamous cell carcinoma
  - Small cell carcinoma

Handbook of Oral Pathology and Oral Medicine, First Edition. S. R. Prabhu.
© 2022 John Wiley & Sons Ltd. Published 2022 by John Wiley & Sons Ltd.
Companion website: www.wiley.com/go/prabhu/oral_pathology

- – Large cell carcinoma
- – Lymphoepithelial carcinoma
- – Sialoblastoma
- Benign epithelial tumours:
  - – Pleomorphic adenoma
  - – Myoepithelioma
  - – Basal cell adenoma
  - – Warthin tumour
  - – Oncocytoma
  - – Canalicular adenoma
  - – Sebaceous adenoma
  - – Lymphadenoma: sebaceous/non-sebaceous
  - – Ductal papilloma/inverted ductal papilloma
  - – Intraductal papilloma
  - – Sialadenoma papilliferum
  - – Cystadenoma

22.2 Pleomorphic Adenoma

22.2.1 Definition/Description

- A common benign salivary gland tumour
- The term 'pleomorphic' refers to both histogenesis and histology of the tumour
- Also known as benign mixed tumour

22.2.2 Frequency

- Common in the major salivary glands:
  - – 50–77% of parotid gland tumours
  - – 53–72% of submandibular gland tumours
  - – 33–41% of minor salivary gland tumours

22.2.3 Aetiology/Risk Factors

- Chromosomal translocation which activates one of the two genes: *PLAG1* or *HMGA2*
- Other chromosomal abnormalities involving oncogenes and tumour suppressor genes
- Prior radiation increases the risk of developing pleomorphic adenoma

22.2.4 Clinical Features

- Most common in middle age
- Slow growth for several years
- Slight female predilection
- Most are in the superficial lobe of the parotid gland in front of the ear and unilateral
- Painless, well-circumscribed, firm, rubbery swellings
- When found in the parotid tail, the tumour may present as an eversion of the ear lobe

- Palate is the most common intraoral site, followed by the upper lip (19–27%) and buccal mucosa (13–17%)
- Smooth (small) or lobulated (large) swellings with mobile overlying skin or mucosa (Figure 22.1a)

22.2.5 Microscopic Features

- Capsule; often incomplete
- Mixture of glandular epithelium and myoepithelial cells
- Islands of epithelium forming ducts and cystic structures (Figure 22.1b)
- Often, mucous producing and keratinizing squamous cells seen
- Myoepithelial cells in large numbers
- Mesenchyme-like/myxomatous background of the stroma (Figure 22.1c)

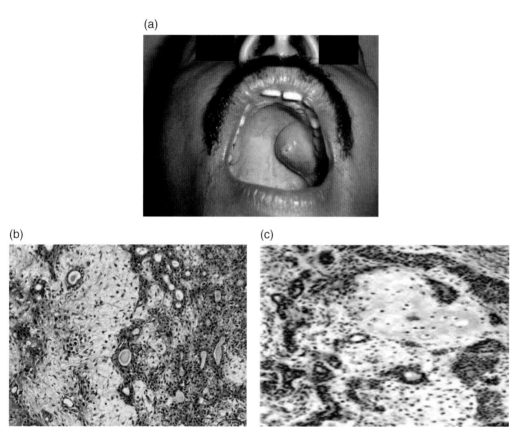

Figure 22.1 Pleomorphic adenoma. (a) Pleomorphic adenoma presenting as a firm well-circumscribed, smooth swelling on the posterior aspect of the left half of the hard palate (source: reproduced with permission from Ramdas, K., Lucas, E., Thomas, G. et al. 2008. *A Digital Manual for the Early Diagnosis of Oral Neoplasia*. Lyon: IARC. Available from http://screening.iarc.fr/atlasoral.php?lang=1). (b) Photomicrographic image showing a minor salivary gland (mucous glands in right upper half of the slide) and a well-defined pleomorphic adenoma (left lower half of the slide). Note islands of epithelium forming ducts and cystic structures. Pleomorphic adenomas in minor salivary glands are usually not encapsulated but are well demarcated (*Source:* by kind permission of Dr. Julia Yu-Fong Chang, Department of Dentistry, National Taiwan University Hospital, Taipei, Taiwan). (c) Photomicrograph shows benign neoplastic lesion in a stroma with myxoid and chondroid tissue (*source:* by kind permission of Abhishek Ranjan Pati, Government Dental College and Research institute, Bangalore, Karnataka, India).

- Accumulation of mucoid/chondroid material
- Rarely, chondroid material may ossify to form bone
- Areas of keratinization occasionally seen

22.2.6 Differential Diagnosis

- Adenoid cystic carcinoma
- Monomorphic adenoma
- Polymorphous low-grade adenocarcinoma
- Fibroma
- Mucocele
- Schwannoma
- Neurofibroma

22.2.7 Diagnosis

- History
- Clinical findings
- Ultrasound, computed tomography, magnetic resonance imaging (to assess the extent of the tumour)
- Microscopic findings (cytology: fine-needle/core needle biopsy or biopsy)

22.2.8 Management

Surgical resection with appropriate margin is considered curative

22.2.9 Prognosis

- Enucleation is associated with 15–25% risk of local recurrence
- Recurrences are usually within 18 months but can be many years later
- Risk of malignant transformation is around 5%
- Risk factors for malignant transformation:
  - Multiple recurrences
  - Submandibular location
  - Older age
  - Larger size
  - Prominent hyalinization
  - Increased mitotic rate (if present, to be sampled tumour more thoroughly)
  - Radiation exposure

22.3 Warthin's Tumour (Papillary Cystadenoma Lymphomatosum)

22.3.1 Definition/Description

A benign tumour characterized by its incorporation of lymphoid tissue in the parotid gland or induction of cystic and oncocytic changes by inflammatory infiltrate

22.3.2 Frequency

- Accounts for 4–25% of all salivary gland tumours
- The second most common benign parotid gland tumour after pleomorphic adenoma
- Almost all tumours are found in the parotid gland

22.3.3 Aetiology

Develop from heterotopic salivary ducts trapped within intraparotid or paraparotid lymphoid tissue

22.3.4 Clinical Features

- Almost always seen in the parotid gland
- Slow-growing, painless, firm or fluctuant to palpation nodular mass
- Usually located near the tail of the parotid gland
- 5–17% may be bilateral
- Rarely in oral cavity, larynx, cervical lymph nodes
- Usually, male smokers age 40+ years
- Male predominance (male to female ratio 10 : 1)

22.3.5 Microscopic Features

- Tumour is part cystic, part solid
- Shows mixture of ductal epithelium and lymphoid stroma (Figure 22.2)
- Folded epithelium lines the cystic spaces with papillary projections into the cystic spaces
- Lymphoid tissue resembles lymph node with lymphoid follicles and germinal centres
- Tumour is encapsulated

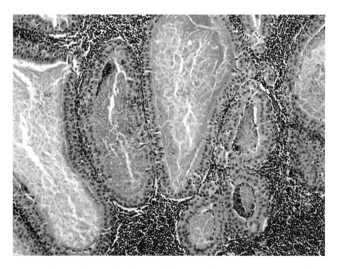

Figure 22.2 Histopathology of Warthin's tumour in the parotid gland, showing a mixture of ductal epithelium and lymphoid stroma (*source:* KGH, https://commons.wikimedia.org/wiki/File:Warthin_tumor_(2).jpg. Licensed under CC BY-SA 3.0).

22.3.6 Differential Diagnosis

- Pleomorphic adenoma
- Adenoid cystic carcinoma
- Monomorphic adenoma
- Polymorphous low-grade adenocarcinoma

22.3.7 Diagnosis

- History
- Clinical findings
- Microscopic findings (fine-needle biopsy)

22.3.8 Management

Surgical removal

22.3.9 Prognosis

- Good
- 2–6% recur
- Malignant change (less than 1%) to lymphoma, adenocarcinoma, mucoepidermoid carcinoma, oncocytic carcinoma, salivary duct carcinoma or Warthin's adenocarcinoma

22.4 Mucoepidermoid Carcinoma

22.4.1 Definition/Description

- A mixed malignant tumour characterized by the presence of squamous cells, goblet mucin-secreting cells, and cells of intermediate type
- Most common neoplasm of salivary glands

22.4.2 Frequency

- Account for 2.8–15.5% of all salivary gland tumours
- 12–29% of malignant salivary gland tumours
- 6.5–41% of minor salivary gland tumours globally

22.4.3 Aetiology

Uncertain:
  - Radiation-induced neoplasm in many patients
  - Translocations of *MECT1* and *MAML2* genes causing a new fusion gene that promotes neoplastic change

22.4.4 Clinical Features

- The most common malignant neoplasm of the major and minor salivary gland in children and adults
- Female predilection; female to male ratio 3 : 2

- Most occur in the parotid gland followed by submandibular and sublingual glands
- The palate is a frequent intraoral site
- Slow growing asymptomatic
- Occasionally facial nerve palsy may occur
- Intraoral (palatal) neoplasm: asymptomatic, often fluctuant and bluish in colour

22.4.5 Microscopic Features

- Mixture of mucous-secreting cells, squamous epithelial (epidermoid) cells, intermediate cells, and clear cells (Figure 22.3)
- Mucous-secreting cells contain foamy cytoplasm and positive to mucin stains
- Epithelial cells show basal and prickle cells but usually do not keratinize
- The neoplasm is histologically graded as: low, intermediate and high-grade types
- Low grade: cystic and minimal cellular atypia and has higher ratio of mucous cells
- High grade: solid tumour with pleomorphism and increased mitotic activity, has a smaller ratio of mucous cells
- Intermediate grade: features fall between low and high degree of neoplasm

22.4.6 Differential Diagnosis

- Benign salivary gland tumours
- Metastatic carcinoma
- Necrotizing sialometaplasia
- Poorly differentiated adenocarcinoma

22.4.7 Diagnosis

- History
- Clinical features
- Microscopic features

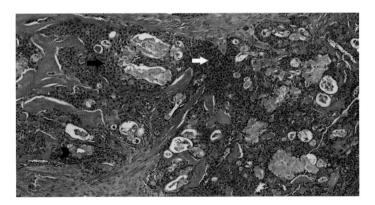

Figure 22.3 Mucoepidermoid carcinoma composed of epidermoid cells (black arrow), intermediate cells (white arrow), and mucous cells (arrowhead). (*Source:* by kind permission of Associate Professor Kelly Magliocca, Department of Pathology and Laboratory Medicine, Winship Cancer Institute at Emory University, Atlanta, GA, USA.)

22.4.8   Management/Prognosis

- Surgical removal of the tumour
- Radiotherapy in selected cases only
- Chemotherapy where tumour is not amenable to surgical and radiotherapy
- The five-year survival rate: 95% in low-grade tumours and 50% in intermediate/high-grade tumours
- High-grade tumours occasionally metastasize

22.5   Adenoid Cystic Carcinoma

22.5.1   Definition/Description

- A malignant tumour of the salivary glands with a deceptively benign histological appearance characterized by indolent, locally invasive growth with high propensity for local recurrence and distant metastasis
- Adenoid cystic carcinoma can also affect nose, antrum, lacrimal glands, breasts, uterine cervix, oesophagus, lungs, and prostate

22.5.2   Frequency

The third most common malignant salivary gland tumour overall: major salivary glands (50%) and minor salivary glands of the oral cavity (35%)

22.5.3   Aetiology

Activation of the oncogenic transcription factor gene *MYB*

22.5.4   Clinical Features

- most common in the fifth and sixth decades of life
- Slight female preponderance
- Slow-growing mass
- Pain is a major symptom followed by swelling
- Swelling is smooth surfaced or ulcerated
- Radiographical evidence of bone destruction may be present
- Propensity to invade along nerves (perineural spread)
- If parotid gland is involved, facial nerve palsy is common

22.5.5   Microscopic Features

- Groups of myoepithelial and ductal cells predominate with three patterns: cribriform, tubular, and solid
- Group of small darkly staining cells surrounding multiple clear spaces (containing mucoid material) form a cribriform or 'Swiss cheese' pattern (classic and common pattern, often diagnostic) Figure 22.4a)
- Other patterns include tubular and sold variants (Figure 22.4b and c)
- Cellular pleomorphism and mitotic activity is common in the solid pattern of the tumour

(a)

(b)

(c)

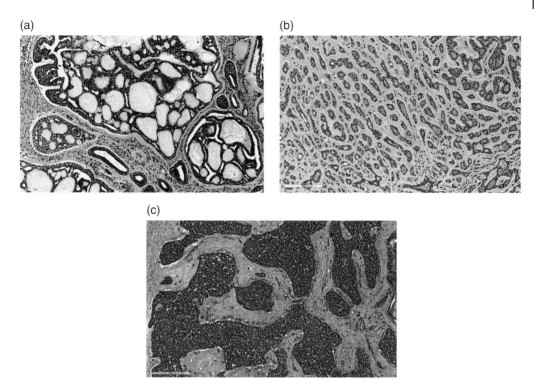

Figure 22.4   Adenoid cystic carcinoma. (a) Common cribriform pattern. Photomicrograph shows cribriform pattern composed predominantly of myoepithelial cells admixed with hyalinized or myxoid globules. Scattered ductal elements are also seen. (b) Tubular variant. Photomicrograph shows tubular pattern composed of inner ductal and outer myoepithelial cells. The ductal cells are cuboidal with eosinophilic cytoplasm. The myoepithelial cells are angulated and basaloid. (c) Solid variant. Photomicrograph shows tumour cells forming solid sheets and nests. (*source:* images by kind permission of Dr Bin Xu, Assistant Attending Pathologist, Department of Pathology, Memorial Sloan Kettering Cancer Centre, New York, USA).

22.5.6   Differential Diagnosis

- Benign salivary gland tumours
- Metastatic carcinoma
- Necrotizing sialometaplasia
- Poorly differentiated adenocarcinoma

22.5.7   Diagnosis

- History
- Clinical findings
- Microscopic findings (fine-needle biopsy)

22.5.8   Management

Surgery and surgery in combination with radiotherapy

22.5.9   Prognosis

- Five-year survival 55–89%
- Local recurrence 16–67%
- Distant metastasis 8–46% (lung is most common site of distant metastasis)

Recommended Reading

Bradley, P.J. and Eisele, D.W. (eds.) (2016). *Salivary Gland Neoplasms*, Advances in Otorhinolaryngology, vol. 78. Basel: Karger.

El-Naggar, A.K, Chan, J K C., Grandis, J R., Takata and Sootweg P. (Eds.) (2017). *Tumours of the salivary glands. World Health Organization.* Classification of Head and Neck Tumours. (4th edn), Lyon IARC press, pp. 159–202.

Mubeen, K., Vijayalakshmi, K.I., Pati, A.R. et al. (2011). Benign pleomorphic adenoma of minor salivary gland of palate. *Journal of Dentistry and Oral Hygiene* 3 (6): 82–88.

Neville, B.W., Damm, D.D., Allen, C.M., and Chi, C.A. (2016). Salivary gland tumours. In: *Oral and Maxillofacial Pathology*, 4e, 440–465. St. Louis, MO: Elsevier.

Odell, E.W. (2017). Salivary gland neoplasms. In: *Cawson's Essentials of Oral Pathology and Oral Medicine*, 9e, 355–365. Edinburgh: Elsevier.

Speight, P.M. and Barrett, A.W. (2002). Salivary gland tumours. *Oral Diseases* 8: 229–240.

To, V.S.H., Chan, J.Y.W., Tsang, R.K.Y., and Wei, W.I. (2012). Review of salivary gland neoplasms. *International Scholarly Research Network Otolaryngology* 2012: 872982.

Zarbo, R. (2002). Salivary gland neoplasia: a review for the practicing pathologist. *Modern Pathology* 15: 298–323.

Part V

Clinical Presentation of Mucosal Disease

23

White Lesions of the Oral Mucosa

23.1 Actinic Cheilitis: Key Features

- Actinic cheilitis is characterized by white lesions on the lower lip
- Caused by chronic and excessive exposure to solar (ultraviolet) radiation
- Also called actinic keratosis of the lip or solar cheilosis
- Common on the vermilion of the lower lip among fair-skinned outdoor workers (e.g. farmers, fishermen)

Handbook of Oral Pathology and Oral Medicine, First Edition. S. R. Prabhu.
© 2022 John Wiley & Sons Ltd. Published 2022 by John Wiley & Sons Ltd.
Companion website: www.wiley.com/go/prabhu/oral_pathology

- Pale opaque lesions with intervening red atrophic areas are suggestive
- In later stages, lesions may accompany white, thickened patches and scaly, crusted lesions. These lesions may carry malignant potential
- Histopathology of actinic cheilosis reveals hyperparakeratosis, parakeratosis with atrophic or acanthotic epithelium. Some degree of epithelial dysplasia may be present. Connective tissue shows variable amount of chronic inflammatory cell infiltrate
- Management includes surgical or laser removal of the keratotic lesion
- Medical treatment includes topical application of 5-fluorouracil cream to the lesion
- Further exposure to chronic solar radiation should be avoided
- Sunscreens (SPF 15 or above) should be used to block ultraviolet light
- Actinic cheilitis is a potentially malignant disorder
- For further details see Chapter 19 (section 19.9)

23.2   Chemical Burn: Key Features

- Chemical burn occurs as a result of exposure of the oral mucosa to caustic chemicals such as aspirin
- Other caustic agents include silver nitrate, pure eugenol, sodium hypochlorite, formocresol, and dental cavity varnishes
- Chemical burn results in the formation of a white pseudomembrane (Figure 23.1)
- Diagnosis is by history and clinical examination
- Treatment for symptoms is effective
- Chemical exposure to be avoided

23.3   Chronic Hyperplastic Candidosis: Key Features

- A white-and-red keratotic fixed mucosal lesion usually at the labial commissural region associated with chronic *Candida albicans* infection
- More common in adult males, those in middle-age or older, and smokers

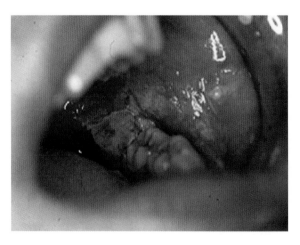

Figure 23.1   Chemical burn. Clinical photograph of aspirin burn involving left lower alveolar and buccal mucosa. Note the wrinkled white pseudomembrane (*source:* by kind permission of Professor Kobkan Thongprasom Faculty of Dentistry, Chulalongkorn University, Bangkok, Thailand).

- Well-demarcated, palpable, raised irregular fixed white (or red-and-white) lesions which cannot be rubbed off
- Common on the labial commissure(s) followed by the dorsum of the tongue
- Lesions are usually painless, occasionally sore
- All white keratotic lesions that cannot be rubbed off should be included in the differential diagnosis
- Histopathology is required to confirm candidal presence and rule out epithelial dysplasia
- Microscopic features include parakeratotic epithelium, candidal hyphae in the spinous layer, and moderate number of leukocytes (microabscesses). Epithelium in the deeper layers shows acanthosis and a small number of cases the basal cell layer may present epithelial dysplasia
- Treated with antifungal agent such as miconazole topical gel. These are not always effective. Systemic antifungal agents (such as fluconazole or ketoconazole) for a prolonged period are necessary (to be followed up with liver function tests). Long-term intermittent antifungal therapy may be required
- Surgery, laser, or cryotherapy are used with some success
- Local and systemic predisposing factors should be addressed
- Cessation of smoking is essential
- Long-term follow-up is required
- This is a potentially malignant disorder; level of risk is low
- For further information see Chapter 19 (section 19.3)

23.4 Darier's Disease: Key Features

- Also known as Darier–White disease, keratosis follicularis
- Darier's disease is a genetic disorder
- It is potentially malignant
- For further information see Chapter 19 (section 19.14)

23.5 Dyskeratosis Congenita: Key Features

- A rare, genetic, progressive bone marrow failure syndrome characterized by the triad of reticulated skin hyperpigmentation, nail dystrophy, and oral leukoplakia
- The mucocutaneous features appear between the ages of 5 and 15 years
- Oral mucosal leukoplakia on buccal mucosa, tongue, and oropharynx occurs in 80% of patients (part of the triad)
- Skin lesions include reticulated tan-to-grey hyperpigmentation or hypopigmented macules
- Nail dystrophy with ridging and longitudinal splitting is seen in 90% of patients
- Other features include haematological abnormalities and symptoms and signs of bone marrow failure
- Specialist referral for biopsy and treatment is essential
- Oral leukoplakia in this disorder is a potentially malignant lesion; oral squamous cell carcinoma (OSCC) develops in up to a third cases
- For full details see Chapter 19 (section 19.11)

23.6   Fordyce Granules: Key Features

- Also known as Fordyce spots
- Asymptomatic yellowish-white granular lesions on the buccal mucosa and lips
- Believed to be due to an ectopic collection of sebaceous glands in the cheek mucosa and lips
- Soft symmetrically distributed, creamy white spots
- When spots coalesce, cream white patches occur, which may be mistaken for leukoplakia
- More prominent in the elderly
- Cannot be rubbed off with gauze
- These lesions should not be mistaken for mucosal disease
- Diagnosis is on clinical grounds
- Biopsy is not required
- More prominent in the elderly
- No treatment is necessary For further information see chapter 12. (Section 12.1)
- Patient assurance is required

23.7   Frictional Keratosis: Key Features

- Reactive keratotic white lesions due to chronic mucosal friction
- 'Linea alba' is the term used to describe the white keratotic line on the buccal mucosa approximating the occlusal plane, it is asymptomatic and occurs bilaterally
- Parafunctional habits with constant rubbing, chewing, or sucking of the oral mucosa against the teeth can cause keratoses of the buccal mucosa (morsicatio buccarum) or tongue (morsicatio linguarum)
- Sharp cusps of teeth rubbing against cheek mucosa or tongue can result in keratotic lesions caused by chronic friction
- The retromolar pad and edentulous alveolar ridge can exhibit benign keratosis due to masticatory forces, occlusal trauma, or ill-fitting dentures or other appliances (Figure 23.2)
- Lesions of frictional keratosis are benign and cannot be rubbed off by gauge
- Histopathology shows surface keratin layer and a prominent granular cell layer. No evidence of epithelial dysplasia

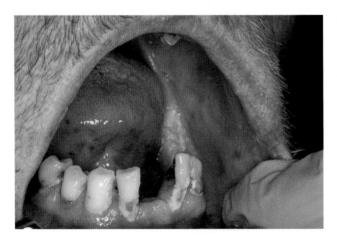

Figure 23.2   Frictional keratosis. Keratotic white lesion on the alveolar ridge due to masticatory friction (*source:* by kind permission from Associate Professor Nagamani Narayana, UNMC, Nebraska, USA).

- Frictional keratosis is not a potentially malignant lesion; lesions resolve after the cause has been eliminated
- No specific treatment is required
- Elimination of the cause is recommended

23.8 Hereditary Benign Intraepithelial Dyskeratosis: Key Features

- An inherited (autosomal dominant) disorder affecting the eye and the oral mucosa
- Eye lesions usually present by the first year of life. They are foamy, gelatinous plaques in the bulbar conjunctiva
- Oral lesions are not noticed until the second decade
- Oral lesions involve the buccal and labial mucosa, floor of mouth, lateral and ventral tongue, and gingiva. They are thick corrugated white lesions mimicking those of white sponge nevus
- Histological features include hyperkeratosis and acanthosis. Dyskeratotic cells are present in the mid to upper one-third of the epithelium, appearing engulfed by adjacent normal keratinocytes, giving a 'cell-within-a-cell' appearance
- There is no known risk of malignant transformation for these lesions
- Referral to a specialist is required
- No specific treatment for oral lesions is required unless they become symptomatic
- Reassurance is recommended

23.9 Leukoedema: Key Features

- Leukoedema is characterized by a grey-white, diffuse milky opalescent film on the buccal mucosa which blanches when stretched
- Leukoedema is bilateral and common in smokers and those of African or Asian descent
- Genetic predisposition may be associated with this condition
- Opalescent film blanches on pressure (diascopy positive)
- This condition can be regarded as a normal variation and does not require any treatment
- Leukoedema does not carry malignant potential
- No specific treatment is required
- If the patient is aware and concerned, reassurance is necessary
- See also Chapter 12 (section 12.3)

23.10 Leukoplakia: Key Features

- A predominantly white plaque of questionable risk having excluded (other) known diseases or disorders that carry no increased risk for cancer
- Predisposing factors include tobacco habit and alcohol consumption. In a small number of cases, *Candida albicans* and human papillomavirus infections may be associated
- Three clinical forms of leukoplakia are recognized: homogeneous, speckled (non-homogeneous) and verrucous (nodular) forms

- Homogenous leukoplakia is characterized by smooth white patches adherent to the underlying tissues. This is the most common variety of leukoplakia; it shows minimal, if any, evidence of malignant potential
- Speckled leukoplakia is a mixture of white and red patches, for which reason it is also called erythroleukoplakia
- Proliferative verrucous leukoplakia is a raised warty/verrucous fixed white lesion
- Leukoplakia cannot be scrapped off by rubbing with gauze
- Diagnosis is by history, clinical examination, and microscopic findings
- Basic microscopic features of leukoplakia include hyperkeratosis (of ortho- or parakeratotic type) and acanthosis of the epithelium, with various degrees of chronic inflammatory infiltrates in lamina propria. These are essentially benign features of keratotic white lesions
- Sometimes various degrees (mild, moderate, or severe) of epithelial dysplasia may occur
- Patient should be referred to a specialist for biopsy and management
- Management of leukoplakia includes surgical or laser removal of the lesions
- Retinoids may have beneficial effects during treatment
- Follow-up is essential
- Tobacco and other predisposing factors need to be eliminated
- Leukoplakia is a potentially malignant disorder
- Mean annual malignant transformation rate for leukoplakia 0.13–34% with a mean annual transformation rate of 3.8% per year
- For further details see Chapter 19 (section 19.2)

23.11   Oral Hairy Leukoplakia: Key Features

- A white keratotic lesion located mainly on the lateral surfaces of the tongue in persons whose immune status is severely compromised
- Caused by Epstein–Barr virus infection in an immunocompromised patient
- For further details see Chapter 15 (section 15.6)

23.12   Oral Lichen Planus: Key Features

- Lichen planus is a chronic mucocutaneous immune mediated disorder that affects the skin nails, hair and the mucous membranes
- Oral lichen planus is the mucosal counterpart of lichen planus that affects oral mucosa either alone or with concomitant skin lesions
- Reticular: lace-like, criss-crossing radiating white striae (Wickham's striae); most common form
- Papular: small white raised papules resembling Fordyce's granules
- Plaque-like: plaques resembling white keratotic lesions (leukoplakia-like)
- Lesions are bilateral and symmetrical
- Reticular, papular and plaque types may be asymptomatic, common on the buccal mucosa (the erosive type is atrophic and not keratotic; not discussed here).
- Asymptomatic lesions generally need no treatment
- There is no cure
- Low- or medium-potency topical corticosteroid topical applications may be necessary for symptomatic lesions

- Recommended treatment: fluocinonide 0.05% gel or betamethasone dipropionate 0.5% ointment or cream to be applied on the lesions twice daily after meals and at bedtime until symptoms resolve (for more details see Chapter 16, section 16.2.8)
- If no improvement is achieved within three weeks of treatment, patient should be referred to specialist
- Associated with increased risk of malignant change and considered a potentially malignant lesion
- For further details see Chapter 16 (section 16.2)

23.13   Oral Squamous Cell Carcinoma: Key Features

- Oral squamous cell carcinoma (OSCC) is a malignant neoplasm arising from squamous cells of the oral epithelium
- Wide range of clinical features
- About 5–8% of cases of early OSCC present as white patches
- In majority of cases, tobacco and alcohol are implicated as aetiological factors
- A small percentage of OSCC are associated with human papillomavirus (types 16 and 18) infection in those who have no alcohol or tobacco habit
- In its early stages may appear as a white patch fulfilling the criteria of leukoplakia. Exophytic squamous cell carcinoma may develop in these patches
- Common locations include buccal mucosa, labial commissures, lateral borders of the tongue, floor of the mouth, palate, and vermilion of the lower lip
- Initially, the white patch is asymptomatic; the lesion may show ulceration and become symptomatic at a later stage
- Histopathology malignancy is based on the degree of differentiation, which include well-differentiated, moderately differentiated, and poorly differentiated squamous cell carcinoma
- Management modalities include surgery, radiotherapy, and chemotherapy
- For further details, see Chapter 20 (section 20.1)

23.14   Pseudomembranous Candidosis: Key Features

- Also known as thrush, pseudomembranous candidosis is the most common candidal infection of the oral mucosa
- The elderly and infants are at increased risk of developing pseudomembranous candidosis
- Predisposing factors include xerostomia, poor oral hygiene, immunodeficiency, diabetes, radiation, and iron-deficiency anaemia
- Asymptomatic or mild symptoms such as burning sensation and bad taste
- White–cream coloured curd-like plaques or flecks loosely adherent to the oral mucosa
- White superficial plaques may be localized or generalized
- Buccal mucosa palate and dorsal tongue are frequently involved
- Plaques can be wiped off with gauge or mirror head exposing the underlying mucosa
- Differential diagnosis of pseudomembranous candidosis includes other white lesions such as leukoplakia, frictional keratosis, chemical or thermal burn, white sponge nevus, lichen planus and mucosal lesions of contact allergy

- Topical antifungal agents such as nystatin, miconazole, or amphotericin B are effective. For adults and children and infants, the following is recommended: oral suspension of 400 000 to 600 000 units for adults and children four times a day that is held in the mouth for as long as possible then swallowed. Infants are treated with 200 000 units three times a day.
- For further details see Chapter 14 (section 14.1)

23.15   Smokeless Tobacco-Induced Keratosis: Key Features

- Also known as tobacco pouch keratosis or snuff-dipper's lesion
- A condition that results from spit tobacco being habitually placed in the mucobuccal fold in the mandibular anterior or posterior regions where the mucosa is in direct contact with snuff or chewing tobacco
- Early lesion tends to have a filmy white to grey opalescent appearance with a wrinkled surface and minimal mucosal thickening (Figure 23.3)
- As lesion progresses, it becomes more keratotic with furrowing of the epithelium and thickening
- Stretching the mucosa may reveal a 'pouch'
- Lesion requires one to five years of the smokeless tobacco habit to develop
- Mandibular vestibule is the common site
- Associated with gingival recession
- Differential diagnosis includes all fixed white lesions
- With discontinuation of smokeless tobacco most lesions resolve within six weeks
- If the lesion does not regress within six weeks without smokeless tobacco use, biopsy should be performed and the lesion to be treated as leukoplakia
- This lesion is not a potentially malignant disorder
- Follow-up is necessary

23.16   Smoker's Keratosis: Key Features

- Smoker's keratosis is an oral white lesion induced by the action of tobacco smoke
- Smoker's keratosis is caused by cigarette, pipe, and cigar smoking
- Reverse smoking is also an important cause
- Mild keratosis may be seen on the lip or labial commissures in cigarette smokers

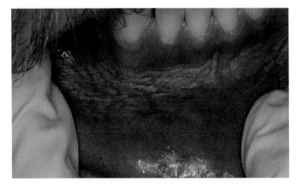

Figure 23.3   Smokeless tobacco-induced keratosis of the lower labial mucosa. Note the typical white wrinkled lesion (*source:* by kind permission of Associate Professor Nagamani Narayana, UNMC, Nebraska, USA).

(a)

(b)

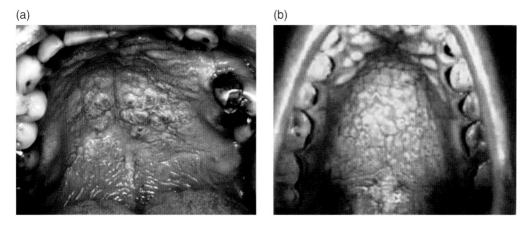

Figure 23.4 (a) Smoker's palate. Note red inflamed orifices of minor salivary glands against the white background. (b) Smoker's keratosis in a reverse smoker. Note extensive keratotic white patch involving the entire palate (*source:* reproduced with permission from Ramdas, K., Lucas, E., Thomas, G. et al. 2008. *A Digital Manual for the Early Diagnosis of Oral Neoplasia.* Lyon: IARC. Available from http://screening.iarc.fr/atlasoral.php?lang=1).

- In pipe and cigar smokers, palatal lesions are characterized by red inflamed orifices of minor salivary glands against the white background is common This is also called smoker's palate, stomatitis nicotina or nicotinic stomatitis (Figure 23.4a)
- In reverse smokers, palatal changes are much more pronounced, causing extensive palatal keratosis that often carries malignant potential (Figure 23.4b)
- Cessation of smoking usually results in disappearance of smokers' keratosis
- Smokers' keratosis is not a potentially malignant disorder. In reverse smokers, however, it is known to carry malignant potential
- For further information on palatal lesions in reverse smokers, see Chapter 19 (section 19.4)

23.17 Sublingual Keratosis: Key Features

- Sublingual keratosis is leukoplakia located in the sublingual region
- Lesion cannot be rubbed off with gauze
- For further details see Chapter 19 (section 19.12)

23.18 Syphilitic Leukoplakia: Key Features

- Syphilitic leukoplakia is a rare mucosal white patch in patients with tertiary syphilis
- Known to carry malignant potential
- For further details see Chapter 19 (section 19.13)

23.19 Verrucous Carcinoma: Key Features

- Verrucous carcinoma is a variant of squamous cell carcinoma
- Caused by tobacco use (snuff dipping in particular), alcohol and occasionally ill-fitting dentures
- Common in males aged above 60 years

- Gingiva, alveolar mucosa, and buccal mucosa are the favoured sites
- Exophytic slow-growing lesion with white pebbly surface is characteristic
- Shows invasive growth in most cases and rarely infiltrative
- Usually does not metastasize to regional lymph nodes or to distant parts of the body
- Surgery and laser therapy are effective
- For further details, see Chapter 20 (section 20.1)

23.20 White Hairy Tongue: Key Features

- A disorder due to the accumulation of keratin on the filiform papillae resulting in a hair-like fashion
- There is no known single cause
- Factors associated with hairy tongue include poor oral hygiene, chronic use of mouthwashes containing oxidizing agents, and excessive smoking
- Mostly asymptomatic; patients may complain of altered taste and gagging
- Hair-like elongated papillae which cannot be readily rubbed off with gauze
- Management includes elimination of causes or predisposing factors
- Restoring oral hygiene improves the condition
- Application of keratolytic trichloroacetic acid may be required for severely elongated papillae

23.21 White Sponge Nevus: Key Features

- White spongy nevus, also known as white folded gingivostomatitis or Cannon's disease, is a hereditary disorder characterized by diffuse white keratotic patches involving oral mucosa
- Clinically seen as folded (spongy) and thickened white mucosa that becomes prominent in the second decade of life (Figure 23.5a and b)
- Buccal mucosa is commonly involved

(a)

(b)

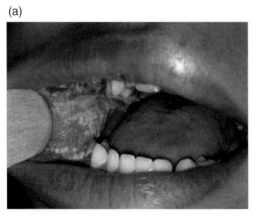
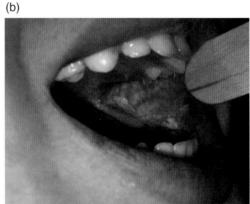

Figure 23.5 (a and b) White sponge nevus. White irregular plaques with well-defined borders and symmetric distribution on the buccal mucosa in a six-year-old girl (*source:* Elfatoiki, S.Z., Capatas, S., Skali, H.D. et al. 2020. Oral white sponge nevus: an exceptional differential diagnosis in childhood. *Case Reports in Dermatological Medicine* 2020: 9296768. doi:10.1155/2020/9296768).

- Other sites of involvement include nasal, oesophageal, and anogenital mucosa
- White patch cannot be rubbed off with gauze
- This condition does not carry any malignant potential
- No treatment is required
- Patient reassurance is recommended

Recommended Reading

Odell, E.W. (2017). Benign chronic white mucosal lesions. In: *Cawson's Essentials of Oral Pathology and Oral Medicine*, 291–297. Edinburgh: Elsevier.

Prabhu, S.R. (2019). Benign mucosal white lesions. In: *Clinical Diagnosis in Oral Medicine: A case based approach*, 1–26. New Delhi: Jaypee Brothers Medical Publishers.

Prabhu, S.R. (2004). White lesions of the oral mucosa. In: *Textbook of Oral Medicine*, 91–100. New Delhi: Oxford University Press.

Prabhu, S.R. and Felix, D.H. (2016). Mucosal white lesions. In: *Handbook of Oral Diseases for Medical Practice* (ed. S.R. Prabhu), 129–154. New Delhi: Oxford University Press.

Scully, F.D.H. (2005). Oral medicine-update for the dental practitioner: oral white patches. *British Dental Journal* 199: 567–572.

24

Red and Purple Lesions of the Oral Mucosa

24.1   Contact Stomatitis: Key Features

- Contact stomatitis refers to an inflammatory reaction of the oral mucosa by contact with irritants or allergens
- It can occur in two forms: irritant contact stomatitis or allergic contact stomatitis
- Allergic contact stomatitis is a rare acute or chronic allergic reaction of the oral mucosa
- Ingredients of dentifrices, mouthwashes, and dental cleaners, food including cinnamaldehyde or cinnamon essential oils that are used as flavouring agents, beverages, candies, latex, and hygiene products are possible causes of irritant or allergic contact stomatitis
- Irritant reactions appear to be more common than allergic reactions
- Symptoms of contact stomatitis include burning sensation, pain, paraesthesia, numbness, bad taste, excessive salivation, and perioral itching
- Presentations of contact stomatitis include localized or diffuse erythematous lesions, erosions/ulcerations, leukoplakia-like lesions, or oral lichenoid reactions
- Patch testing is useful to distinguish irritant reactions from allergic reactions

Handbook of Oral Pathology and Oral Medicine, First Edition. S. R. Prabhu.
© 2022 John Wiley & Sons Ltd. Published 2022 by John Wiley & Sons Ltd.
Companion website: www.wiley.com/go/prabhu/oral_pathology

- Removal of the causative agent is essential in the management of contact stomatitis
- Intraoral topical steroids are prescribed for severe cases

24.2 Desquamative Gingivitis: Key Features

- Desquamative gingivitis is not a specific diagnosis but is a descriptive term for non-specific gingival manifestation
- Associated with different dermatological and vesiculoerosive diseases
- Gingival condition is characterized by atrophy, erosion, and desquamation seen as diffuse erythema of the marginal and keratinized gingiva
- Represents a manifestation of one of several different diseases, such as mucous membrane pemphigoid, pemphigus vulgaris, systemic lupus erythematosus, lichen planus, linear immunoglobulin A disease, dermatitis herpetiformis, and psoriasis, erythema multiforme, or contact allergic reactions
- Desquamation of the free and keratinized gingival epithelium; shiny, smooth epithelium is fragile and peels off readily
- Labial/buccal surfaces commonly involved; vesicles may precede desquamation
- Symptoms include chronic pain/burning sensation, intolerance to spicy food
- Rarely asymptomatic
- White streaks on the red background (if due to lichen planus)
- Symptomatic treatment with topical corticosteroid application is required
- Identification and treatment of the underlying disorder is important.
- For further details see Chapter 5 (section 5.5)

24.3 Erythema Migrans: Key Features

- Irregular, pink or red depapillated map-like areas, which change in shape, and increase in size
- When on the tongue, also known as geographic tongue or benign migratory glossitis
- For further details see Chapter 12 (section 12.5)

24.4 Erythema Multiforme: Key Features

- An acute, self-limited, and sometimes recurring mucocutaneous condition
- Considered to be a type-IV hypersensitivity reaction associated with certain infections, medications, or other various triggers
- Two forms: minor and major
- Minor: only skin involvement with less severe symptoms
- Major: skin, oral, nasal, and genital involvement and symptoms are severe
- 'Target 'lesions or 'iris' lesions (well-defined red macules with a bluish cyanotic centre); appear on the extremities and spread centrally
- Oral lesions include inflamed red patches, multiple irregular blisters, and shallow ulcers occur anteriorly on the labial, buccal and lingual mucosa
- Lips may show bleeding tendencies, labial ulcers ooze fibrin and form haemorrhagic crusts
- Lesions may be self-healing within two to four weeks but may recur at an interval of several months

- Minor erytheme multiforme is treated with adequate hydration, liquid diet, analgesics, and topical corticosteroid agents
- Major erytheme multiforme require systemic corticosteroids, parenteral fluid replacement and antipyretics
- If evidence of an antecedent viral infection or trigger exists, systemic antiviral drugs during the disease or as a prophylactic measure
- For further details see Chapter 16 (section 16.6)

24.5   Erythematous Candidosis: Key Features

- Erythematous candidosis is characterized by red lesions caused by candidal albicans
- Prolonged use of broad-spectrum antibiotics and poorly maintained denture hygiene are the main causes
- Acute antibiotic (acute atrophic) candidosis:
  - Also known as acute atrophic candidosis
  - History of the use of broad-spectrum antibiotics
  - Burning mouth sensation is common
  - Loss of filiform papillae resulting in red or 'bald' areas on the tongue on the dorsum of the tongue are characteristic
  - Can also occur on the palate
- Denture-induced stomatitis (chronic atrophic candidosis, denture sore mouth):
  - History of the continuous use of removable denture (maxillary denture in particular)
  - Varying degree of erythema confined to the denture-bearing maxillary mucosal surface
  - Palatal erythema may be focal and pin-pointed, diffuse, or nodular in appearance
  - Usually asymptomatic
  - Occasional petechiae may be seen on the affected mucosa
  - Diagnosis is by history, clinical examination, and smear for microbiology
  - Management includes antifungal treatment (topical or if required systemic), denture and oral hygiene maintenance and attention to underlying disorders
- For further details see Chapter 14

24.6   Erythroplakia: Key Features

- A red patch or a plaque that cannot be clinically or pathologically diagnosed as any other definable lesion
- Aetiology is unknown; a considerable number of patients have tobacco, betel quid and alcohol habits
- Middle-aged/older people with male preponderance
- Asymptomatic, with occasionally a burning sensation
- Favoured sites include floor of the mouth, lateral and ventral surfaces of the tongue, soft palate, and buccal mucosa
- Characterized by well-demarcated erythematous patch with a soft velvety texture
- Occasionally combined with a white lesion (erythroleukoplakia)
- Erythroplakia is a potentially malignant lesion
- 50% of erythroplakia lesions turn out to be malignant in the first biopsy

- The remaining 50% show dysplasia of varying degree
- Surgical excision or laser ablation is the recommended treatment
- Long-term follow-up is required
- Cessation of tobacco, betel quid and alcohol use is required
- For further details, see Chapter 19 (section 19.1)

24.7 Haemangioma: Key Features

- Haemangioma can be grouped as congenital haemangioma and vascular malformations. The former is a hamartomatous lesion characterized by endothelial proliferation
- Both types develop during infancy and childhood
- Haemangiomas usually involute as child grows whereas vascular malformations persist and grow larger as the child grows
- Haemangioma on the face or the mucous membrane may present as flat or raised red lesions
- Flat red lesions are usually due to capillary haemangioma and the elevated lesions are caused by cavernous haemangioma with large, dilated sinuses filled with blood
- When traumatized, lesions bleed heavily
- Haemangioma is diascopy positive (blanches on pressure)
- Congenital haemangiomas usually involute over time
- No treatment is required unless traumatized. These cases require observation
- Sclerotherapy, cryosurgery, laser therapy, and microembolization followed by resection are some of the treatment methods in use
- For details see Chapter 18 (section 18.4)

24.8 Hereditary Haemorrhagic Telangiectasia: Key Features

- Hereditary haemorrhagic telangiectasia is a genetic disorder that is characterized by abnormal blood vessel formation in the skin and mucous membranes
- This condition is also called Osler–Weber–Rendu syndrome
- Multiple bright red papules or nodular lesions on lips, tongue, and palate which disappear on digital pressure (Figure 24.1)

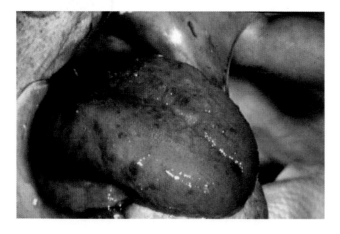

Figure 24.1 Hereditary haemorrhagic telangiectasia. Node multiple, nodular red/purple-coloured lesions on the tongue.

- Bleed when traumatized
- Other features include nosebleeds and gastrointestinal haemorrhage
- Skin lesions are usually located on the fingertips
- Patient may be anaemic due to gastrointestinal bleeding
- Observation; no treatment is necessary

24.9 Infectious Mononucleosis: Key Features

- Infectious mononucleosis, also known as glandular fever, is an acute infection with Epstein–Barr virus (human herpesvirus type 4) in children or young adults
- Common mode of transmission is through saliva
- In children it may not produce minimal symptoms but in young adults, clinical features include fever, sore throat, and enlarged lymph nodes
- The disease is self-limiting; most recover within two weeks
- Oral manifestations of infectious mononucleosis include palatal petechiae, uvular oedema and tonsillar exudate
- Generalized lymphadenopathy, skin rash and sore throat are common
- Antibody tests (monospot test, Paul Bunnell test) are positive
- For further details see Chapter 15 (section 15.5)

24.10 Kaposi's Sarcoma: Key Features

- Kaposi's sarcoma is an angioproliferative neoplasm caused by Kaposi sarcoma-associated herpesvirus, which is a human herpesvirus type 8
- A common neoplasm in patients who are HIV positive
- Purple-coloured macular/papular or nodular lesions are common on the gingiva and palate
- Lesions do not blanch on pressure
- Diagnosis is based on medical history, clinical examination, and histological evaluation of the lesion
- Management of oral Kaposi's sarcoma includes intralesional injections of chemotherapeutic agents (vinblastine sulphate, for example) or surgical removal
- Early lesions may spontaneously regress with antiretroviral therapy
- Oral hygiene should be emphasized for patients with gingival lesions
- For further details see Chapter 20 (section 20.3)

24.11 Linear Gingival Erythema: Key Features

- Linear gingival erythema, also known as 'red-band gingivitis', is seen as a 2–3 mm wide red band along the gingival margin in people who are HIV positive (Figure 24.2)
- Aetiology is not known, often candidal association has been reported
- Gingival bleeding is a common feature
- Diagnosis is based on the medical history (HIV) and clinical appearance
- Treatment includes periodontal debridement, rinses with a 0.12% chlorhexidine gluconate suspension and improved home oral hygiene
- Often does not respond to treatment

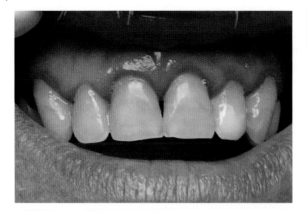

Figure 24.2   Linear gingival erythema in a patient who is HIV positive, presenting as a red band along gingival margins.

24.12   Lupus Erythematosus: Key Features

- Lupus erythematosus is an autoimmune connective tissue disorder characterized by skin lesions and rarely lichen planus-like oral lesions
- For further details see Chapter 19 (section 19.8)

24.13   Median Rhomboid Glossitis: Key Features

- Seen as an erythematous patch in the mid-line of the dorsum of the tongue at the junction of the anterior two thirds with the posterior one third
- Believed to be due to chronic candidal infection
- Lesion is usually diamond shaped
- Asymptomatic in most cases
- Surface may be nodular or lobulated
- Autoinoculation on the palatal vault resulting in an erythematous lesion may occur in some cases
- Topical application of antifungal agent is recommended
- For further details see Chapter 14 (section 14.1)

24.14   Mucosal Ecchymosis, Haematoma, and Petechiae: Key Features

- Ecchymosis is a bruise
- Occurs due to haemorrhage and accumulation of blood in the connective tissue
- Causes of ecchymosis include trauma or deficiency of platelets and/or clotting factors and viral infections
- An ecchymosis is typically flat and red, purple, or blue in colour
- Ecchymosis due to trauma will resolve spontaneously and no treatment is necessary
- A haematoma is the result of haemorrhage with pooling of blood in the connective tissue; causes a purple or black thickening or swelling of the mucosa
- No treatment is necessary once a diagnosis is made; it will resolve spontaneously in several weeks to over one month

- Petechiae are round, red, pinpoint areas of haemorrhage
- Petechiae are usually caused by trauma, viral infection such as infectious mononucleosis, streptococcal pharyngitis, or a bleeding disorder such as idiopathic thrombocytopenia
- Petechiae do not require treatment; they resolve over a few weeks
- Investigation of the cause of petechiae is indicated

24.15 Plasma Cell Gingivitis: Key Features

- Plasma cell gingivitis is a rare inflammatory condition characterized by dense plasma cell infiltrate in the gingival connective tissue secondary to hypersensitive reaction
- Hypersensitivity to a variety of agents used in chewing gums or toothpastes
- Allergens also include mint, cinnamon, cloves, cardamom, red chilli peppers, khat, colocasia leaves or pumice used in prophy paste
- Asymptomatic in some cases
- Appears as a diffuse reddening and oedematous swelling of the gingiva with a sharp demarcation along the mucogingival border
- Anterior gingival segment is commonly involved
- Gingiva bleeds readily
- Management includes identification and elimination of allergen
- Topical or systemic immunosuppressive agents (betamethasone rinses, fluocinonide gel, topical triamcinolone is effective)
- For further details, see Chapter 5 (section 5.3)

24.16 Port-Wine Nevus: Key Features

- A port-wine stain is usually a capillary vascular malformation that presents commonly as a large flat patch of purple or dark red skin or mucous membrane (rare) with well-defined borders
- Port-wine nevus can be one of the presenting intraoral features of Sturge–Weber syndrome (also known as encephalotrigeminal angiomatosis)
- Port-wine nevus is a rare, congenital, neuro-oculocutaneous disorder which is characterized extraorally by unilateral port wine stains on the face, glaucoma, seizures and mental restriction, and intraorally by ipsilateral gingival haemangioma which frequently affects the maxilla or mandible

24.17 Radiation Mucositis: Key Features

- Radiation mucositis is caused by radiation treatment of the head and neck region
- Early response to radiotherapy results in erythema of the oral mucosa, particularly during the first week of radiation
- Erythematous mucositis is followed by erosions and ulcers
- Pain is a major feature
- Mucositis resolves after the cessation of radiation
- Symptomatic treatment for oral lesions is recommended
- For further details see Chapter 16 (section 16.14)

24.18   Thermal Burn: Key Features

- Thermal burn (erythema) occurs due to accidental ingestion of extremely hot beverages or food
- Occasionally iatrogenic (during dental treatment)
- Common in children
- Lesions appear red or white depending on the tissue response
- If desquamation occurs erosions are the result
- Palate, buccal mucosa and tongue are usual sites of lesions of thermal burn
- No treatment is required for most lesions
- If pain is intense, topical anaesthetic agent can be applied

Recommended Reading

Joseph, T.I., Vargheese, G., Georg,e, D. et al. (2012). Drug induced oral erythema multiforme: a rare and less recognized variant of erythema multiforme. *Journal of Oral and Maxillofacial Pathology* 16 (1): 145–148.

Odell, E.W. (2017). Tongue disorders. In: *Cawson's Essentials of Oral Pathology and Oral Medicine*, 9e, 283–289. Edinburgh: Elsevier.

Prabhu, S.R. (2019). Benign mucosal red lesions. In: *Clinical Diagnosis in Oral Medicine: A case based approach*, 29–64. New Delhi: Jaypee Brothers Medical Publishers.

Prabhu, S.R. (2016). Mucosal red lesions. In: *Handbook of Oral Diseases for Medical Practice*, 177–185. New Delhi: Oxford University Press (India).

Prabhu, S.R. (2004). Red lesions of the oral mucosa. In: *Textbook of Oral Medicine*, 117–122. New Delhi: Oxford University Press (India).

Scully, C. and Felix, D.H. (2005). Oral medicine-update for the dental practitioner. Oral red and hyperpigmented pztches. *British Dental Journal* 199: 639–645.

25

Blue, Black, and Brown Lesions of the Oral Mucosa

25.1 Addison's Disease: Key Features

- Addison's disease is a primary adrenal deficiency caused by infiltrative or autoimmune processes
- One of the most important signs of Addison's disease is mucocutaneous hyperpigmentation related to melanogenesis action of adrenocorticotrophic hormone (ACTH)
- Hyperpigmentation may involve skin, oral cavity, conjunctiva, and genitalia
- Brown patches of gingiva, vermilion border of the lips, buccal mucosa, palate, and tongue may represent the first signs of Addison's disease (Figure 25.1)
- Patient with Addison's disease presents systemic findings such as abdominal pain, nausea, vomiting, weight loss, and hypotension
- Serum cortisol levels and measurement of ACTH are confirmatory
- Corticosteroid replacement is the treatment of choice

25.2 Amalgam Tattoo: Key Features

- Amalgam tattoo is a pigmented lesion of the oral mucosa caused by accidental implantation of amalgam during restorative procedures
- Amalgam tattoo presents as a localized blue-grey lesion on the gingival or alveolar mucosa (Figure 25.2)

Handbook of Oral Pathology and Oral Medicine, First Edition. S. R. Prabhu.
© 2022 John Wiley & Sons Ltd. Published 2022 by John Wiley & Sons Ltd.
Companion website: www.wiley.com/go/prabhu/oral_pathology

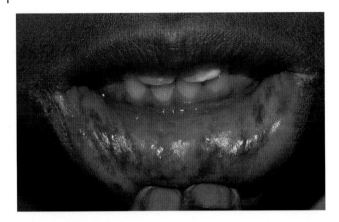

Figure 25.1 Classic brown pigmentation of the labial mucosa in a patient with Addison's disease (*source:* by kind permission of Dr Albert C. Yan, MD, Paediatric Dermatology, Children's Hospital of Philadelphia, USA).

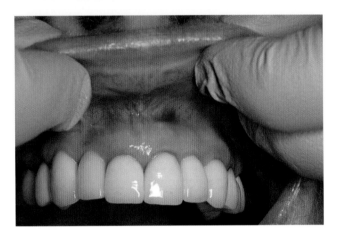

Figure 25.2 Amalgam tattoo. Note bluish-grey lesion on the mucosa (*source:* by kind permission of Dr Nagamani Narayana, University of Nebraska School of Dentistry, UNMC, Nebraska, USA).

- Other oral mucosal areas may also be involved
- Size of the pigmented lesions varies depending on the amount of amalgam embedded in the tissues
- If the amalgam particles are large, they may be detected on the periapical radiography
- There is no inflammatory response of the mucosa to amalgam
- History reveals amalgam restorations or traumatic extraction of the amalgam-filled tooth
- No treatment is required

25.3   Black/Brown Hairy Tongue: Key Features

- Black or brown hairy tongue refers to a condition where the filiform papillae are elongated with black or brown discoloration (Figure 25.3)
- Causes or predisposing conditions of black hairy tongue include poor oral hygiene, smoking, radiation, xerostomia, the use of antibiotics (tetracyclines), antacids, chlorhexidine rinses, iron salts, and overgrowth of fungal or bacterial organisms
- The condition is asymptomatic. Some individuals may complain of dry mouth, bad taste, oral malodour or gagging sensation

Figure 25.3 Black and brown hairy tongue (*source:* by kind permission of Dr Nagamani Narayana, University of Nebraska School of Dentistry, UNMC, Nebraska, USA).

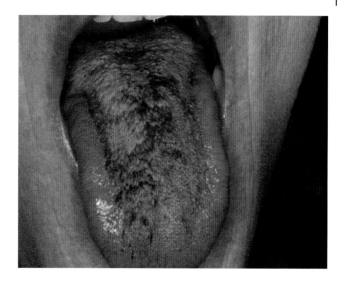

Figure 25.4 Brown pigmentation of the left buccal mucosa in a patient who is HIV positive and receiving zidovudine.

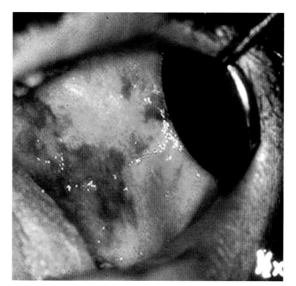

- Elimination of causative or predisposing factors, oral hygiene maintenance, and tongue cleaning (by gentle scraping or brushing before sleep) are effective
- Some patients may require topical application of keratolytic agents such as podophyllin

25.4 Drug-Induced Pigmentation: Key Features

- Several medications are known to cause oral pigmentation based on the type and duration of drug used
- Drugs which can cause mucosal pigmentation include:
  - antimalarials (chloroquine), antiretroviral drugs (zidovudine used for HIV)
  - antibiotics (minocycline)

- oral contraceptives
  - antifungal drugs (ketoconazole)
  - immunosuppressants (cyclophosphamide)
  - bleomycin and 5-fluorouracil used as chemotherapeutic drugs for malignant lesions
- Most of the above-listed medications cause melanocyte stimulation
- The lesions are patchy and usually blue-black or blue-grey in colour
- Hard palate, tongue, and buccal mucosa are commonly involved sites (Figure 25.4)
- No treatment is required for mucosal pigmentation
- Change or reduction of the medication may be required

25.5   Heavy Metal Pigmentation: Key Features

- Condition caused by ingestion or exposure to heavy metals such as mercury, bismuth, lead, or silver
- Clinically seen as a bluish line along the gingival margins or pigmented spots in the gingival papillae similar to amalgam tattoo
- Rarely the bluish-black pigmentation is diffuse and patchy
- No treatment is required for pigmented lesions

25.6   Laugier–Hunziker Syndrome: Key Features

- Laugier–Hunziker syndrome is an acquired pigmentary condition affecting lips, oral mucosa, and acral area, frequently associated with longitudinal melanonychia
- A rare, acquired disorder with adult female predilection
- Characterized by the presence of lenticular macules of variable colour located on the lip and other parts the oral mucosa (Figure 25.5)
- In more than 60% of cases, nail changes (melanonychia) are seen
- Known to be an entirely benign disease with no systemic manifestations
- Treatment is for aesthetic purposes only

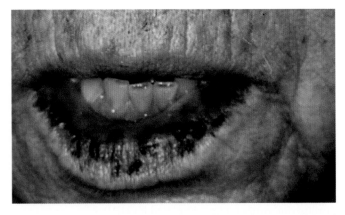

Figure 25.5   Laugier–Hunziker syndrome. Brown pigmentated macules on the labial mucosa similar in appearance to that of Peutz–Jeghers syndrome (*Source:* credit: Mohammed2018. licensed under the Creative Commons Attribution-Share Alike 4.0 International licence).

25.7   Melanoma: Key Features

- Melanoma is a malignant lesion caused by uncontrolled proliferation of melanocytes
- Although rare in the mouth, palate and gingiva are common intraoral sites for melanoma.
- Melanoma may present as an asymptomatic brown or black patch with irregular borders
- In some patients, melanoma may present as a rapidly growing black mass with ulceration, pain, bone destruction, and bleeding
- Some melanomas may not show discolouration. These are called amelanotic melanomas
- Regional lymph node metastasis is a common feature
- Treatment should be offered by the specialists as soon as the diagnosis is confirmed by histology
- Management includes radical surgical resection
- Prognosis is poor
- Early detection improves the prognosis
- For further details see Chapter 20 (section 20.2)

25.8   Melanotic Macule: Key Features

- Oral melanotic macule is a pigmented lesion commonly found on the lower lip
- Other less common sites include gingiva, buccal mucosa, and hard palate
- Caused by increased melanin production
- Melanotic macule is a brown lesion, usually single and smaller than 1 cm, with clearly demarcated borders (Figure 25.6)
- Melanotic macule is a benign lesion
- No treatment may be necessary

25.9   Peutz–Jeghers Syndrome: Key Features

- Peutz–Jeghers syndrome is a rare genetic disorder characterized by pigmented mucocutaneous macules and gastrointestinal polyposis
- Multiple small melanotic spots are found on and around the lips (Figure 25.7); also found on the skin and other mucosal surfaces

Figure 25.6   Melanotic macule on the lower lip. (*Source:* By kind permission of Professor David Wilson, Adelaide Australia)

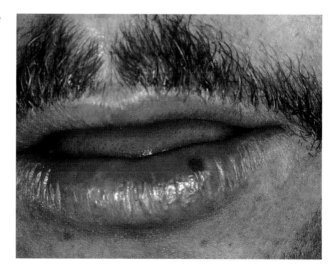

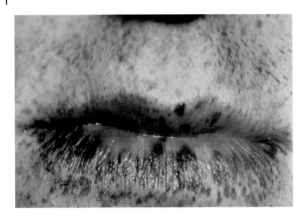

Figure 25.7 Perioral pigmentation in a patient with Peutz–Jeghers syndrome. (*Source:* By kind permission of Professor David Wilson, Adelaide Australia)

- Increased risk for malignancies of the small intestines, colon, stomach, and breast
- No treatment is required for pigmented lesions

25.10 Physiological Pigmentation: Key Features

- Physiological pigmentation of the oral mucosa is common in people of African and Asian origin
- Gingival surface is the most favoured site
- Usually a dark brown, ribbon-like band is seen bilaterally on the attached gingiva (Figure 25.8)
- In some instances, dark brown patches are seen on the buccal mucosa, hard palate, tongue, or lips, which are asymptomatic
- No treatment is required

25.11 Mucosal Nevi: Key Features

- Mucosal nevi are rare developmental pigmented lesions found on the mucosa
- Focal oral pigmentation caused by an accumulation of nevus cells in the epithelial and or connective tissue

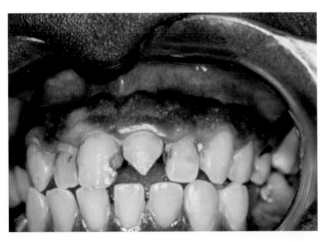

Figure 25.8 Physiological pigmentation of the gingiva in an African individual.

- A mucosal nevus appears as a solitary, flat, dark brown lesion (Figure 25.9)
- When the nevus is light brown in colour and dome shaped, it is called a intramucosal or compound nevus
- Intramucosal nevi are common
- Buccal mucosa and hard palate are the favoured sites for oral nevi
- Excision biopsy is recommended because occasionally oral nevi may represent precursor lesions for oral melanomas

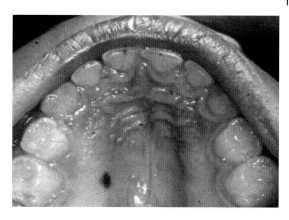

Figure 25.9 Brown oval-shaped pigmented nevus on the hard palate. (*Source:* By kind permission of Professor David Wilson, Adelaide Australia)

25.12 Smoker's Melanosis: Key Features

- Smoker's melanosis refers to smoking-related pigmentation of the oral mucosa
- Heavy smoking: increased production of melanocytes provides a biological defence against the adverse effects of tobacco smoke
- Anterior gingival surface is commonly affected with brown/black pigmentation similar to physiological pigmentation
- In heavy smokers, buccal mucosa may be involved (Figure 25.10)
- Differential diagnosis includes lesions such as Addisonian pigmentation, racial pigmentation, medication-related pigmentation, pigmentation in fibrous dysplasia, cafe-au-lait pigmentation of neurofibromatosis, and trauma-associated pigmentation
- Cessation of smoking is recommended
- If pigmented areas show ulceration or surface elevation, biopsy is essential

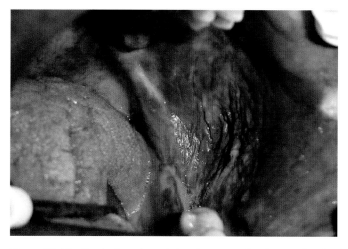

Figure 25.10 Smoker's melanosis in a heavy smoker (*source:* Rosebush, M.S., Anderson, K.M., Rawal, Y.B. 2014. Common lesions of varied aetiology. In: *Diagnosis and Management of Oral Lesions and Conditions: A resource handbook for the clinician*, ed. C.A. Migliorati, F.S. Panagakos, doi: 10.5772/57597. London: IntechOpen. doi: 10.5772/57597).

Recommended Reading

Cawson, R.A. and Odell, E.W. (2017). Benign mucosal pigmented lesions and disorders. In: *Cawson's Essentials of Oral Pathology and Oral Medicine*, 9e, 131–151. Edinburgh: Churchill Livingstone.

Lewis, M.A.O. and Jordan, R.C.K. (2012). Pigmentation. In: *Oral Medicine*, 2e, 147–165. London: CRC Press.

Prabhu, S.R. (2019). Benign mucosal pigmented lesions and disorders. In: *Clinical Diagnosis in Oral Medicine: A case based approach* (ed. S.R. Prabhu), 131–151. New Delhi: Jaypee Brothers Medical Publishers.

Prabhu, S.R. (2016). Mucosal pigmented lesions. In: *Handbook of Oral Diseases for Medical Practice*, 186–196. New Delhi: Oxford University Press.

Rosebush, M.S., Anderson, K.M., and Rawal, Y.B. (2014). *Common lesions of varied aetiology*. In: *Diagnosis and Management of Oral Lesions and Conditions: A resource handbook for the clinician* (eds. C.A. Migliorati and F.S. Panagakos). London: IntechOpen https://doi.org/10.5772/57597 https://www.intechopen.com/books/diagnosis-and-management-of-oral-lesions-and-conditions-a-resource-handbook-for-the-clinician/common-lesions-of-varied-etiology (accessed 12 March 2021).

Scully, C. and Felix, D.H. (2005). Oral medicine-update for the dental practitioner. Oral red and hyperpigmented pztches. *British Dental Journal* 199: 639–645.

Shah, S.S., Oh, C.H., Coffin, S.E., and Yan, A.C. (2005). Addisonian pigmentation of the oral mucosa. *Cutis* 76: 97–99.

Wilson, D.F., Moore, S.R., and Logan, R.M. (2004). Pigmented lesions of the oral mucosa. In: *Textbook of Oral Medicine*, 107–116. New Delhi: Oxford University Press.

26

Vesiculobullous Lesions of the Oral Mucosa

26.1   Angina Bullosa Haemorrhagica: Key Features

- Angina bullosa haemorrhagica is a common disorder characterized by the formation of blood blisters on the soft palate
- Cause unknown
- A large blood-filled blister on the soft palate that may burst leaving an empty epithelial sac (Figure 26.1)
- Condition is more common in those who use inhalers for asthma
- Resolves within a week
- This is a self-limiting lesion
- Patient reassurance is recommended

26.2   Bullous Lichen Planus: Key Features

- A rare form of lichen planus of the oral mucosa
- Characterized by bullous lesions which soon rupture leaving erosions or ulcers
- Lesions show white striations surrounding the bullous lesions
- Lesions are painful
- Buccal or labial mucosae are involved

Handbook of Oral Pathology and Oral Medicine, First Edition. S. R. Prabhu.
© 2022 John Wiley & Sons Ltd. Published 2022 by John Wiley & Sons Ltd.
Companion website: www.wiley.com/go/prabhu/oral_pathology

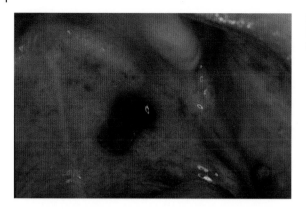

Figure 26.1 Angina bullosa haemorrhagica. Note a large ruptured blood blister on the soft palate.

- Lesions are bilateral
- Topical corticosteroid application is effective; rarely systemic corticosteroids may be necessary

26.3 Dermatitis Herpetiformis: Key Features

- A chronic blistering skin condition characterized by multiple blisters filled with fluid clinically mimicking those of herpesvirus infection (hence the name)
- This disorder may be associated with coeliac disease
- An autoimmune disorder
- Skin lesions appear as vesicular rash with intense itchy sensation
- Oral vesicles occur on palatal mucosa
- Dapsone or sulphonamides are effective

26.4 Erythema Multiforme: Key Features

- Erythema multiforme is a mucocutaneous disorder of unknown cause
- This disorder usually follows a viral infection or systemic drug exposure
- Oral mucosal involvement exhibits generalized erythema
- Sometimes accompanied with erosions or bullous lesions
- Crusting of the lips is characteristic
- Severe form of erythema multiforme is called Stevens–Johnson syndrome; oral, conjunctival, and genital mucosae are involved
- History and clinical examination
- Biopsy is confirmatory
- Discontinuation of the medication and low doses of systemic steroids
- Topical application of local anaesthetic agents or the use of antihistaminic elixir rinse is of use in control of pain
- For further details see Chapter 16 (section 16.6)

26.5 Hand, Foot and Mouth Disease: Key Features

- Hand, foot, and mouth disease occurs in children particularly in locations where the infection is epidemic
- Causative virus A16 and rarely A5 and A9 and A10

- Incubation 3–10 days
- Small blisters on the dorsal and lateral aspects of the fingers and toes and rashes on the hands and feet are consistent clinical features
- Systemic findings include fever, malaise, and lymphadenopathy, and are generally mild
- Oral aphthous-like ulcers surrounded by erythema develop on the tongue and buccal mucosa
- This is a self-limiting disease, which resolves within a week
- Symptomatic treatment may be necessary
- For further details see Chapter 15 (section 15.9)

26.6   Herpes Zoster (Shingles): Key Features

- Herpes zoster infection, also known as shingles, is caused by the reactivation of varicella (herpes zoster) virus in adults
- Reactivation of the varicella zoster (herpes zoster) virus occurs in those who have had chickenpox in childhood
- This virus remains dormant in the sensory ganglia until reactivated
- Common in immunocompromised individuals
- Most commonly involves thoracic dermatomes
- Trigeminal involvement occurs in 30% of cases, usually involving the mandibular division
- During the prodromal phase, the pain in the region is deeply seated and unilateral often mimicking pain of dental origin. This is followed by vesicles seen unilaterally along the distribution of the branches of the involved nerve
- On the skin these vesicles rupture and form crusts whereas intraorally crusting does not occur
- Shallow ulcers result from the rupture of vesicles
- If the maxillary division is involved, ulcerations are found on the hard and soft palate
- Shingles is a very painful condition
- Systemic symptoms may include fever and malaise
- Complication of herpes zoster may cause postherpetic neuralgia
- Antiviral agents: acyclovir (800 mg five times daily for five days) is effective in reducing the severity of symptoms
- For further details, see Chapter 15 (section 15.4)

26.7   Mucous Membrane Pemphigoid: Key Features

- Mucous membrane pemphigoid is an autoimmune disease characterized by formation of blisters at the basement membrane zone of the mucous membranes
- Autoantibodies are directed against epithelial basement membrane of the oral mucosa
- Usually affects women in their fifth or sixth decade
- Gingiva and palate are preferred sites of involvement. Blisters rupture leaving ulcers with yellowish slough on their surfaces
- Other areas involved include conjunctiva, larynx, and genital mucosa
- Conjunctival involvement may lead to scarring. Skin involvement is rare. On the gingiva, causes desquamative gingivitis
- Confirmation is by histological and immunofluorescence examination of the biopsy specimen
- Topical application of corticosteroids or tacrolimus yields good results
- For further details see Chapter 16 (section 16.5)

26.8   Pemphigus Vulgaris: Key Features

- Pemphigus is an autoimmune disorder characterized by bullous lesions involving the skin and mucous membranes
- Antibodies against epithelial intercellular attachments (desmosomes) cause acantholysis leading to blister formation
- There are different types of pemphigus, which vary in severity, including pemphigus vulgaris, pemphigus vegetans and paraneoplastic pemphigus
- Pemphigus vulgaris is the most common type, involving the oral mucosa
- Middle-aged and elderly women are commonly predisposed to pemphigus
- Gentle digital sliding pressure on the uninvolved adjacent skin causes stripping of the epithelium (Nikolsky's sign)
- Oral bullous lesions are short lived; once they have ruptured, lesions leave erosions and ulcers
- Soft palate, buccal mucosae, lips, and gingiva are common sites of oral involvement
- Histological and immunofluorescence examination of the biopsy specimen are confirmatory
- Systemic corticosteroids and immunosuppressant therapy are required to control the condition
- For further details see Chapter 16 (section 16.4)

26.9   Primary Herpetic Gingivostomatitis: Key Features

- Primary herpes simplex virus infection results in primary herpetic gingivostomatitis
- Caused by herpes simplex virus type 1
- Usually affects children
- Multiple vesicles occur on the gingival and other mucosal surfaces which rupture leaving shallow painful ulcers
- Systemic manifestations are minimal
- Cervical lymph nodes are enlarged
- If symptomatic and severe, systemic antiviral agents (acyclovir) are recommended
- For further details see Chapter 15 (section 15.1)

26.10   Herpes Labialis: Key Features

- Also known as secondary (recurrent) herpetic stomatitis
- Reactivation of herpes simplex virus causes secondary infection
- Usually recurrent
- Found on the lip at the mucocutaneous junction of the mouth (cold sore)
- Secondary or recurrent herpetic infection is caused by the reactivation of herpes simplex virus (type 1 in most cases), which remains dormant in the sensory ganglia after the primary infection
- Predisposing factors for the reactivation of the dormant virus include sunlight or cold, psychological stress, menstruation, trauma, the common cold and immune suppression
- Recurrent herpetic infection has a prodromal phase. During this phase, an itching and tingling sensation occurs a day before the appearance of multiple vesicles on the lip and sometimes on the side of the nose. Vesicles rupture and heal without scarring
- Intraoral involvement of recurrent herpetic infection is rare in immunocompetent individuals

- Application of 5% acyclovir cream or 1% penciclovir during the prodromal phase is effective in lessening the clinical course
- For further details see Chapter 15 (section 15.2)

Recommended Reading

Odell, E.W. (2017). Diseases of the oral mucosa: non-infective stomatitis. In: *Cawson's Essentials of Oral Pathology and Oral Medicine*, 9e, 255–279. Edinburgh: Elsevier.

Prabhu, S.R. (2019). Benign mucosal blisters, erosions, and ulcers. In: *Clinical Diagnosis in Oral Medicine: A case based approach*, 154–201. New Delhi: Jaypee Brothers Medical Publishers.

Prabhu, S.R. (2004). Ulcerative and erosive lesions of the oral mucosa. In: *Textbook of Oral Medicine*, 124–136. New Delhi: Oxford University Press.

Prabhu, S.R. and Felix, D.H. (2016). Mucosal, blisters and ulcers. In: *Handbook of Oral Diseases for Medical Practice* (ed. S.R. Prabhu), 129–154. New Delhi: Oxford University Press.

Scully, C. and Felix, D.H. (2005). Oral medicine-update for the dental practitioner: mouth ulcers of more serious connotation. *British Dental Journal* 199: 339–343.

27

Ulcerative Lesions of the Oral Mucosa

27.1 Oral Ulcers in Agranulocytosis: Key Features

- A haematological disorder characterized by severe reduction in granulocytes, particularly neutrophils
- Drugs or infections are major causes. In some cases, cause is not detectable (idiopathic)
- The disease is of sudden onset
- Systemic infection results in sore throat, chills, and fever
- Respiratory and gastrointestinal symptoms develop soon after the onset of neutropenia
- Oral manifestations include development of painful ulcers covered by grey-white pseudomembrane. These ulcers have no halo around them
- Mastication is painful
- Necrotizing ulcerative gingivitis can occur in neutropenia
- Agranulocytosis oral lesions should be differentiated from those of stomatitis, cyclic neutropenia, acute necrotizing gingivitis, Wegener's granulomatosis, leukaemia, and infectious mononucleosis

Handbook of Oral Pathology and Oral Medicine, First Edition. S. R. Prabhu.
© 2022 John Wiley & Sons Ltd. Published 2022 by John Wiley & Sons Ltd.
Companion website: www.wiley.com/go/prabhu/oral_pathology

- Complete blood count and bone marrow aspiration tests are confirmatory
- Treatment should be offered by a specialist: discontinuation of drugs, white blood cell transfusion, administration of granulocyte colony stimulating factor, appropriate broad-spectrum antibiotics, antipyretics, and maintenance of oral hygiene with chlorhexidine mouth wash and hydrogen peroxide rinses are recommended
- Invasive periodontal debridement to be avoided

27.2 Oral Ulcers in Behçet's Disease: Key Features

- A systemic disorder characterized by oral recurrent aphthous stomatitis, genital ulceration, uveitis, arthritis and other systemic manifestations
- Common in Asia and the Middle East; uncommon in western populations
- Exact cause is not known; possibly due to non-infectious inflammation of blood vessels (vasculitis)
- Genetic predisposition noted
- A chronic disorder; occasionally life threatening
- Affects mostly adult men 20–40 years of age
- Oral recurrent aphthous ulcers, genital recurrent ulcers and uveitis are common features
- Arthritis is limited to weight-bearing bones
- Skin lesions include erythema nodosum
- Sensory and motor disturbances (due to vasculitis in the central nervous system) may occur
- History, clinical findings, and a positive pathergy test are highly suggestive of the diagnosis
- Differential diagnosis of oral ulcers of Behçet's disease include erythema multiforme, Crohn's disease, Reiter's syndrome, mucous membrane pemphigoid, and erosive lichen planus
- Management involves a multidisciplinary approach: cyclosporin, tacrolimus, and systemic corticosteroids are useful as systemic therapy. Thalidomide and topical tacrolimus are effective for oral lesions
- Prognosis of oral lesions is fair
- In treated patients, disease may eventually burn out
- Complications of the disease may include blindness, rupture of blood vessels, thrombosis and embolism (For further details see Chapter 16)

27.3 Oral Ulcers in Coeliac Disease: Key Features

- Coeliac disease, (also known as gluten-sensitive enteropathy) is characterized by atrophy of the jejunal mucosa due to its sensitivity to dietary gluten in wheat and cereal products
- An important cause of malnutrition, affecting about 1% of the population
- Majority of patients have the predisposing human leukocyte antigen DQ2
- Disease may be asymptomatic in the early stages
- Systemic features include malabsorption (leading to vitamin and mineral deficiencies), abdominal pain and diarrhoea
- Oral manifestations include glossitis (due to anaemia), angular cheilitis, bleeding tendencies, oral mucosal recurrent aphthous ulcers, enamel hypoplasia (seen as spotty hypoplastic mottling), and delayed eruption usually of permanent teeth

- Serologic screening tests, such as assays for antigliadin antibody and anti-endomysium antibody are helpful tools in diagnosis
- Histological confirmation of the intestinal damage in serologically positive individuals is confirmatory
- Avoidance of gluten in the food is required for successful management/treatment
- Oral manifestations respond to treatment of the underlying disorder

27.4   Chronic Ulcerative Stomatitis: Key Features

- A rare autoimmune mucosal disorder characterized by lichen planus-like lesions
- Affects predominantly females
- Clinically and histologically similar to lichen planus
- Shallow ulcers, erosions, and erythema seen on tongue, buccal mucosa, and gingiva
- Symptomatic, with pain and burning sensation
- Differential diagnosis includes oral involvement of lichen planus, lupus erythematosus, mucous membrane pemphigoid, pemphigus vulgaris, and linear immunoglobulin A disease
- Direct immunofluorescence shows autoantibodies to squamous epithelial nuclear proteins (chronic ulcerative stomatitis protein)
- Hydroxychloroquine is effective
- Local or systemic corticosteroids are often used (but less effective)

27.5   Oral Ulcers in Crohn's Disease: Key Features

- Also known as regional enteritis, Crohn's disease is an idiopathic, chronic, relapsing, inflammatory immunologically mediated condition. Crohn's disease is a form of inflammatory bowel disease
- Global estimation of inflammatory bowel disease: 400–500 people per 100 000. Prevalence is increasing
- Aetiology of Crohn's disease is unknown, possibly immunologically mediated, and genetic factors are frequently associated
- Disease first becomes evident in teens with a second peak after 60 years of age
- Abdominal cramping, pain, nausea, diarrhoea, and occasional fever, weight loss, and anaemia are common
- Oral lesions of Crohn's disease include diffuse mucosal nodules, cobble stone appearance of the (buccal) mucosa, deep mucosal linear ulcers in the buccal vestibule, aphthous-like ulcers, gingival erythematous macules and patches, and occasional association of pyostomatitis vegetans
- Differential diagnosis of oral lesions of Crohn's disease include major recurrent aphthous ulcers, blastomycosis, tuberculous ulcers, and ulceration of tertiary syphilis
- History (of intestinal and oral symptoms), oral lesions and histopathology indicating a non-caseating granulomatous inflammation are confirmatory
- Management of Crohn's disease involves a multidisciplinary approach: systemic corticosteroids are effective.
- Oral lesions are treated with intralesional corticosteroid injections and administration of non-steroidal anti-inflammatory drugs
- Prognosis of oral lesions is linked to intestinal response to treatment; usually fair

27.6 Oral Ulcers in Cyclic Neutropenia: Key Features

- Characterized by a fall in the circulating neutrophils at a regular interval of three to four weeks
- A rare disease
- Possibly a hereditary autosomal dominant disorder
- A childhood disorder in most cases
- Systemic features include fever, malaise, cervical lymphadenopathy, and arthralgia
- Oral manifestations include ulcerative lesions covered by pseudomembrane and surrounded by an erythematous halo similar to aphthous ulcers
- Corticosteroids, granulocyte colony-stimulating factor, or splenectomy are used in controlling the disorder

27.7 Cytomegalovirus Ulcers: Key Features

- Cytomegalovirus (herpesvirus type 5) can cause acute primary as well as recurrent infection
- In primary disease, symptoms are similar to those of infectious mononucleosis
- In patients who are HIV positive, cytomegalovirus infections cause ulcerative lesions in the mouth
- Ulcers are non-specific in their surface characteristics; they are usually solitary, large, and shallow
- Histopathological examination of the ulcer is necessary to identify the presence of the virus infected cells
- Antiviral agents (acyclovir) are effective

27.8 Eosinophilic Ulcer: Key Features

- A rare ulcerative condition possibly caused by local trauma and characterized by ulcerative granuloma with marked eosinophilia
- Single or multiple ulcers with a sudden onset; tongue is the common site
- Ulcers are painful, irregular, and covered with a whitish-yellow pseudomembrane
- Differential diagnosis includes major aphthous ulcers, traumatic ulcers, necrotizing sialometaplasia, squamous cell carcinoma, and ulcers of Wegener's granulomatosis
- Histopathology is diagnostic
- Ulcers are self-healing
- Short course of low doses of corticosteroids are useful

27.9 Gangrenous Stomatitis: Key Features

- Also known as noma or cancrum oris
- A rapidly progressive ulcerative disease caused by *Fusobacterium nucleatum*, *Prevotella intermedia*, *Borrelia vincentii*, *Streptococcus* species, and *Staphylococcus aureus*
- Rare disease but common in African children
- Predisposing factors include severe protein malnutrition, poor oral hygiene, leukaemia, uncontrolled severe diabetes mellitus and immune defects

- Clinically acute necrotizing ulcerative gingivitis is the first sign, followed by the spread of ulcerative lesions to the surrounding mucosa and bone
- Common sites are gingiva, buccal mucosa, labial mucosa, and bone
- Ulcers are covered with yellowish-white or brown membrane with fibrin and debris on their surface
- Halitosis is intense
- Fever, malaise, headache, and cervical lymphadenopathy are common
- History and clinical findings are highly indicative of diagnosis
- Appropriate antibiotics, antipyretics and debridement of debris are effective
- Nutritional supplements are necessary to address malnutrition
- Surgical correction for destructive necrosis of facial tissues is required

27.10   Necrotizing Sialometaplasia: Key Features

- An uncommon ulcerative lesion of the salivary glands believed to be caused by local ischaemic necrosis
- Sudden onset
- Posterior palate is the common site
- Nodular painful lesion with a craterlike ulcer mimicking a malignant ulcer
- Differential diagnosis includes squamous cell carcinoma, mucoepidermoid tumour, and adenoid cystic carcinoma of the minor salivary glands
- Histopathological examination of the tissue is confirmatory
- Lesion usually heals within four to eight weeks

27.11   Necrotizing Ulcerative Gingivitis: Key Features

- Necrotizing ulcerative gingivitis is a non-contagious anaerobic infection characterized by the rapid onset of painful gingivitis followed by interproximal and marginal necrosis and ulceration. Also known as Vincent's infection
- An infectious disease caused by mixed bacterial flora. Microorganisms involved include *F. nucleatum, B. vincentii, P. intermedia*, *Porphyromonas gingivalis,* and *Selenomonas sputigena*
- Malnutrition, viral infections, immune defects (HIV), stress, lack of sleep, and smoking are predisposing factors
- Necrotic, crater-like 'punched-out' ulcerations of the interdental papilla covered by grey pseudomembranous slough are typical of the disease
- Other features include spontaneous haemorrhage, halitosis, fever, lymphadenopathy, and malaise
- Affects children, young adults, and those who are HIV positive
- Diagnosis includes history, clinical examination, and microbial culture (smears from the ulcers show fusospirochaetal bacteria and leukocytes)
- Management includes debridement of necrotic debris under local anaesthesia, mouth rinses with chlorhexidine, warm salt water, or diluted hydrogen peroxide
- Systemic antibiotics: metronidazole or amoxicillin (for those with systemic signs of infection or immunocompromised status), analgesics/antipyretics for pain and fever
- Soft nutritious diet, fluid intake, and bed rest, oral hygiene instruction, and tobacco counselling

- Prognosis is good
- Signs and symptoms resolve within a week of adequate therapy
- For further details see Chapter 5 (section 5.3)

27.12   Oral Ulcers in Reactive Arthritis: Key Features

- Oral manifestations: stomatitis, erosion/ulcers
- Also known as Reiter's disease, reactive arthritis is an immunologically mediated disease characterized by arthritis, urethritis, conjunctivitis, and occasional stomatitis
- Immunological reaction is triggered by micro-organisms such as enterococci and sexually transmitted chlamydia
- Prevalence is approximately 10%
- Young adults are affected, with equal sex frequency
- Non-gonococcal urethritis, conjunctivitis, and arthritis are consistent features
- 40% of patients develop oral lesions such as erosion, red patches, or ulcerations on the buccal, palatal or labial mucosa
- History, clinical examination, and serology are important diagnostic tools
- Antibiotics, non-steroidal anti-inflammatory drugs, and immunosuppressive agents are effective
- Topical corticosteroid application is useful for oral lesions

27.13   Recurrent Aphthous Ulcers: Key Features

- Also known as recurrent aphthous stomatitis, canker sores
- A common condition characterized by multiple recurrent, small, round ulcers with circumscribed margins, erythematous halos, and yellow or grey floors
- Exact cause not known; genetic predisposition has been noted (family history in about 30% of patients); immune dysfunction may be a factor (antibody-dependent cellular cytotoxicity reaction)
- Predisposing factors include stress, anxiety, hormonal changes (during menstruation for example), dietary factors and trauma, iron, and folate deficiency (20% of patients), neutropenia, sodium lauryl sulfate in oral health products, cessation of smoking, Crohn's disease, coeliac disease, Behçet's disease, immune deficiency (e.g. HIV positivity), bone marrow suppression, food allergy and vitamin B12 and zinc deficiency
- Three main clinical types:
  - Minor:
    o The most common type
    o Single/multiple (up to five) small round or oval ulcers 2–4 mm in diameter with yellow/grey floor and surrounded by an erythematous halo
    o Commonly found on non-keratinizing mucosa; rarely on the keratinizing mucosa
    o Self-limiting; heal in seven to ten days with no scarring and recur at intervals of one to four months
  - Major:
    o Usually single, rarely multiple (two to three in number) and larger ulcer (1 cm or greater in diameter)
    o Ulcers are deep with ragged edges and elevated margins (mimicking squamous cell carcinoma)

- ○ Ulcers are more painful than minor types and may involve any mucosal surface (keratinizing and non-keratinizing)
- ○ Heal slowly often with scarring in 10–40 days
- ○ Ulcers recur more frequently
  - – Herpetiform:
    - ○ Usually, 1–2 mm in diameter and seen in clusters, could be 10–100 in number
    - ○ Ulcers occur on non-keratinizing or keratinizing mucosa
    - ○ They heal within 7–14 days leaving no scar
    - ○ Recur very frequently
    - ○ Management includes topical corticosteroid treatment (gels, creams, or ointments four to six times a day), tetracycline-based oral rinse, intralesional corticosteroid injections (for major aphthae)
    - ○ Systemic corticosteroids and other immunomodulating drugs (dapsone, hydroxychloroquine, topical tacrolimus, amlexanox) are useful. Colchicine (0.6–1.2 mg/d) and thalidomide treatment is sometimes beneficial
    - ○ Underlying systemic disorders, if present, should be addressed
- For further details see Chapter 16 (section 16.1)

27.14 Squamous Cell Carcinoma Presenting as an Ulcer: Key Features

- Tobacco habits and excessive alcohol consumption have been considered as the most common aetiological factors for oral squamous cell carcinoma
- Squamous cell carcinoma of the oral mucosa has a number of different clinical presentations
- Presentations include appearances such as white patch (leukoplakia), red patch (erythroplakia), tumour mass, papillary (verrucous) growth or ulcer
- Squamous cell carcinoma that presents as a non-healing ulcer (as well as other forms) infiltrates deep into the connective tissue and clinically shows as a firm indurated area with associated loss of tissue mobility
- Borders of the ulcer are raised and everted
- For further details see Chapter 20 (section 20.1)

27.15 Syphilitic Ulcers: Key Features

- Syphilis is a sexually transmitted disease caused by the bacterium *Treponema pallidum*
- Oral mucosal lesions can occur in three clinical forms: primary, secondary, and tertiary
- Oral manifestations:
  - – Primary syphilis:
    - ○ Lesion is called 'chancre'
    - ○ Chancre develops two to eight weeks after infection
    - ○ Lips and tip of the tongue are commonly involved
    - ○ Chancre starts as a firm painless nodule, surface breaks and becomes an indurated raised ulcer after a few days
    - ○ Regional lymph nodes are enlarged (rubbery consistency)

- Secondary syphilis:
    - Symptoms appear within one to four months after infection
    - Fever, malaise, generalized lymphadenopathy are common
    - Pinkish symmetrically distributed macular skin lesions on the trunk
    - Ulcers on tongue, tonsils and lips covered by greyish membrane
    - Mucosal 'snail's track' ulcers and mucous patches are characteristic
    - Papillary lesions called condyloma lata develop in some cases
    - This is a highly infectious stage
- Tertiary syphilis:
    - Nearly 30% of patients develop tertiary stage disease
    - Oral lesions: syphilitic leukoplakia and gumma
    - Leukoplakia seen on the dorsum of the tongue may carry malignant potential
    - Gumma is a necrotic lesion seen on the palate, tongue, or tonsils
    - Palatal gumma may perforate the palate
    - Management is by specialists
- For further details, see Chapter 13 (section 13.2)

27.16   Traumatic Ulcer: Key Features

- Traumatic ulcers are common
- Usually single and can occur as an acute or chronic ulcer
- Cause is known: physical, thermal, or chemical
- Trauma prone areas: lip, buccal mucosa, lateral surfaces of the tongue or mucosa adjacent to denture flange
- Acute traumatic ulcer is tender, with yellowish-grey floor covered with fibrin; borders are not indurated (Figure 27.1a)
- Chronic traumatic ulcer has milder symptoms, and may show indurated borders mimicking carcinoma (Figure 27.1b)
- Elimination of the cause is effective
- Traumatic ulcer heals within one week or ten days
- After elimination of the cause, if ulcer does not heal in 10 days, biopsy is required to rule out other causes (such as malignancy or syphilitic ulcer)

27.17   Tuberculous Ulcer: Key Features

- Tuberculosis (TB) is a chronic granulomatous specific infection caused by *Mycobacterium tuberculosis*
- Types: primary and secondary
    - Primary: usually involves lungs (pulmonary TB) of previously unexposed people
    - Secondary: usually infects people who have been previously infected or immunocompromised or immunosuppressed. This causes miliary TB (detectable on chest radiography)
- Oral lesions include chronic non-healing ulcer, non-healing socket, or stomatitis
- Oral mucosal sites include tongue (mid-dorsal surface or lateral borders), gingiva, lips, buccal mucosa, and soft and hard palate
- Oral tuberculous ulcer:
    - Caused by secondary infection of the mucosa from pulmonary TB

Figure 27.1   Traumatic ulcer.
(a) Acute; note the yellowish-grey
floor of the ulcer and lack of
induration of the border. (b). Chronic;
note the indurated borders
mimicking squamous cell carcinoma.
(*Source:* images by kind permission of
Dr Nagamani Narayana, University
of Nebraska School of Dentistry,
UNMC, Nebraska, USA.)

(a)

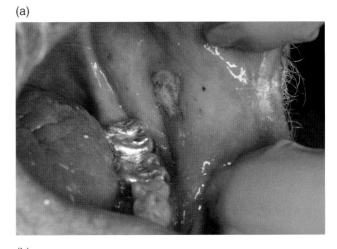

(b)

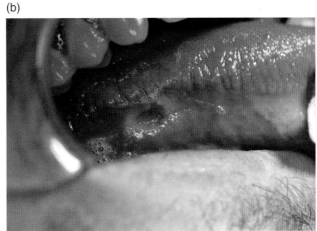

- – Typically, solitary painless angular ulcer with overhanging indurated edges
- – Cervical lymph nodes may be enlarged
- – Primary TB of oral mucosa is extremely rare
- – Systemic chemotherapy: isoniazid, rifampin, streptomycin, and other anti-tuberculous drugs
- – Oral lesions respond to systemic therapy
- For details see Chapter 13 (section 13.4)

27.18   Oral Ulcer in Ulcerative Colitis: Key Features

- Ulcerative colitis is an inflammatory condition that affects any part of the colon
- Oral manifestations include in any of the following forms:
  - – Aphthous-like ulceration
  - – Superficial haemorrhagic ulcers
  - – Angular stomatitis
  - – Pyostomatitis vegetans
- Oral lesions usually respond to systemic treatment of ulcerative colitis

Recommended Reading

Odell, E.W. (2017). Diseases of the oral mucosa: non-infective stomatitis. In: *Cawson's Essentials of Oral Pathology and Oral Medicine*, 9e, 255–279. Edinburgh: Elsevier.

Prabhu, S.R. (2019). Benign mucosal blisters, erosions, and ulcers. In: *Clinical Diagnosis in Oral Medicine: A case based approach*, 154–201. New Delhi: Jaypee Brothers Medical Publishers.

Prabhu, S.R. (2004). Ulcerative and erosive lesions of the oral mucosa. In: *Textbook of Oral Medicine*, 124–136. New Delhi: Oxford University Press.

Prabhu, S.R. and Felix, D.H. (2016). Mucosal, blisters and ulcers. In: *Handbook of Oral Diseases for Medical Practice* (ed. S.R. Prabhu), 129–154. New Delhi: Oxford University Press.

Scully, C. and Felix, D.H. (2005). Oral medicine-update for the dental practitioner: mouth ulcers of more serious connotation. *British Dental Journal* 199: 339–343.

28

Papillary Lesions of the Oral Mucosa

CHAPTER MENU

28.1   Condyloma Acuminatum: Key Features
28.2   Multifocal Epithelial Hyperplasia (Heck's Disease): Key Features
28.3   Oral Proliferative Verrucous Leukoplakia: Key Features
28.4   Squamous Papilloma: Key Features
28.5   Squamous Cell Carcinoma: Key Features
28.6   Verruca Vulgaris (Oral Warts): Key Features
28.7   Verrucous Carcinoma: Key Features

28.1   Condyloma Acuminatum: Key Features

- A sexually transmitted disease caused by human papillomavirus
- Human papillomavirus types 6 and 11 transmitted to the oral cavity via orogenital contact
- Lesions of condyloma acuminatum are pink or white exophytic papillary growths located commonly on the lingual frenum or soft palate
- Other mucosal surfaces may also be involved
- Usually, lesions are solitary and up to 3 cm in size
- Surgical removal is the treatment of choice
- See also Chapter 15 (section 15.11)

28.2   Multifocal Epithelial Hyperplasia (Heck's Disease): Key Features

- A human papillomavirus type 13 and 32 infection involving oral soft tissues
- Predominantly seen in children
- Slightly raised multiple asymptomatic whitish-pink papules and plaques seen on the buccal and labial mucosa
- No treatment is required; lesions regress spontaneously
- For aesthetic reasons, surgical removal is recommended
- See also Chapter 15 (section 15.12)

Handbook of Oral Pathology and Oral Medicine, First Edition. S. R. Prabhu.
© 2022 John Wiley & Sons Ltd. Published 2022 by John Wiley & Sons Ltd.
Companion website: www.wiley.com/go/prabhu/oral_pathology

28.3   Oral Proliferative Verrucous Leukoplakia: Key Features

- Proliferative verrucous leukoplakia is a slow-growing, progressive, verrucous white lesion of the oral mucosa that is potentially malignant
- Exact cause is not known
- This lesion occurs in smokers as well as non-smokers
- Elderly women are commonly affected
- Initially lesion may appear as a flat white patch (leukoplakia) which over time becomes a verrucous lesion
- Buccal mucosa, gingiva and tongue are the favoured sites
- If untreated, the lesion progresses to verrucous carcinoma or squamous cell carcinoma
- Surgical removal
- Difficult to completely eradicate these lesions
- Spread to other sites and recurrence is common
- For further details see Chapter 19 (section 19.2)

28.4   Squamous Papilloma: Key Features

- Oral squamous papilloma is a cauliflower-like, pedunculated or sessile, normal pink or whitish lesion that occurs on the oral mucosa
- Human papillomavirus types 6 and 11 are aetiologically associated with oral papilloma
- Oral papilloma is a painless papillary lesion commonly located on the hard and soft palate and uvula
- Tongue and lips are also involved but less frequently
- Papilloma is usually less than 1 cm in diameter and exhibits papillary projections which are white or normal pink colour
- When traumatized the lesion may bleed
- Surgical removal is the treatment of choice
- For further details see Chapter 15 (section 15.10)

28.5   Squamous Cell Carcinoma: Key Features

- Tobacco habits and excessive alcohol consumption are aetiologically associated with majority of oral squamous cell carcinoma
- Oral squamous cell carcinoma presents in different clinical forms; warty appearance is one of its clinical forms
- Lesions are white, exophytic, warty, and cauliflower like in appearance
- Surgery and radiotherapy are effective modes of treatment
- For further details see Chapter 20 (section 20.1)

28.6   Verruca Vulgaris (Oral Warts): Key Features

- Verruca vulgaris is a mucocutaneous warty lesion usually found in lips, palate or attached gingiva
- Human papillomavirus (types 2, 4, 6, or 11) is the causative agent
- Skin lesions are common

- In the majority of cases, oral lesions are caused by autoinoculation of the virus from the lesions on the fingers
- Lesions of verruca vulgaris are nodular or cauliflower-like, pedunculated, white or pink lesions
- Multiple lesions may be found in immunocompromised patients
- Surgical removal
- Cryosurgery or laser surgery is also effective
- See also Chapter 15 (section 15.13)

28.7 Verrucous Carcinoma: Key Features

- Verrucous carcinoma is a well-differentiated squamous cell carcinoma with a relatively better prognosis than that of squamous cell carcinoma
- Tobacco habits (smoking and chewing) seem to be associated with verrucous carcinoma in majority of cases
- Human papillomavirus association has also been reported
- Verrucous carcinoma appears as a painless, thick, white, cauliflower-like lesion
- Common intraoral sites of involvement include buccal mucosa, mandibular alveolar ridge, gingiva, and the tongue
- Lip and floor of the mouth are also occasionally involved
- Verrucous carcinoma generally does not metastasize to the regional lymph nodes, but they may be tender due to inflammation
- Surgery is the primary mode of treatment
- For further details see Chapter 20 (section 20.1)

Recommended Reading

Eversole, L.R. (2000). Papillary lesions of the oral cavity: relationship to human papillomaviruses. *Journal of the California Dental Association* 28 (12): 922–927.

Mainville, G.N. (2019). Non-HPV papillary lesions of the oral mucosa: clinical and histopathologic features of reactive and neoplastic conditions. *Head and Neck Pathology* 13: 71–79.

Prabhu, S.R (ed.) (2016). Mucosal warts and wart-like lesions. In: *Handbook of Oral Diseases for Medical Practice*, 197–200. New Delhi: Oxford University Press.

Zain, R.B., Kallarakkal, T.G., Ramanathan, A. et al. (2016). Exophytic verrucous hyperplasia of the oral cavity – application of standardized criteria for diagnosis from a consensus report. *Asian Pacific Journal of Cancer Prevention* 17 (9): 4491–4501.

Part VI

Orofacial Pain

29

Orofacial Pain

CHAPTER MENU

29.1   Odontogenic Orofacial Pain

29.1.1   Pulpitis/Dentine Hypersensitivity

- Reversible:
  - Intermittent dental pain in response to stimuli such as hot, cold or sweet foods or drinks
  - Pain resolves once stimulus is removed
  - Cause: reversible pulpitis/dentine hypersensitivity
  - Analgesia is not required
  - Tooth desensitization or dental restorative procedures recommended
- Irreversible:
  - Severe pain in the tooth exposed to stimuli such as hot, cold or sweet food or drinks
  - Persistent dull throbbing pain even after the stimulus is removed
  - Pain may become continuous
  - Cause: irreversible pulpitis
  - Analgesics such as non-steroidal anti-inflammatory drugs (NSAIDs) are effective
  - Antibiotics are not required
  - Dental restorative procedures are recommended
  - Endodontic treatment or extraction of the offending tooth

For further details see chapter 3.

29.1.2   Apical Periodontitis or Infected Root Canal

- Dull throbbing pain not associated with any stimulus (such as hot, cold or sweet food or drinks) but may be painful on biting
- Analgesics (NSAIDs) are effective

Handbook of Oral Pathology and Oral Medicine, First Edition. S. R. Prabhu.
© 2022 John Wiley & Sons Ltd. Published 2022 by John Wiley & Sons Ltd.
Companion website: www.wiley.com/go/prabhu/oral_pathology

- Antibiotics are not usually required for localized infection (unless there are signs of spread of the infection)
- Endodontic treatment or extraction of the offending tooth

For further details see chapter 3

29.1.3   Fractured or Cracked Tooth

- Tenderness of the tooth to pressure and on biting
- Cause: cracked tooth or localized dental infection
- Analgesics (NSAIDs) are effective
- Antibiotics are not usually required for localized infection (unless there are signs of spread of infection)
- Restoration, endodontic treatment or extraction of the offending tooth

For further details, see chapter 4

29.1.4   Spreading Odontogenic Infection Without Severe or Systemic Features

- Dental pain associated with localized facial swelling
- Cause: localized dental (periapical) infection
- Management:
  - Culture and sensitivity testing
  - Endodontic/periodontal treatment or extraction of tooth
  - Drainage of pus
  - Oral antibiotic therapy (after the sample has been obtained for culture and sensitivity tests):
    ○ Metronidazole 400 mg (children: 10 mg/kg up to 400 mg) orally, 12-hourly for five days *plus*
    ○ Phenoxymethylpenicillin 500 mg (children: 12.5 mg/kg up to 500 mg) orally six-hourly for five days *or*
    ○ Amoxicillin 500 mg (children: 15 mg up to 500 mg) orally eight-hourly for five days
  - For patients allergic to penicillins:
    ○ Clindamycin 300 mg (children: 7.5 mg/kg up to 300 mg) orally eight-hourly for five days
  - Systemic analgesia for mild to moderate pain (ibuprofen 400 mg six to eight hourly for no more than five days)

For further details see Chapter 6

29.1.5   Cellulitis/Ludwig Angina with Systemic Features

- Severe dental pain associated with diffuse facial swelling, trismus, difficulty swallowing, neck swelling, fever, malaise etc.
- Cause: spreading infection (cellulitis/Ludwig's angina) with systemic features
- Immediate hospitalization
- Surgical intervention and intravenous antibiotic administration
- Management:
  - Urgent hospitalization (under the care of oral and maxillofacial surgeon)
  - Maintain patent airway
  - Drainage of pus by incising affected facial spaces and placing drains
  - Obtaining blood or other samples for culture and sensitivity tests
  - Intravenous antibiotic therapy:
    ○ Benzylpenicillin intravenously 2.4 g (children: 50 mg/kg up to 2.4 g) 4-hourly, *plus*
    ○ Metronidazole 500 mg (children: 12.5 mg/kg up to 500 mg) intravenously 12-hourly

- NSAIDs for pain (ibuprofen 400 mg orally six- to eight-hourly for five days plus paracetamol 1000 mg orally four- to six-hourly for a short duration)
- Stop antibiotic therapy once drains do not produce pus, or signs and symptoms have subsided, and the white blood cell count has returned to normal

For further details see Chapter 6

29.1.6 Dry Socket

- Tooth socket pain (one to four days after extraction)
- Cause: Dry socket (alveolar osteitis)
- Analgesics (NSAIDs) are effective
- Antibiotics are not usually required
- Removal of debris from the socket with warm sterile saline, socket irrigation, and obtundent dressing of the socket

29.2 Neuropathic Orofacial Pain

29.2.1 Trigeminal Neuralgia

- Unilateral, intense, stabbing, electric shock-like pain in the area of the face where the branches of the trigeminal nerve are distributed
- Cause unknown
- Possible cause: cerebral vessels become less flexible with atherosclerosis and age and press upon roots of trigeminal nerve in the posterior cranial fossa, causing neuronal discharge
- Sites of pain: eyes, lips, nose, scalp, forehead, lower and upper jaw
- Elderly (50–70 years of age) commonly affected
- Paroxysmal attacks of a few seconds (less than two minutes)
- Distribution of pain: along one or more divisions of the trigeminal nerve
- Sudden intense stabbing or burning type of pain
- Pain often triggered by talking, washing, eating, shaving, or brushing teeth
- Pain does not cross to the contralateral side
- Asymptomatic between attacks
- Pain does not affect sleep
- Less severe form is called atypical trigeminal neuralgia
- Management:
  - Consult a specialist first
  - First-line therapy is carbamazepine 200–1200 mg/day and oxcarbazepine 600–1800 mg/day. The typical starting dose is 100–200 mg twice daily then gradually increased to 200 mg
  - Second-line therapy: lamotrigine 400 mg/day
  - Other useful medications include phenytoin, clonazepam, gabapentin, pregabalin, topiramate, levetiracetam, and valproate, as well as tocainide 12 mg/day
  - Local anaesthetics such as alcohol, glycerol, phenol, tetracaine, or bupivacaine injections are used in diagnosis and treatment
  - Analgesic effect of botulinum neurotoxin type A has also been reported
  - Percutaneous trigeminal ganglion balloon compression rhizotomy is usually reserved for patients who cannot tolerate the above-mentioned treatments or are refractory to it

29.2.2   Glossopharyngeal Neuralgia

- Cutting, stabbing, and shooting pain, or sharp sensations in the throat, triggered by swallowing or coughing
- Less common
- Usually secondary to tumours
- Triggers include swallowing, talking, yawning, and coughing
- Activation of the dorsal motor nucleus of the vagus nerve (cranial nerve X) during a glossopharyngeal neuralgia episode may result in bradycardia and syncope
- Anticonvulsants (as for trigeminal neuralgia) are recommended (but less effective)
- Specialist consultation is essential

29.2.3   Post-herpetic Neuralgia

- Burning sensation or excruciating pain in dermatome supplied by the nerve
- The damage of the nerve caused by reactivation of varicella in the affected dermatomic area of the skin to send abnormal electrical signals to the brain. These signals may convey excruciating pain, and may persist or recur for months or years, or even for life
- Usually occurs about three months after the rashes of shingles have resolved
- Elderly people (who have had shingles) are affected
- Tricyclic antidepressants (e.g. amitriptyline, nortriptyline, desipramine, and maprotiline), gabapentin, pregabalin, opioids, and topical lidocaine patches are effective
- Specialist consultation is essential
- Management:
  - Amitriptyline:
    - Start with a single nightly dose of 10 mg for elderly (25 mg for patients under 50 years) and titrate upwards in weekly increments of 10 mg or 25 mg, respectively
  - Gabapentin:
    - A reasonable first choice when a tricyclic antidepressant is contraindicated
    - Start with a single bedtime dose of 300 mg (100 mg for frail elderly patients) and escalate as tolerated to a maximum of 3600 mg (1200 mg three times a day, or 800 mg four times a day)
    - Avoid abrupt withdrawal
  - 5% lidocaine plasters:
    - Applied over the painful area and used in a 12 hours on, 12 hours off regimen
    - Capsaicin 0.075% (over the counter). Topical application four times a day (to be used only after the lesions have healed)

For further details see Chapter 15

29.2.4   Burning Mouth Syndrome

- Burning sensation: tongue is the common site followed by palate and labial mucosa (also called glossodynia) in the absence of any known organic cause
- An oral sensory disorder with no detectable oral disease or cause
- A chronic neuropathic pain syndrome
- Female preponderance, older women
- Burning sensation mild in the morning; increases as the day progresses
- Other associated symptoms: dry mouth, oral malodour, and metallic taste

- A diagnosis of exclusion: allergy, mucocutaneous conditions, systemic disorders, and adverse effects of drugs
- Management:
  - Tricyclic antidepressants and psychotic medications:
    ○ Clonazepam tablets 0.5 mg (100 tablets); half to one tablet three times daily and then adjust the dose after three-day interval. The patient should not be titrated to a dosage of greater than 2.0 mg daily
    ○ Chlordiazepoxide tablets 5 mg. (50 tablets); 5–10 mg three times daily
    ○ Diazepam tablets 2 mg (50 tablets); 2–4 mg three times daily
    ○ Amitriptyline tablets. 25 mg (50 tablets); 25 mg at bedtime for one week and then 50 mg at bedtime. Increase to 75 mg at bedtime after two weeks and maintain at that dosage or titrate as appropriate
  - Topical capsaicin preparations to improve the burning sensation:
    ○ Capsaicin cream 0.025% (one tube); apply sparingly to affected site(s) four times daily. Wash hands after each application
- Other measures:
  - Blood examination should include: complete blood count, differential white blood cells, fasting blood sugar, haemoglobin, iron, ferritin, folic acid, and vitamin B12 estimation and thyroid profile
  - Reassurance that the disorder is not infectious, or potentially malignant
  - Patient should be informed of the rationale for the treatment with tricyclic antidepressant or psychotic medications
  - Patient must be made aware of the adverse effects of the drugs
  - Patient's medical practitioner should be informed of use of these medications
  - Stress management is essential

29.3 Other Conditions with Orofacial Pain

29.3.1 Acute Necrotizing Ulcerative Gingivitis

- Severe pain in the necrotic and ulcerative gingival interdental papillae associated with bleeding and intense halitosis
- Cause: fusospirochaetal infection of the gingiva causing necrotizing ulcerative gingivitis
- Analgesics (NSAIDs) for pain
- Chlorhexidine mouth rinses for oral hygiene
- Thorough gingival debridement, hydrogen peroxide mouth rinses, and antibiotics for anaerobic and aerobic micro-organisms
- Management:
  - Debridement under local anaesthesia
  - Removal of pseudomembrane using cotton pellet dipped in chlorhexidine
  - Antibacterial mouthwash: chlorhexidine 0.12% twice daily
  - Control pain with analgesics: ibuprofen 400–600 mg three times daily
  - Antibiotics if patient is immunocompromised (e.g. AIDS, leukaemia, cyclic neutropenia) or, in case of systemic involvement (e.g. fever, malaise, and lymphadenopathy):

      ○ Amoxicillin 250 mg three times daily for seven days
      and/or
      ○ Metronidazole 250 mg three times daily for seven days
- Assess treatment outcomes in 24 hours, then every other day until signs and symptoms are resolved and gingival health and function are restored
- Patient counselling should include instruction on proper nutrition, oral care, appropriate fluid intake, and smoking cessation

For further details see Chapter 5

29.3.2 Temporomandibular Joint Disorders

- Pain involving the temporomandibular joint (TMJ) and surrounding muscles of mastication as well as dysfunction of the joint
- A common condition, signs of which appear in up to 60–70% of the population
- Causes are multifactorial and include anatomical, pathophysiological, and psychosocial factors
- Parafunctional behaviours (e.g. bruxism, teeth grinding, clenching, and abnormal posture, stress and anxiety) contribute to masticatory muscle pain and spasm
- Cognitive and psychiatric disturbance (e.g. depression and anxiety, and autoimmune disorders, fibromyalgia and other chronic pain conditions) are also frequently associated
- Intra-articular causes include internal joint derangement, osteoarthritis, capsular inflammation, hypermobility and traumatic injury, and rheumatoid arthritis and ankylosing spondylitis
- Symptoms and signs include:
  - Acute periauricular unilateral or bilateral pain associated with trismus
  - Restriction of mandibular opening (normal 35–45 mm)
  - Headache
  - Neck pain
  - Clenching/bruxism
  - TMJ sounds
  - Tenderness of the joint and associated muscles
  - Reduced mouth opening
  - Clicking and crepitus during mouth movements
  - Magnetic resonance imaging is the gold standard to assess soft tissue structures, articular disc displacement, and the presence of joint effusion with a high degree of specificity and sensitivity
- Management:
  - Application of cold or warm compresses
  - Rest to the jaws, soft food
  - Analgesics (NSAIDs)
  - Occlusal splint therapy to reduce joint load
  - Intramuscular botox injections have been shown to be efficacious in myofascial causes of TMJ pain and tension-type headache
  - Short-term use of analgesics (ibuprofen and paracetamol), muscle relaxants, anxiolytics, anti-convulsants, steroids, and antidepressants

29.3.3 Atypical Facial Pain (Persistent Idiopathic Facial Pain)

- Facial pain that cannot be attributed to any demonstrable organic cause including dental pain
- Cause is not fully understood
- Often psychogenic factors or depression are associated with this disorder; over 50% of patients are depressed

- Malar region, orbit, and temple are the common sites of pain
- Pain is deep-seated, severe, continuous, and usually throbbing in nature
- The pain may be bilateral and mainly affects middle-aged women
- Patients are able to identify the exact location of pain either extra orally and/or in the dentoal-veolar complex (in a tooth, teeth or edentulous mucosa)
- In the absence of an organic cause of facial pain, antidepressants are effective
- Analgesics are usually not effective

29.3.4 Migraine

- A chronic neurological disorder characterized by recurrent moderate to severe headaches
- The underlying causes of migraine are unknown. In about two thirds of cases, migraines run in families, and they rarely occur due to a single gene defect. Triggers may include cheese, wine and coffee
- Typically, the headache is unilateral and pulsating or throbbing in nature, lasting 2–72 hours
- Associated symptoms may include nausea (in 90% of cases), vomiting (in 30% of cases), photophobia (increased sensitivity to light), phonophobia (increased sensitivity to sound)
- Pain is generally aggravated by physical activity
- Up to one third of people with migraine headaches perceive an aura characterized by blurred vision, flashing lights, numbness, tingling sensation, and odd smells. These are transient visual, sensory, or motor disturbances, which signal that a headache will soon occur
- Other symptoms may include nasal stuffiness, diarrhoea, frequent urination, pallor, or sweating. Swelling or tenderness of the scalp and neck stiffness may occur
- Topiramate, propranolol, metoprolol, angiotensin-converting enzyme inhibitors, and amitriptyline are used with good results
- Botox has also been found to be useful in sufferers of chronic migraines

29.3.5 Sinusitis

- Inflammation of the paranasal sinuses. Inflammation of the maxillary sinus causes maxillary sinusitis
- Causes: infection by bacteria (e.g. *Haemophilus influenzae*, *Streptococcus pneumoniae*, *Staphylococcus aureus* and *Moraxella catarrhalis*), allergy, and systemic autoimmune disorders
- Headache, facial pain, and nasal obstruction. Pain may worsen when the affected person bends over or when lying down
- Thick nasal discharge (usually green in colour) may contain pus (purulent) and/or blood
- Halitosis, postnasal drip, and cough are present
- Usually self-limiting
- Antibiotics are used to speed the recovery
- Topical decongestants are useful in relieving a stuffy nose
- Complications may include orbital cellulitis, cavernous sinus thrombosis, meningitis, and brain abscesses

29.3.6 Temporal Arteritis (Giant Cell Arteritis)

- Also known as giant cell arteritis, temporal arteritis is an autoimmune disorder involving the temporal artery in the elderly
- Cause not known. Immunological (autoimmune) background has been suggested
- A disease predominantly of elderly white women

- Features include scalp tenderness, headaches, thickened, tender temporal arteries
- Pulseless temporal arteries, ulcers on the scalp, visual disturbances
- Blindness in advanced cases
- Erythrocyte sedimentation rate and C-reactive protein are elevated in active disease
- Treat with systemic corticosteroids
- Advanced cases may need immunosuppressants such as methotrexate or azathioprine

29.3.7 Cardiogenic Jaw Pain

- When pain of cardiac origin presents in the orofacial and neck region, commonly involved areas include neck, throat, ear, teeth, and mandible
- Cause: cardiac ischaemia
- Pain may last for minutes or hours
- Pain is precipitated by exertion and relieved with rest
- Pain is relieved using sublingual nitroglycerine spray or tablet
- Oxygen administration and immediate referral to a cardiologist is recommended

29.3.8 Sialolithiasis (Salivary Calculus)

- Salivary calculi (stones) in the submandibular duct can cause obstruction of the flow of saliva resulting in swelling and pain of the submandibular region
- Swelling and pain in the submandibular region usually occur at mealtimes when the salivary flow is stimulated
- Stone(s) in the duct are palpable and elicit tenderness
- Radiographical views confirm the presence of salivary stones in the duct
- Parotid gland sialolithiasis also occurs but is less common

For further details see Chapter 21

Recommended Reading

Green, K. (2017). Diagnosing trigeminal neuralgia. In: *Diagnosing Dental and Orofacial Pain* (eds. A.J., A.J. Moule and M.L. Hicks), 109–112. Oxford: Wiley Blackwell.

Lamey, P.J. and Lewis, M.A.O. (1997). Burning mouth syndrome. In: *A Clinical Guide to Oral Medicine*, 2e (eds. P.J. Lamey and M.A.O. Lewis), 13–18. London: BDJ Books.

Moule, A.J. and Krishnan, U. (2017). Diagnosing dental pain. In: *Diagnosing Dental and Orofacial Pain* (eds. A.J. Moule and M.L. Hicks), 61–68. Oxford: Wiley Blackwell.

Oral and Dental Expert Group (2019). *Therapeutics Guidelines: Oral and Dental (Version 3)*. Melbourne: Therapeutic Guidelines Ltd.

Prabhu, S.R. (2019). Dental and orofacial pain. In: *Clinical Diagnosis in Oral Medicine: A Case Based Approach*, 285–310. New Delhi: Jaypee Brothers Medical Publishers.

Prabhu, S.R. (2016). Orofacial pain of non-dental origin. In: *Handbook of Oral Diseases for Medical Practice* (ed. S.R. Prabhu), 43–58. New Delhi: Oxford University Press.

Sadr, A., Manickam, S., and Prabhu, S.R. (2016). Orofacial pain of dental origin. In: *Handbook of Oral Diseases for Medical Practice* (ed. S.R. Prabhu), 29–42. New Delhi: Oxford University Press.

Scully, C. and Felix, D. (2006). Oral medicine update for the dental practitioner: orofacial pain. *British Dental Journal* 28: 75–83.

Part VII

Miscellaneous Topics of Clinical Relevance

30

Oral Manifestations of Systemic Disorders

CHAPTER MENU

30.1 Gastrointestinal and Liver Disorders
30.2 Cardiovascular Disease
30.3 Respiratory Disease
30.4 Kidney Diseases
30.5 Endocrine and Metabolic Disorders
30.6 Nervous System Disorders
30.7 Haematologic Disorders
30.8 Immune System Disorders

30.1 Gastrointestinal and Liver Disorders

30.1.1 Gastroesophageal Reflux Disease

- Gastroesophageal reflux disease is a condition in which acidic gastric fluid flows backwards into the oesophagus, resulting in heartburn
- Oral manifestations include erosion of the palatal aspects of the maxillary anterior teeth and premolars
- Erosive lesions appear smooth, shiny, yellow, and sensitive to cold
- Other symptoms include xerostomia, burning mouth syndrome, and halitosis

30.1.2 Bulimia and Anorexia

- Bulimia, also called bulimia nervosa, is an eating disorder characterized by episodes of binge eating followed by inappropriate methods of weight control, such as self-induced vomiting (purging), abuse of laxatives and diuretics, or excessive exercise. The insatiable appetite of bulimia is often interrupted by periods of anorexia
- Oral manifestations of bulimia include dental erosion, xerostomia, increased dental caries rate; parotid enlargement is often reported

Handbook of Oral Pathology and Oral Medicine, First Edition. S. R. Prabhu.
© 2022 John Wiley & Sons Ltd. Published 2022 by John Wiley & Sons Ltd.
Companion website: www.wiley.com/go/prabhu/oral_pathology

30.1.3 Crohn's Disease

- Crohn's disease is an inflammatory disease of any part of the gastrointestinal tract, predominantly affecting the small intestine
- Oral manifestations of Crohn's disease include diffuse labial, gingival or mucosal swelling, cobble-stoning of buccal mucosa and gingiva, aphthous ulcers, mucosal tags, angular cheilitis, and oral granulomas
- Oral lesions usually resolve with systemic treatment of the underlying disease
- See also Chapter 16 (section 16.10) and Chapter 27 (section 27.5)

30.1.4 Ulcerative Colitis

- Ulcerative colitis is an inflammatory condition that affects any part of the colon
- Oral manifestations of ulcerative colitis include aphthous ulceration or superficial haemorrhagic ulcers, angular stomatitis, and pyostomatitis vegetans
- Oral lesions usually respond to systemic treatment of ulcerative colitis

30.1.5 Coeliac Disease

- Coeliac disease, (also known as gluten-sensitive enteropathy) is characterized by atrophy of the jejunal mucosa due to its sensitivity to dietary gluten
- Oral manifestations of celiac disease include glossitis, angular cheilitis, bleeding tendencies, oral mucosal ulcers, dental enamel hypoplasia, delayed eruption, and oral mucosal signs of anaemia
- Oral manifestations respond to the treatment of the underlying disorder
- Avoidance of gluten in the food is required for successful management
- See also Chapter 27 (section 27.3)

30.1.6 Irritable Bowel Syndrome

- Irritable bowel syndrome is characterized by constipation, diarrhoea, abdominal pain (in the left iliac fossa), and the frequent passage of stools
- Psychogenic facial pain and temporomandibular joint symptoms are sometimes present

30.1.7 Alcoholic Liver Disease

- Alcoholic liver disease is liver damage as a result of alcohol abuse
- Oral manifestation includes jaundice of the oral mucosa, advanced periodontal disease, parotid enlargement, sweet and musty oral malodour, and bleeding tendencies

30.1.8 Liver Cirrhosis

- Liver cirrhosis is characterized by replacement of liver tissue by fibrosis, scar tissue, and nodules, leading to loss of liver function
- Oral manifestations include jaundice of the oral mucosa (soft palate and sublingual region), bleeding tendencies, and poor oral hygiene

30.2 Cardiovascular Disease

30.2.1 Angina Pectoris and Myocardial Infarction

- Angina pectoris (angina) and myocardial infarction are caused by ischaemia of the heart muscle usually caused by obstruction or spasm of the coronary arteries
- During the attack of angina or myocardial infarction, in addition to the chest pain, the patient may complain of acute pain in the jaw
- Jaw pain may resolve as soon as the chest pain is brought under control

30.2.2 Congenital Heart Disease

- Congenital heart disease is a general term for any defect of the heart, heart valves, or central blood vessels that is present at birth
- Oral manifestations may include, delayed tooth eruption, frequent positional anomalies of teeth, and hypoplastic enamel
- Patients are at a higher risk for dental caries and periodontal disease

30.2.3 Rheumatic Fever/Infective Endocarditis

- Rheumatic fever is a non-contagious acute fever marked by inflammation and pain in the joints caused by a streptococcal infection
- Infective endocarditis (bacterial endocarditis) is an infection (usually by *Staphylococcus aureus*) of the endocardial surface of the heart, which may include one or more heart valves, the mural endocardium, or a septal defect
- There are no specific oral manifestations of these conditions. However, many countries (except the UK) recommend that patients with previous history of infective endocarditis receiving invasive dental treatment are given antibiotic prophylaxis prior to invasive dental procedures (e.g. tooth extraction, implant placement, subgingival probing and scaling, endodontic treatment, placement of matrix and orthodontic bands, and intraligamentary and local anaesthetic injections)

30.2.4 Hypertension

- Hypertension refers to abnormally high blood pressure
- There are no specific oral manifestations of hypertension
- The dental practitioner should be aware of oral adverse effects of antihypertensive drugs. These include xerostomia, gingival hyperplasia (with nifedipine), salivary gland swelling (with clonidine), and increased postoperative bleeding (e.g. for those patients on aspirin or thrombolytic therapy). Calcium channel blockers can cause mucosal lichenoid reactions and gingival swellings

30.3 Respiratory Disease

30.3.1 Chronic Obstructive Pulmonary Disease

- Chronic obstructive pulmonary disease (COPD) is a lung disease characterized by chronic obstruction of lung airflow that interferes with normal breathing and is not fully reversible. The

terms 'chronic bronchitis' and 'emphysema' are no longer used but are now included within the COPD diagnosis
- Chronic bronchitis (blue bloaters) and emphysema (pink puffers) are two of the most common conditions that contribute to COPD
- There are no significant oral manifestations in COPD; however, blue bloaters may show signs of cyanosis of the lips

30.3.2 Lung Abscess and Bronchiectasis

- A lung abscess is a pus-filled cavity in the lung surrounded by inflamed tissue
- Bronchiectasis refers to permanent abnormal widening of the bronchi or their branches, causing a risk of infection
- Periodontal disease and halitosis are common in these diseases

30.3.3 Pulmonary Tuberculosis

- Pulmonary tuberculosis refers to primary infection of the lungs by *Mycobacterium tuberculosis*
- Primary tuberculosis infection of the oral soft tissues is extremely rare; however, secondary involvement of oral tissues can occur
- Lesions of secondary infection of the oral tissues (from pulmonary tuberculosis for example) may include chronic painless tuberculous ulcers on the dorsum or lateral borders of the tongue
- Ulcers disappear once systemic infection is treated with antituberculosis medication

30.3.4 Cystic Fibrosis

- Cystic fibrosis is a hereditary disorder affecting the exocrine glands. It causes the production of abnormally thick mucus, leading to the blockage of the pancreatic ducts, intestines, and bronchi and often resulting in respiratory infection
- In cystic fibrosis, disorders of the salivary glands can give rise to xerostomia
- Increased calculus formation, enamel defects, gingivitis, and swelling of the lips are reported in these patients

30.4 Kidney Diseases

30.4.1 Chronic Kidney Failure

- Chronic kidney failure refers to a gradual loss of kidney function over time
- Oral findings of chronic kidney failure may include:
  - Ammoniacal salivary odour
  - Metallic taste
  - Mucosal pallor due to anaemia
  - Necrotising ulcerative gingivitis
  - Orange-coloured mucosa due to deposition of carotene-like pigments
  - Xerostomia with or without candidosis
  - Uraemic stomatitis; in severe cases with a burning sensation and ulceration, petechiae, and gingival bleeding

30.4.2 Nephrotic Syndrome

- Nephrotic syndrome is a clinical disorder characterized by heavy proteinuria, hypoalbuminaemia, and oedema
- Oral manifestations include:
  - Facial oedema
  - Gingival inflammation
  - Mucosal pallor
  - Oral ulceration in those on cyclosporin
  - Symptoms and signs of kidney failure

30.4.3 Patients on Kidney Dialysis

- Dental considerations: recommendations (adopted from Klassen and Krasko (2002):
  - Record the patient's medical history and medication list on the dental chart and review these documents at each visit
  - The dialysis unit should notify the dentist once dialysis has been initiated
  - Perform dental treatment of haemodialysis patients on non-dialysis days to ensure the absence of circulating heparin
  - Use local anaesthetics with reduced epinephrine in all dialysis patients, as most are hypertensive
  - Withhold anticoagulants for a period agreed upon with the nephrologist
  - Be aware that meticulous local haemostatic measures, including mechanical pressure, packing, suturing, and topical thrombin, may be required, given the platelet dysfunction that often occurs in patients with renal failure
  - Avoid compression of the arm with the arteriovenous graft or fistula. Never use this arm for blood pressure measurements, intravenous administration of medication or phlebotomy
  - Lidocaine, narcotics (except meperidine) and diazepam can be used safely in patients with renal failure. Dose adjustment is needed for aminoglycosides and cephalosporins. Tetracycline is generally not recommended in patients with end-stage renal failure. Many nephrologists agree to the use of nonsteroidal anti-inflammatory drugs, as dialysis patients usually have little salvageable renal function
  - See the patient for dental check-ups as regularly as would be the case if they were not undergoing dialysis
  - For patients being considered for transplantation, complete all necessary dental care before the surgery
  - Use antibiotic prophylaxis, if recommended by the patient's nephrologist, before extractions, periodontal procedures, placement of dental implants, reimplantation of avulsed teeth, endodontic instrumentation, or surgery (beyond the apex only), subgingival placement of antibiotic fibres or strips, initial placement of orthodontic bands and intraligamentary injections of local anaesthetic. Advise the patient about the need for the antibiotic, such that it can be prescribed and taken just before the dental visit
  - Advise patients to avoid chewing on ice; instead, recommend that they suck on the ice or chew sugar-free gum
  - Recommend that alcohol-free mouthwashes be used to reduce oral dryness. Alternatively, recommend a saliva substitute
  - Follow universal precautions. The importance of doing so should not be underestimated, as the incidence of hepatitis B and C may be higher among dialysis patients

30.5 Endocrine and Metabolic Disorders

30.5.1 Hyperthyroidism

- Hyperthyroidism occurs when the thyroid makes too much thyroid hormone (T4, T3, or both)
- Increased risk for periodontal disease and premature eruption of teeth are occasionally reported in patients with hyperthyroidism

30.5.2 Hypothyroidism

- In hypothyroidism, the thyroid gland is underactive and fails to secrete enough hormones into the bloodstream
- Untreated neonatal (congenital) hypothyroidism may result in an altered development of the jaws, malocclusion, delayed tooth eruption, and a protruding tongue (cretinism)
- In older children, hypothyroidism may result in macroglossia, glossitis, salivary gland swelling, an increased risk of dental caries, and periodontal disease
- Adults with hypothyroidism may show delayed tooth eruption, an enlarged tongue, periodontal disease, alteration in taste sensation, and delayed wound healing

30.5.3 Hypopituitarism

- Hypopituitarism is an underactive pituitary gland that results in deficiency of one or more pituitary hormones
- Delayed eruption of teeth is a feature of hypopituitarism

30.5.4 Hyperpituitarism (Acromegaly)

- Hyperpituitarism refers to an excessive secretion or production of one or more of the hormones produced by the pituitary gland
- Acromegaly is a disorder that results from excess growth hormone in adulthood after the growth plates have closed. Growth hormone is the secretion of pituitary gland
- Mandibular prognathism, malocclusion, diastema, enlarged tongue, and ankylosis of roots are common in acromegaly

30.5.5 Diabetes Insipidus

- Diabetes insipidus is a rare condition caused by a reduction in, or failure to respond to, antidiuretic hormone. This results in large amounts of urine and excessive thirst
- In patients with diabetes insipidus, osseous infiltrates are often found on the skull and jaws (identified on conventional dental radiography)
- Loose teeth are often reported
- Children with diabetes insipidus drink large amounts of water (fluoridated at optimal level) due to excessive thirst, which can lead to dental fluorosis

30.5.6 Addison's Disease (Adrenal Insufficiency)

- Addison's disease is a disorder that occurs when the adrenal glands do not produce enough hormones due to damage to the adrenal cortex
- Pigmentation of the oral mucosa is a feature

- Pigmented lesions are brown, diffuse, and patchy in distribution, commonly found on the dorsum of the tongue and buccal mucosa

30.5.7 Cushing's Disease (Adrenocortical Excess)

- Cushing's disease is a form of Cushing's syndrome. It is characterized by increased secretion of adrenocorticotropic hormone from the anterior pituitary gland resulting in frequent weight gain, truncal obesity, striae, hypertension, glucose intolerance, and infections
- Facial features in Cushing's syndrome/disease include a red round face (plethora; 'moon face') and frontal balding

30.5.8 Diabetes Mellitus

- Diabetes mellitus is a disorder in which pancreas does not produce enough insulin or the body respond normally to insulin, causing blood sugar (glucose) levels to be abnormally high
- Poorly controlled diabetics have an increased risk for periodontal disease and impaired salivary gland function
- Patients with diabetes may present with candidiasis, taste dysfunction, salivary dysfunction, burning mouth syndrome, and generalized atrophy of the tongue
- Delayed wound healing is a major consequence of diabetes

30.5.9 Hypocalcaemia

- Hypocalcaemia is defined as a total serum calcium concentration less than 8.8 mg/dl (less than 2.20 mmol/l) in the presence of normal plasma protein concentrations or as a serum ionized calcium concentration less than 4.7 mg/dl (less than 1.17 mmol/l)
- Tetany is caused by severe hypocalcaemia, characterized by paraesthesia of the lips, tongue, fingers, and feet, carpopedal spasm, generalized muscle aching, and spasms of the facial musculature
- Chvostek's sign (involuntary twitching of the facial muscles elicited by a light tapping of the facial nerve just anterior to the external auditory meatus) is a facial manifestation in tetany

30.5.10 Hypercalcaemia

- Hypercalcemia can result when too much calcium enters the extracellular fluid or when there is insufficient calcium excretion from the kidneys
- May cause symptoms associated with the musculoskeletal, neurological, cardiovascular, and gastrointestinal systems
- In patients with hypercalcaemia, jawbone demineralization, loss of lamina dura, and osteitis fibrosa cystica (Von Recklinghausen's disease of bone) may be seen

30.6 Nervous System Disorders

30.6.1 Stroke

- A stroke is a sudden interruption in the blood supply of the brain
- Most strokes are caused by an abrupt blockage of arteries leading to the brain (ischaemic stroke)

- Other strokes are caused by bleeding into brain tissue when a blood vessel bursts (haemorrhagic stroke)
- Oral and facial manifestations in stroke include slurred speech, difficulty swallowing, unilateral paralysis of the oral and facial musculature, deviation of the tongue and loss of sensory stimuli of the oral tissues. These symptoms may occur after an episode of stroke

30.6.2 Epilepsy

- Epilepsy is a central nervous system (neurological) disorder in which brain activity becomes abnormal, causing seizures or periods of unusual behaviour, sensations, and sometimes loss of awareness
- Facial twitching is a feature of petit-mal seizures
- Those patients with epilepsy taking phenytoin may present hyperplasia of the maxillary and mandibular anterior gingival tissues
- In patients with epilepsy, oral soft tissue injuries (e.g. ulcers of the tongue) caused by trauma received during seizures may be detected

30.6.3 Parkinson's Disease

- Parkinson's disease is a progressive neurodegenerative disorder caused by the loss of dopaminergic neurons in the substantia nigra pars compacta
- The cardinal motor signs are tremor, rigidity, bradykinesia/akinesia, and a gait disorder characterized by a flexed posture and short, shuffling steps
- Other than excessive salivation, there are no specific oral manifestations of Parkinson's disease

30.6.4 Multiple Sclerosis

- Multiple sclerosis is a chronic, typically progressive disease involving damage to the sheaths of nerve cells in the brain and spinal cord, whose symptoms may include numbness, impairment of speech and of muscular coordination, blurred vision, and severe fatigue
- Patients may complain of facial anaesthesia or lower lip numbness and xerostomia. They may also experience facial pain, and the disorder can trigger trigeminal neuralgia or facial palsy

30.6.5 Myasthenia Gravis

- Myasthenia gravis is marked by muscular weakness without atrophy, and caused by a defect in the action of acetylcholine at neuromuscular junctions
- Oral manifestations include facial weakness, a sensation of stiffness of the mouth, an inability to whistle, 'myasthenic snarl' (giving patient's smile an appearance of a snarl), chewing difficulty, regurgitation of fluids through the nose, and choking
- Patients also experience inability to keep the head in balance

30.6.6 Bell's Palsy

- Bell's palsy refers to paralysis of the facial nerve producing distortion on one side of the face
- Characterized by an acute onset of unilateral, lower motor neuron weakness of the facial nerve in the absence of an identifiable cause

- Signs of Bell's palsy include unilateral sagging of the mouth, taste impairment, saliva dribbling and watery eyes, an inability to whistle and close the lips, or blow out the cheeks
- The palpebral fissures are wide
- Unilateral lacrimation (the production of crocodile tears) in the first month following a Bell's palsy episode occurs when the patient eats
- Loss of taste is common

30.7 Haematological Disorders

30.7.1 Anaemia

- Anaemia is characterized by decreased red cells or haemoglobin in the blood, resulting in decreased oxygen in peripheral tissues
- Anaemias are divided into various groups based on cause, such as iron deficiency anaemia, megaloblastic anaemia (from decreased vitamin B12 or folic acid), or aplastic anaemia (where red blood cell precursors in the bone marrow are depleted)
- In all forms of anaemia, the oral mucosa shows pallor
- Megaloblastic anaemia: atrophic glossitis is common. The dorsum of the tongue is smooth, bald and red. There may be accompanying erythematous candidosis
- Iron deficiency anaemia: the dorsum of the tongue appears bald and red. Patients often complain of a burning sensation
  - In Plummer–Vinson syndrome, oral ulcerations, erythroplakia patches or squamous cell carcinomas may occur. Pharyngeal involvement is also common
- Haemolytic anaemia: mucosal pallor and jaundice due to haemolysis is common
  - Dental radiography may show increased radiolucency with lamellar striations due to hyperplasia of the bone marrow in response to increased haemolysis
- Sickle cell anaemia: increased widening, and fewer trabeculations and signs of osteoporosis of the jaw bones may be evident on radiographs
  - Trabeculae between the teeth appear horizontal, giving a 'stepladder' appearance, and lamina dura may be more distinct and dense
  - Vaso-occlusive events may precipitate ischaemic necrosis in the bone
  - Delayed eruption of teeth and dental hypoplasia are often reported
- Thalassaemia major: bi-maxillary protrusion and alveolar enlargement gives rise to characteristic chipmunk facies

30.7.2 Thrombocytopenia

- Thrombocytopenia is a blood disease characterized by an abnormally low number of platelets in the bloodstream
- The normal number of platelets is usually 150 000–450 000 cells/litre of blood
- When the platelet number drops below 150 000 cells/litre of blood, the patient is said to be thrombocytopenic
- In thrombocytopenia, oral mucous membranes may show purpuric spots, often accompanied by purpuric spots on the skin
- Spontaneous gingival bleeding is also a feature of a severe form of thrombocytopenia

30.7.3 Haemophilia

- An inherited disorder almost exclusively of males in which the ability of blood to clot normally is impaired due to deficiency of, or defects in, coagulation factors such as VIII (for haemophilia A), IX (for haemophilia B) and XI (for haemophilia C)
- Spontaneous bleeding from oral soft tissues may occur in the severe form of the disorder
- Excessive bleeding from trauma or surgery, including tooth extraction, is common

30.7.4 Leukaemia

- Progressive proliferation of abnormal white blood cells found in hemopoietic tissues, and usually in the blood in increased numbers
- Leukaemia is classified in several ways: acute and chronic, and the predominant proliferating cell types such as myelocytic, granulocytic, and lymphocytic
- Patients with acute or chronic leukaemia may reveal ulceration of the mucosa, gingival enlargement (due to leukaemic infiltrate) bleeding, petechiae and ecchymosis of the mucous membrane
- Gingival enlargement is common in myelogenous leukaemia
- Lymphadenopathy is common in all forms of leukaemia
- Acute oral infections are common. These infections must be promptly treated, and their recurrence prevented

30.7.5 Multiple Myeloma

- Multiple myeloma is a malignancy of the antibody-producing plasma cells, which grow in an uncontrolled and invasive manner
- Oral symptoms may include paraesthesia and pain in the jaw bones
- Oral manifestations include enlargement of the tongue due to amyloid deposition
- Radiography of the jaw bones or the skull show characteristic single or multiple 'punched out' radiolucencies

30.7.6 Non-Hodgkin Lymphoma

- Lymphoma is a group of haematological malignancies that develop from lymphocytes and are usually associated with Epstein–Barr virus
- The two main categories of lymphomas are the non-Hodgkin lymphoma (90% of cases) and Hodgkin lymphoma (10%):
  - Hodgkin lymphoma is marked by the presence of Reed–Sternberg cells
  - Non-Hodgkin lymphoma is usually devoid of multinucleated Reed–Sternberg cells
- Salivary glands and mandible may be swollen
- Involvement of the gingiva, palate, alveolar ridge, buccal sulcus, and floor of the mouth have also been reported
- Petechiae, fungal infections, viral infections, mucosal ulcers, and oral paraesthesia are common

30.7.7 Burkitt's Lymphoma

- Burkitt lymphoma is a type of non-Hodgkin lymphoma that most often occurs in young people accounting for 40–50% of childhood non-Hodgkin lymphoma
- This neoplasm is common in central Africa and is associated with Epstein–Barr virus, and is common among children

- Jaw lesions show extensive osteolytic changes. The earliest sign is loosening of the teeth. Teeth float in the tumour mass
- Expansion of the jaw and protrusion of the tumour mass into the mouth is rapid
- Bilateral or involvement of all four quadrants of the jaws by the tumour may occur
- Early radiographical signs show a loss of lamina dura and enlargement of the crypts of developing teeth in children
- Focal areas of radiolucency and the displacement of teeth are also common findings on the extraoral radiographical views

30.8 Immune System Disorders

30.8.1 Allergic Contact Stomatitis

- Allergic contact stomatitis is an uncommon allergic reaction affecting the oral mucosa caused by contact with an allergen, usually flavourings, metals, or other components in oral hygiene products, foods, dental restorations, and medications
- Allergic contact stomatitis can manifest as lichenoid patches of the mucosa, or as swelling of the tongue or lips due to inflammatory oedema
- Allergies to lip stick, toothpaste, food items, chewing gums containing artificial cinnamon, and spices have been reported to cause allergic contact mucositis

30.8.2 Angioedema

- Angioedema is an acute or chronic disorder that affects the mucous membranes and deepest layers of the skin, together with underlying tissue
- It is marked by rapid swelling, large welts, and pain
- Characterized by the rapid swelling of the dermis subcutaneous tissue, mucosa and submucosal tissues
- Clinical features of allergic angioedema include acute and pronounced labial and periorbital swelling
- Swelling can also extend to the tongue, pharynx, and neck, causing fatal respiratory obstruction

30.8.3 Sjögren's Syndrome

- Sjögren's syndrome is an autoimmune disorder that is characterized by dry eyes, dry mouth and other disorders of the connective tissue such as rheumatoid arthritis, lupus erythematosus, scleroderma or polymyositis
- Oral manifestations in Sjögren's syndrome include disturbances in taste sensation, a fissured tongue, candidal infections and extensive dental decay due to xerostomia
- A risk of developing lymphoma of the parotid glands exists at a later stage of the primary disease
- For further details see Chapter 21 (section 21.3)

30.8.4 Temporal Arteritis

- Temporal arteritis, also called as giant cell arteritis, is an autoimmune disorder causing inflammation (vasculitis) of the temporal artery
- Symptoms and signs include scalp tenderness, headaches, pulseless temporal arteries, ulcers on the scalp, visual disturbances, blindness, and thickened, tender temporal arteries

30.8.5 Granulomatosis with Polyangiitis (Wegener's Granulomatosis)

- Granulomatosis with polyangiitis is a rare autoimmune disorder characterized by vasculitis and affects the ears, nose, sinuses, kidneys, and lungs
- Nasal and oral manifestations include bloody nasal discharge, a depressed nasal bridge, ulcers on the palate and pharynx (painless or painful), strawberry gingivitis, underlying bone destruction with loosening of the teeth, and non-specific ulcerations throughout oral mucosa

30.8.6 Behçet's Disease

- Behçet's disease is a rare autoimmune vasculitic disorder characterized by a triple-symptom complex of recurrent oral aphthous ulcers, genital ulcers, and uveitis
- Aphthous-like oral ulcers are common
- For further information see Chapter 16 (section 16.9)

30.8.7 HIV/AIDS

- The human immunodeficiency virus (HIV) is the virus that causes acquired immunodeficiency syndrome (AIDS). The late stage of HIV infection is called AIDS. Not all people who are HIV positive develop AIDS
- Specific conditions in the mouth caused by HIV infection have not been reported
- Conditions seen in people who are HIV positive occur due to immunocompromised status
- Oral conditions include:
  - Candidiasis
  - Herpes simplex virus infections
  - Ulcerative gingivitis/ulcerative periodontitis
  - Linear gingival erythema
  - Hairy leukoplakia
  - Kaposi sarcoma
  - Hodgkin and non-Hodgkin lymphoma
  - Cytomegalovirus infections
  - Human papillomavirus infections
  - Aphthous-like ulcerations
  - Salivary gland swelling

Reference

Klassen, J.T. and Krasko, B.M. (2002). The dental health status of dialysis patients. *Journal of the Canadian Dental Association* 68 (1): 34–38.

Recommended Reading

Ac, C., Neville, B.W., Krayer, J.W., and Gonsalves, W.C. (2010). Oral manifestations of systemic disease. *American Family Physician* 82: 1381–1388.

Islam, N.M., Bhattacharya, I., and Cohen, D.M. (2011). Common oral manifestations of systemic disease. *Otolaryngologic Clinics* 44: 161–182.

Porter, S., Mercadente, V., and Fedele, S. (2018). Oral manifestations of systemic disease. *BDJ Team* 5: 18012.

31

Systemic Diseases Associated with Periodontal Infections

31.1 Cardiovascular Disease

- Periodontal disease predisposes individuals to cardiovascular disease:
  - Oral bacteria such as *Streptococcus sanguis* and *Porphyromonas gingivalis* induce platelet aggregation, which leads to thrombus formation
  - One or more periodontal pathogens have been found in 42% of atheromas in patients with severe periodontal disease
  - Lipopolysaccharides from periodontal organisms being transferred to the serum as a result of bacteraemia or bacterial invasion may have a direct effect on endothelia so that atherosclerosis is promoted
  - Periodontitis as an infection may stimulate the liver to produce C-reactive protein (a marker of inflammation), which in turn will form deposits on injured blood vessels

31.2 Coronary Heart Disease (Atherosclerosis and Myocardial Infarction)

- Atherosclerosis is a progressive disease process that involves the large- to medium-sized muscular and large elastic arteries which in advanced cases is characterized by the formation of atheroma
- Atheroma are elevated focal intimal plaques with a necrotic central core containing lysed cells, cholesterol ester crystals, lipid-laden foam cells, and surface plasma proteins, including fibrin and fibrinogen

Handbook of Oral Pathology and Oral Medicine, First Edition. S. R. Prabhu.
© 2022 John Wiley & Sons Ltd. Published 2022 by John Wiley & Sons Ltd.
Companion website: www.wiley.com/go/prabhu/oral_pathology

- Reports indicate that atherosclerotic plaques are commonly infected with Gram-negative periodontal pathogens, including *Aggregatibacter actinomycetemcomitans* and *P. gingivalis*
- The presence of atheroma tends to make the patient prone to thrombosis
- A myocardial infarction is the damaging or death of an area of the heart muscle resulting from a reduced blood supply to that area
- Myocardial infarction is almost always caused by the formation of an occlusive thrombus at the site of rupture of an atheromatous plaque in a coronary artery

31.3 Stroke

- Stroke is a cerebrovascular disease that affects blood vessels supplying blood to the brain
- It occurs when a blood vessel in the brain bursts or is clogged by local thrombus formation or by aggregates of bacteria and fibrin from other sources such as the heart
- Reports indicate that inflamed periodontium releases inflammatory cytokines, lipopolysaccharides, and bacteria into the systemic circulation, and they may promote atherosclerosis and affect blood coagulation, the function of platelets, and prostaglandin synthesis, thereby contributing to the onset of stroke

31.4 Infective Endocarditis

- Infective endocarditis is an infection of the heart valves or the endothelium of the heart, usually with streptococci and staphylococci and rarely with fungi
- Occurs when bacteria in the bloodstream lodge on abnormal heart valves or damaged heart tissue
- Associated with periodontal infections and invasive dental treatment procedures
- Bacteraemia from oral procedures may 'prime' the endothelial surface of the heart valves over many years, and promotes early valve thickening, and allows bacterial adherence and colonization over days to weeks
- Oral streptococci have been implicated in the causation of infective endocarditis
- Untreated, infective endocarditis is fatal

31.5 Bacterial Pneumonia

- Pneumonia is an infection of pulmonary parenchyma caused by a wide variety of infectious agents, including bacteria, fungi, parasites, and viruses
- Bacterial pneumonia results from aspiration of oropharyngeal flora into the lower respiratory tract
- Potential respiratory pathogens include *S. pneumoniae*, *Mycoplasma pneumoniae*, *Haemophilus influenzae*, *A. actinomycetemcomitans* and anaerobes such as *P. gingivalis* and *Fusobacterium* species. These pathogens colonize the oropharynx and are aspirated into the lower airways, causing pneumonia
- Elderly individuals are predisposed for aspiration pneumonia

31.6 Low Birth Weight

- Low birth weight is defined as a body weight of the newborn at birth less than 2500 g
- Risk factors for low birthweight infants include prematurity, older (over 34 years) and younger (less than 17 years) maternal age, low socioeconomic status, inadequate prenatal care, drug, alcohol, and/or tobacco abuse, hypertension, genitourinary tract infection, diabetes, and multiple pregnancies
- Oral infections also seem to increase the risk for or contribute to low birth weight in newborns
- During pregnancy, the ratio of anaerobic Gram-negative bacterial species to aerobic species increases in dental plaque in the second trimester
- Reports indicate that four organisms namely *Bacteroides forsythus*, *P. gingivalis*, *A. actinomycetemcomitans*, and *Treponema denticola*, associated with mature plaque and progressing periodontitis, are detected at higher levels in mothers of preterm or low birth weight infants than in controls

31.7 Diabetes Mellitus

- Diabetes mellitus is a clinical syndrome characterized by hyperglycaemia due to an absolute or relative deficiency of insulin
- Classified according to its aetiology as type 1, type 2, gestational, and other specific types
- Type 1 results from the destruction of beta-cells within the islets of Langerhans of the pancreas resulting in a complete insulin deficiency; it can be immune mediated or have an idiopathic aetiology
- Type 2 ranges from an insulin resistance, which progresses into an insulin deficiency due to a secondary failure in the pancreatic beta-cells
- Gestational diabetes is defined as any degree of glucose intolerance with onset or first recognition during pregnancy
- Severe periodontal disease often coexists with severe diabetes mellitus and diabetes can be a risk factor for severe periodontal disease
- Gingival recession, swelling, inflammation, spontaneous bleeding, and generalized alveolar bone loss may be associated with advanced diabetes mellitus
- Periodontal disease either predisposes or exacerbates the diabetic condition
- Periodontal disease increases the severity of diabetes mellitus and complicates metabolic control
- The mechanism of links between these two conditions is not completely understood, but involves aspects of immune functioning, neutrophil activity, and cytokine biology
- Control of the chronic Gram-negative periodontal infection is beneficial and should be part of the standard treatment of patients with diabetes

Recommended Reading

Li, X., Kolltveit, K.M., Tronstad, L., and Olsen, I. (2000). Systemic diseases caused by Oral infection. *Clinical Microbiology Reviews* 13: 547–558.

Preshaw, P.M., Alba, A.L., Herrera, D. et al. (2012). Periodontitis and diabetes: a two-way relationship. *Diabetologia* 55 (1): 21–31.

32

Other Signs and Symptoms Related to the Oral Environment

32.1   Halitosis

- Halitosis refers to frequent or persistent bad breath (oral malodour)
- Causes include:
  - Poor oral hygiene
  - Periodontal necrotizing disease
  - Pericoronitis
  - Smoking
  - Ingested food (e.g. garlic and onion)
  - Hydrogen sulphide-producing bacteria on the tongue
  - Tonsillitis
  - Mucosal ulcers
  - Blood clot in the tooth socket
  - Dry mouth
  - Sinusitis
  - Oral cancer
  - Systemic conditions (e.g. diabetes, uraemia, respiratory, hepatic, and gastrointestinal diseases)
- Patients complain of malodour in the exhaled breath
- Some who do not have halitosis may imagine it because of psychogenic factors
- Often, patients cover the mouth or nose while talking, or avoid people; they may chew gums, or use mints, or brush teeth frequently
- Those with systemic disorders may present symptoms related to the underlying disease

Handbook of Oral Pathology and Oral Medicine, First Edition. S. R. Prabhu.
© 2022 John Wiley & Sons Ltd. Published 2022 by John Wiley & Sons Ltd.
Companion website: www.wiley.com/go/prabhu/oral_pathology

- Usually, oral malodour is from oral or pharyngeal sources whereas nasal malodour is from nasal passage or sinus
- When malodour is from both oral and nasal origin, the source may be systemic
- Identifiable causes must be addressed in the management of these conditions

32.2   Taste Disorders

- Disorders of taste include:
  - Unpleasant taste (cacogeusia)
  - Absence of taste (ageusia)
  - Diminished taste (hypogeusia)
  - Distorted taste (dysgeusia)
  - Heightened taste (hypergeusia)
- The basic taste sensations are sweet, salty, sour, and bitter
- Unpleasant taste is usually caused by:
  - Poor oral hygiene
  - Oral and nasal infections
  - Starvation
  - Dry mouth
  - Use of medications or certain foods
  - Diabetes
  - Gastrointestinal, respiratory, hepatic, and renal diseases
- Disorders that can result in taste dysfunction include:
  - Lingual, facial or chorda tympani nerve damage
  - Dry mouth
  - Smoking
  - Drugs
  - Irradiation
  - Psychotic disorders
  - Ageing
  - Nutritional disorders
  - Brain tumours
  - Head injuries
  - Multiple sclerosis
  - Bell's palsy
- Those who have lost the sense of taste also complain of loss of smell (anosmia)
- Loss of smell with taste dysfunction is a frequent symptom of viral infection of the upper respiratory tract
- Metallic taste is a common complaint in patients with poor oral hygiene and blood in the mouth, as in gingival inflammatory conditions
- Medications such as antibiotics, allopurinol (used to treat gout), lithium (used to treat certain psychiatric conditions), chemotherapeutic agents (to treat cancer) and some cardiac medications are also known to cause metallic taste
- Detection and attention to the underlined cause is essential in treating patients with taste disorders
- Medical consultation may be necessary for some patients

32.3   Dry Mouth (Xerostomia)

- Dry mouth, also known as xerostomia, is the subjective sensation of dryness in the mouth caused by lower salivary flow or the complete lack of saliva
- It is a symptom, not a disease
- Reduced salivary flow (hyposalivation) is common among the elderly, dehydrated individuals, smokers, and those on medication
- Patients may complain of difficulty in mastication and swallowing
- In patients with dry mouth the residual saliva is ropy
- Mucosa appears dry and examining gloves of the examiner may stick to the patient's mucosal surface
- Dorsal surface of the tongue may be smooth, shiny, and fissured
- Risk of candidal infections, dental caries, and dental plaque formation increases in patients with dry mouth
- Dry mouth can be a feature of several systemic diseases and conditions. These include:
  - Sjögren's syndrome
  - Diabetes mellitus
  - Parkinson's disease
  - Encephalitis
  - Brain tumours
  - Plummer–Vinson disease
  - Hypertension
  - HIV infection
  - Systemic rheumatic diseases
  - Sarcoidosis
  - Alzheimer's disease
  - Cystic fibrosis
  - Chronic tuberculosis
  - Primary biliary cirrhosis
  - Hacmolytic anaemia
  - Malignant lymphoma
  - Systemic lupus erythematosus
  - Scleroderma,
  - Dermatomyositis
  - Pernicious anaemia
  - Hypothyroidism
  - Amyloidosis
  - Radiotherapy and chemotherapy
  - Salivary gland excision
  - Vitamin A deficiency
  - Menopause
  - Stress, anxiety
  - Dehydration
  - Neurological disorders
  - Senility
  - Oral sensory dysfunction

- Iron deficiency
- Folic acid deficiency
- Uraemia
- Polyuria
- Diarrhoea
- Mouth breathing
- Bone marrow transplantation
- Endocrine disorders
- Pancreatic insufficiency
- Classes of drugs that can cause dry mouth include:
  - Anxiolytics, anticonvulsants
  - Antidepressants
  - Antiemetics
  - Antihistamines
  - Antiparkinsonian drugs
  - Antipsychotics
  - Bronchodilators
  - Decongestants
  - Diuretics
  - Muscle relaxants
  - Analgesics
  - Amphetamines
  - Antihypertensive drugs
- Management of dry mouth includes:
  - Frequent use of ice chips/sips of water
  - Use of artificial saliva and sugarless candies (as stimulant)
  - Discontinuation of xerostomic medication (in consultation with medical practitioner), or systemic pilocarpine (a sialagogue)
- Because of the increased risk of dental caries and plaque build-up in patients with dry mouth, topical fluoride applications and chlorhexidine mouth rinse are recommended

32.4   Sialorrhea

- Sialorrhea, also known as drooling or ptyalism, is a symptom that occurs when there is excess saliva in the mouth beyond the lip margin
- In normally developing babies, drooling is common; it subsides between the ages 15–36 months with establishment of salivary continence
- After the age of four years, drooling is considered abnormal
- In children, the most common cause of pathological hypersalivation (drooling) is cerebral palsy and mental restriction
- In adults, Parkinson's disease is the most common cause
- It is also common in individuals with schizophrenia on clozapine medication
- Impairment in social functioning (embarrassment and isolation), aspiration, skin breakdown, bad odour, and infection are associated with hypersalivation
- Anticholinergic medications, such as glycopyrrolate and scopolamine, are effective in reducing drooling

- The injection of botulinum toxin type A into the parotid and submandibular glands is safe and effective in controlling drooling, but the effects fade in several months, and repeat injections are necessary
- Other effective treatment modalities include surgical intervention, including salivary gland excision, salivary duct ligation, and duct rerouting

32.5   Trismus

- Trismus is defined as painful restriction in opening the mouth
- Normal mouth-opening ranges from 35 to 45 mm and lateral movement is 8–12 mm
- Reports suggest mild trismus as 20–30 mm interincisal opening, moderate as 10–20 mm and severe trismus as less than 10 mm
- Common causes of trismus include:
  - Temporomandibular joint disorders
  - Trauma to the jaws and temporomandibular joint
  - Pericoronitis
  - Tonsillar infections
  - Spreading orofacial infections (cellulitis/Ludwig's angina)
  - Parotid abscess
  - Meningitis
  - Tetanus (lockjaw)
  - Surgical extraction of third molars
  - Submucous fibrosis
  - Scleroderma
  - Nasopharyngeal or infratemporal tumours
  - Head and neck radiotherapy
  - Patients who are hysterical
  - Developmental defects of the temporomandibular joint
- Diagnostic methods include detailed history, clinical examination, and radiography
- Management includes treatment of the underlying condition and control of symptoms with pain medications, muscle relaxants, warm compresses, and splints
- Specialist referral is needed for patients with underlying systemic conditions

32.6   COVID-19 Infection

- COVID-19 is an infectious disease caused by a novel severe acute respiratory syndrome coronavirus 2 (SARS-CoV-2)
- Infection initially started in Wuhan province in China and has now affected populations in more than 200 countries worldwide and has been declared a pandemic by the World Health Organization
- The virus can spread from person to person through:
  - Contact with an infectious person (including in the 48 hours before they had symptoms)
  - contact with droplets from an infected person's cough or sneeze
  - touching objects or surfaces (like doorknobs or tables) that have droplets from an infected person, and then touching mouth or face
- Symptoms of COVID-19 infection include:

- fever (37.5 degrees or higher)
- cough
- sore throat
- shortness of breath (difficulty breathing)
- runny nose
- loss of taste
- loss of smell
- Other reported symptoms include fatigue, muscle pain, joint pain, headache, diarrhoea, nausea/vomiting, and loss of appetite
- In more severe cases, infection can cause pneumonia with severe acute respiratory distress
- Most human cases of COVID-19 are mild (80%), while 20% of infected patients may develop severe disease, and 5% may become critically ill and develop pneumonia or acute respiratory distress syndrome
- Those who are likely to be at higher risk of serious illness if they are infected with the virus are:
  - people 65 years and older with chronic medical conditions
  - people with compromised immune systems (e.g. cancer)
  - people with diagnosed chronic medical conditions
  - People 70 years and older
- The time between the exposure to the virus and first appearance of symptoms is typically 5–6 days, although it may range from 2 to 14 days
- Infection with COVID-19 is diagnosed by finding evidence of the virus in respiratory samples, such as swabs from the back of the nose and throat or fluid from the lungs
- Oral manifestations associated with COVID-19:
  - Chemosensory disorders: dysgeusia and anosmia; the global prevalence of taste disorders in patients with COVID-19 is 45%
  - There is a low certainty of evidence regarding oral mucosal lesions in patients with COVID-19. Some of the reported signs and symptoms include:
    o Non-specific oral ulcerations
    o Oral dryness
    o Desquamative gingivitis
    o Petechiae
    o Vesiculobullous lesions
    o Mucosal burning
    o Depapillation of the dorsal surface of the tongue
    o Commissural cheilitis
    o Co-infections such as candidiasis
- A cause and effect relationship between COVID-19 infection and the appearance of oral lesions has not been established
- Immune suppression and stress may play a role in their appearance

Recommended Reading

Dhanrajani PJ, Jonaidel O (2002). Trismus: aetiology, differential diagnosis, and treatment. *Dent Update*.29(2):88–92, 94.

Díaz Rodríguez, M., Jimenez Romera, A., & Villarroel, M. (2020). Oral manifestations associated with COVID-19. *Oral diseases*, 10.1111/odi.13555. Advance online publication. https://doi.org/10.1111/odi.13555

Hopcraft M S, C Tan C (2010). Xerostomia: An update for clinicians. Australian Dental Journal 55: 238–244.

Iranmanesh, B., Khalili, M., Amiri, R., Zartab, H., & Aflatoonian, M. (2021). Oral manifestations of COVID-19 disease: A review article. *Dermatologic therapy*, 34(1), e14578. https://doi.org/10.1111/dth.14578

Kumbargere Nagraj S, Eachempati P, Uma E, Singh VP, Ismail NM, Varghese E. (2019) *Interventions for managing halitosis*. Cochrane Database of Systematic Reviews 2019, Issue 12. Art. No.: CD012213. DOI: 10.1002/14651858.CD012213.pub2.

Potulska A, Friedman A. Controlling sialorrhoea (2005): a review of available treatment options. Expert Opin Pharmacother. 6(9):1551–4. doi: 10.1517/14656566.6.9.1551. PMID: 16086642.

Villa, A., Connell, C. L., & Abati, S. (2014). Diagnosis and management of xerostomia and hyposalivation. *Therapeutics and clinical risk management*, 11, 45–51. https://doi.org/10.2147/TCRM.S76282

33

Outline of Diagnostic Steps and Procedures Employed in Oral Pathology and Oral Medicine

---

CHAPTER MENU

33.1   History
33.2   Clinical Examination
33.3   Clinical Differential Diagnosis
33.4   Diagnosis

33.1   History

33.1.1   General Framework of History Taking

- Patient identification and biographical data:
  - Name
  - Date of birth/age
  - Occupation (past or present)
  - Marital status/living arrangement
  - Address/telephone number of the family physician
- Reason for seeking care and history of present health concern:
  - Chief complaint (presenting complaint)
  - History of presenting complaint
    - ○ Onset
    - ○ Duration
- Past medical/dental history:
  - Allergies (reaction)
  - Serious or chronic illness
  - Recent hospitalizations
  - Recent surgical/dental procedures
  - Emotional or psychiatric problems (if pertinent)
  - Current medications: prescriptions, over the counter, herbal remedies
  - Medication history: now and past, prescribed, and over-the-counter medicines, allergies

Handbook of Oral Pathology and Oral Medicine, First Edition. S. R. Prabhu.
© 2022 John Wiley & Sons Ltd. Published 2022 by John Wiley & Sons Ltd.
Companion website: www.wiley.com/go/prabhu/oral_pathology

- Family history:
  - Pertinent health status of family members
  - Pertinent family history of heart disease, lung disease, cancer, hypertension, diabetes, tuberculosis, arthritis, neurological disease, obesity, mental illness, genetic disorders
- Social history: smoking, alcohol, recreational drugs, accommodation and living arrangements, marital status, occupation, and hobbies
- Systems review: cardiovascular system, respiratory system, gastrointestinal system, nervous system, musculoskeletal system, genitourinary system
- Consent: preferably in writing

33.2 Clinical Examination

33.2.1 Extraoral Examination

- Visual inspection/observation:
  - General appearance of the patient
  - Facial and neck swellings
  - Pallor
  - Symmetry
- Palpation:
  - Cervical lymph nodes (submental, submandibular, jugulodigastric and jugulo-omohyoid nodes in particular)
  - Temporomandibular joint
  - Muscles of mastication
  - Major salivary glands

33.2.2 Intraoral Examination

- Soft and hard tissues
- Visual inspection:
  - Lips
  - Labial mucosa
  - Buccal mucosa and vestibular sulcus
  - Gingiva and alveolar mucosa
  - Hard palate
  - Soft palate and uvula
  - Fauces and oropharynx
  - Tongue (dorsum, lateral borders, and ventral surface)
  - Floor of the mouth
  - Minor salivary glands

33.2.3 Palpation

- Digital, bi-digital, bimanual, bilateral
- Percussion/probing (where applicable):

– Periodontium
– Dentition/occlusion
– Teeth, tooth mobility and tooth vitality tests

33.2.4   Assessment of Oral Problem

• Problem-specific examination:
  – Examination of swellings and ulcers:
    ○ Swelling:
      ○ Anatomical site
      ○ Shape and size
      ○ Single or multiple
      ○ Colour
      ○ Surface texture
      ○ Tenderness
      ○ Fluctuation
      ○ Sensation/pulsation
    ○ Ulcer:
      ○ Anatomical site
      ○ Size
      ○ Shape
      ○ Single/multiple
      ○ Edge of the ulcer
      ○ Base of the ulcer
      ○ Presence/absence of induration
      ○ Pain/tenderness
• Sensory and motor disturbances:
  – Testing cranial nerve function for sensory/motor disturbances
  – Paraesthesia
  – Paralysis
• Other:
  – Diascopy for suspected vascular lesions
  – Gentle scraping (with gauge) of white lesions
  – Testing Nikolsky's sign for vesiculobullous lesions
  – Testing taste sensation
  – Measuring salivary flow

33.3   Clinical Differential Diagnosis

33.3.1   Definition/Description

• Differential diagnosis refers to creating a list of possible diagnoses
• Differential diagnosis should be approached on the basis of exclusion
• Differential diagnosis forms the basis for ordering tests and procedures to narrow the diagnosis

33.4 Diagnosis

33.4.1 Biopsy

- Fine-needle aspiration
- Core needle
- Exfoliate cytology
- Incision/excision/punch/brush biopsy:
  - Tissue is used for histopathologic diagnosis and immunostaining investigations
  - Routinely, tissues are fixed with neutral formalin 10%, embedded in paraffin, and then manually sectioned with a microtome to obtain 4–5 μm-thick paraffin sections
  - Sections are dewaxed and stained with haematoxylin and eosin (H&E) or special stains and for immunostaining techniques

33.4.2 Histopathology

- Routine histological stains used:
  - Basic dye haematoxylin (blue-black) and acidic dye eosin (red)
  - Periodic acid–Schiff stain:
    - Special stain used for staining carbohydrates, and glycosaminoglycans (e.g. salivary mucins, glycogen, and candidal hyphae)
    - Stains pink
- Immunostaining methods are used to detect:
  - Autoantibody bound to desmosomes as in pemphigus
  - Autoantibody bound to hemidesmosomes as in mucous membrane pemphigoid
  - Presence of cytokeratins in undifferentiated oral squamous cell carcinomas
- Immunostaining methods include immunofluorescent (IF) and immunohistochemical (IHC) staining methods
- Immunofluorescence (IF) staining uses a fluorescent dye to visualize antibody binding
- Two immunofluorescence methods are available:
  - Direct immunofluorescence (DIF)
  - indirect immunofluorescence (IIF)
- IHC is a method for detecting antigens in cells of a tissue section by exploiting the principle of antibodies binding specifically to antigens in biological tissues
- Special tests (Molecular biological tests):
  - Polymerase chain reaction:
    - Used for detecting pathogens (mycobacteria in tuberculosis or to detect RNA genetic material of HIV or HIV DNA in white blood cells infected with the HIV for example) or mutations in genes
  - In situ hybridization:
    - A technique that is used to detect/localize nucleotide sequences in cells, tissue sections, and even whole tissue
    - Fluorescence in situ hybridisation is a molecular testing method that uses fluorescent probes to evaluate genes and/or DNA sequences on chromosomes
    - Some common applications in oral pathology are in virology, such as in detection of cytomegalovirus, Epstein–Barr virus, and human herpesvirus type 8 within cells

33.4.3 Microbiology

- Swabs/smears/oral rinse for identification of pathogens (fungal/viral/bacterial) and for culture and antibiotic sensitivity
- Swabs/smears/oral rinse for identification of pathogens:
  - Examples: direct Gram-stained smears for pseudomembranous candidosis and necrotizing ulcerative gingivitis
  - H&E-stained smears can reveal virally infected epithelial cells in herpes infections
- Culture and antibiotic sensitivity for pyogenic bacteria
  - Examples: osteomyelitis, cellulitis, and acute parotitis

33.4.4 Blood Tests

- Haematology:
  - Haemoglobin estimation, red blood cell count, haematocrit, mean corpuscular volume, white blood cell count, differential white cell count, platelet count, and erythrocyte sedimentation rate
  - Coagulation studies (clotting time/bleeding time/clotting factor estimation)
  - International normalized ratio
  - Iron studies (ferritin)
  - Vitamin B12 and folate
- Serology:
  - Autoantibodies such as rheumatoid factor, antinuclear factor, DNA binding antibodies, SS-A and SS-B for Sjogren's syndrome
  - Viral antibody titres for herpes simplex virus infections, herpes zoster, and other viral infections
  - Paul Bunnel or monospot test for infectious mononucleosis
  - Syphilis serology
- Clinical chemistry (biochemistry):
- Skeletal serum alkaline phosphatase test Paget's disease, hyperparathyroidism
- Blood sugar estimation for diabetes

33.4.5 Imaging

- Plain radiography:
  - The most common dental imaging modality. These include:
    - Bite-wing radiography
    - Periapical radiography
    - Orthopantomography
- Skull radiography:
  - Occipital mental view
  - Posteroanterior mandibular view
- Digital imaging:
  - This method substitutes the conventional film with a digital sensor
- Cone beam computed tomography (CBCT) for skeletal abnormalities, impacted teeth, root abnormalities and dentoalveolar trauma

- Computed tomography (CT) for the assessment of bone tumours, osteomyelitis, and osteonecrosis
- Magnetic resonance imaging for imaging of the temporomandibular joint, squamous cell carcinoma, salivary gland tumours, osteomyelitis
- Diagnostic ultrasound for soft tissue swellings in the neck and salivary glands

33.4.6 Other Tests

- Urine test for diabetes
- Bence Jones protein estimation for myeloma

33.4.7 Referral Letter

- Patient's details: name/date of birth
- Description of patient's presenting complaint/history of presenting complaint
- Results of examination, radiographic findings, and findings of special tests
- Provisional diagnosis

Recommended Reading

Avon, S.L. and Klieb, H. (2012). Oral soft tissue biopsy: an overview. *Journal of the Canadian Dental Association* 78: c75.

Lamey, P.J. and Lewis, M.A. (1997). Special investigations. In: *A Clinical Guide to Oral Medicine*, 2e, 75–82. BDJ Books.

Logan, R.M. and Goss, A.N. (2010). Biopsy of the oral mucosa and the use of histopathology services. *Australian Dental Journal* 55: 9–13.

Odell, E.W. (2017). Principles of investigation, diagnosis, and treatment. In: *Cawson's Essentials of Oral Pathology and Oral Medicine*, 9e, 1–20. Edinburgh: Elsevier.

Index

Page numbers in *italics* refer to illustrations; those in **bold** refer to tables

Handbook of Oral Pathology and Oral Medicine, First Edition. S. R. Prabhu.
© 2022 John Wiley & Sons Ltd. Published 2022 by John Wiley & Sons Ltd.
Companion website: www.wiley.com/go/prabhu/oral_pathology